Managing PCOS For Dummies®

Recognising PCOS Symptoms

Polycystic ovary syndrome, or PCOS, is described as a syndrome rather than a disease because it shows up as a group of signs and symptoms that can occur in any combination. Here are some of the symptoms:

- **Period disruption.** Periods can be heavier, lighter, irregular, or absent altogether.
- **Weight gain.** This is mostly due to high levels of insulin circulating in the blood (refer to Chapter 2 for why this causes weight gain).
- **Acne and oily skin.** Women with PCOS tend to have higher levels of testosterone.
- **Different hair growth patterns.** Your body may get hairier in certain places but hair may thin on your head.
- **Sleep problems and fatigue/exhaustion.** This can be due to fluctuating hormone levels and also increased anxiety.
- **Depression, anxiety, irritability, and mood swings.** These symptoms are probably due to disrupted hormone levels.
- **Fertility problems.** PCOS can disrupt ovulation.
- **Metabolic Syndrome.** This is a cluster of symptoms which includes insulin resistance (where insulin produced by the body does not work efficiently), high blood pressure, and high cholesterol levels. It can lead to diabetes and heart disease.

Tips for PCOS Sufferers

This entire book comprises tips for PCOS sufferers, but here's a snapshot:

- Lose weight if you're overweight by cutting your intake to 1,500 calories per day.
- Eat regular meals (but don't pile your plate), and have a couple of small snacks during the day. Don't let yourself get hungry.
- Follow a low-GI diet by substituting low-GI carbs for the high-GI ones (Chapter 4 has the low-down on eating low-GI).
- Keep the fat level down in your diet, and cut down particularly on saturated and trans fats (including fatty meat, butter, cakes, pastry, and biscuits).
- Use as little salt as possible and look at labels of processed food to try to keep below 6 grams a day.
- Eat at least five helpings of fruit and veg every day.
- Get some physical activity every day. Half an hour is great, but an hour is even better to help keep your weight under control. Chapter 10 is full of exercise tips for PCOS sufferers.
- Enjoy a variety of food, but keep it healthy.
- Enjoy your true friends and family, and keep them close to you!

For Dummies: Bestselling Book Series for Beginners

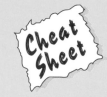

Cheat Sheet

Guideline Daily Amounts (GDA) of Key Nutrients for Women

Nutrient	GDA	GDA for weight loss
Energy (calories)	2,000	1,500
Total fat (g)	70	50
Saturated fat (g)	20	15
Total sugars (g)	90	70
Dietary fibre (g)	24	24
Sodium (g)	2.4	2.4
Salt (g)	6	6

Substituting Not-So-Good Carbs for Good Carbs

Meal	Instead of:	Have:
Breakfast	Cornflakes	Muesli
	Instant porridge oats	Unprocessed oats made into porridge
	White toast	Granary toast
Lunch	Jacket potato with filling	Baked sweet potato with filling
	White baguette	Pitta bread
	Brown bread sandwiches	Wholegrain bread sandwiches
Dinner	Curry with white rice	Curry with basmati rice
	Shepherd's pie	Spaghetti bolognese
	Stir-fry with instant rice	Stir-fry with noodles
Desserts	Bread and butter pudding made with white bread	Bread and butter pudding made with fruit loaf
	Fruit crumble made with white flour	Fruit crumble made with oat topping
Snacks	Muffins/cakes/biscuits	Cakes, biscuits, or muffins made with fruit, oats, and wholegrains
	White bread and jam	Fruit loaf with ricotta
	White crackers and cheese	Wholegrain crispbread with avocado or hummus dip

For Dummies: Bestselling Book Series for Beginners

Managing PCOS
FOR
DUMMIES®

by Gaynor Bussell

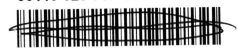

BICENTENNIAL
1807
WILEY
2007
BICENTENNIAL

John Wiley & Sons, Ltd

Managing PCOS For Dummies®

Published by
John Wiley & Sons, Ltd
The Atrium
Southern Gate
Chichester
West Sussex
PO19 8SQ
England

E-mail (for orders and customer service enquires): cs-books@wiley.co.uk

Visit our Home Page on www.wiley.com

For general information on our other products and services, please contact our Customer Care Department within the U.S. at 800-762-2974, outside the U.S. at 317-572-3993, or fax 317-572-4002.

For technical support, please visit www.wiley.com/tec

Wiley also publishes its books in a variety of electronic f
not be available in electronic books.

British Library Cataloguing in Publication Data: A catalog
the British Library

ISBN-13: 978-0-470-05794-0 (P/B)

Printed and bound in Great Britain by Bell & Bain Ltd, Gl

10 9 8 7 6 5 4 3

WILEY

About the Author

Gaynor Bussell is a Registered Dietitian, a Nutrition Consultant, and a member of various professional nutrition organisations, including the Nutrition Society and the British Dietetic Association.

Gaynor began specialising in women's health after taking a short career break to have her two daughters. She worked as a women's health dietitian for over six years at University College Hospital in London, specialising particularly in PMS, menopause, preconception health, eating disorders and, of course, PCOS. She also covered the osteoporosis clinic at this hospital. During this time Gaynor became dietary adviser to a women's health charity.

Since then Gaynor has worked at various women's health clinics including those at Hammersmith and Queen Charlotte's. She was also the dietitian for a private residential eating disorders centre. Gaynor continues to see private patients who have women's health issues and/or eating disorders. She also continues to work with various women's health organisations and charities, and writes and gives talks on various aspects of women's health.

Gaynor currently works as a consultant for the Food and Drink Federation (FDF) where her role includes acting as the interface on nutritional matters between industry and UK and EU authorities and sitting on a number of decision-making committees.

Author's Acknowledgements

Thanks to the excellent team at Wiley, in particular Rachael Chilvers and Alison Yates who kept me encouraged and did not shout too much when deadlines were missed!

Thanks to my family: David and my two daughters, Sally and Jenny. Thanks guys about being good-natured and understanding about my 'being on a roll' so that dinner didn't get served until 10 p.m., again!

Thanks to my work colleagues at the Food and Drink Federation who allowed me to take the time out to write the book and always took an interest in how things were coming along.

Finally, thanks to the team at Next Generation gym. You sorted out my mouse-strained shoulder and gave me excellent workout plans. It was great to go to you as a bolt hole when I needed to think, de-stress, and pound the life out of a treadmill!

Publisher's Acknowledgements

We're proud of this book; please send us your comments through our Dummies online registration form located at www.dummies.com/register/.

Some of the people who helped bring this book to market include the following:

Acquisitions, Editorial, and Media Development

Project Editor: Rachael Chilvers

Development Editor: Tracy Barr

Copy Editor: Martin Key

Proofreader: Andy Finch

Content Editor: Steve Edwards

Technical Editors: Nigel Denby, RD, Dr Sarah Brewer

Recipe Tester: Emily Nolan

Nutritional Analyst: Patty Santelli

Executive Editor: Jason Dunne

Executive Project Editor: Martin Tribe

Cover Photos: © Getty Images/Gus Wedge

Cartoons: Rich Tennant (www.the5thwave.com)

Composition Services

Project Coordinator: Jennifer Theriot

Layout and Graphics: Joyce Haughey, Stephanie D. Jumper, Laura Pence, Heather Ryan

Proofreader: Susan Moritz

Indexer: Aptara

Brand Reviewer: Janet Sims

Publishing and Editorial for Consumer Dummies

    Diane Graves Steele, Vice President and Publisher, Consumer Dummies

    Joyce Pepple, Acquisitions Director, Consumer Dummies

    Kristin A. Cocks, Product Development Director, Consumer Dummies

    Michael Spring, Vice President and Publisher, Travel

    Kelly Regan, Editorial Director, Travel

Publishing for Technology Dummies

    Andy Cummings, Vice President and Publisher, Dummies Technology/General User

Composition Services

    Gerry Fahey, Vice President of Production Services

    Debbie Stailey, Director of Composition Services

Contents at a Glance

Table of Contents

Introduction

· ·

*W*hen you're diagnosed with polycystic ovary syndrome (PCOS), you may feel pretty low – PCOS isn't a nice condition and doesn't yet have a cure. However, the good news is that you can keep the symptoms more or less completely at bay. This doesn't happen simply by taking a pill or two; you have to put in the effort yourself, and you aren't going to see results overnight. That's not a message that everyone likes to hear in today's instant gratification society. The rewards are huge though – you get your life back and you feel so fit and well that you don't want to return to your old lifestyle.

Put simply, you need to live a healthy life to keep PCOS under control. Lose any excess weight, get fit, tone up, and eat food that's going to do the best for your body. All this doesn't need to be dull and boring: Being physically active can be fun and it certainly lifts the mood and gives you a buzz. Have a peek at the recipes in this book and you soon realise that the diet for PCOS is tasty, easy to make, and sure to be liked by your friends and family, too, so no excuse for social exclusion!

About This Book

When you're first told that you have a particular medical condition, you're given a whole heap of advice from different people, including your friends and your Aunty Nelly! And, more than likely, different bits of advice are contradictory. You may have looked up PCOS on the Internet, or leafed through a few books about it. You may even have read articles about it in popular magazines, or read about some celebrity who cured herself by eating nothing but peanut butter sandwiches. Well, what's a girl to do?

This book gives you down-to-earth and up-to-date advice. It tells you what's worked and what hasn't for PCOS sufferers, and takes you through what you can be doing for yourself to help reduce your PCOS symptoms, mostly in the area of diet and exercise. I also briefly cover the medical treatments available for PCOS, but only so that you're aware of what's available and what route your doctor or specialist may want to take you down.

Conventions Used in This Book

The following conventions are used throughout this book to help keep things consistent and easy to understand:

✔ All Web addresses appear in monofont.

✔ Both metric and imperial measurements appear in the recipes. Follow either system – just don't switch halfway through a recipe or it'll end in tears! American measurements are also included (as cups). For certain ingredients that are known by more than one name, both names are used with one in brackets, such as 'courgette (zucchini)'.

✔ All the recipes are followed by the nutrient breakdown per serving.

✔ A little tomato symbol next to a recipe means that it's suitable for vegetarians.

✔ The following terms are used as a shortened abbreviation:

  • 'Calories' is used to mean kilo calories (kcals).

  • 'Carbs' is used to mean carbohydrates.

  • 'Sat fat' is used to mean saturated fat.

✔ Nutritionists commonly use metric terms such as gram (g), milligram (mg), and microgram (mcg) to describe quantities of protein, fat, carbohydrate, vitamins and minerals, and other nutrients. This book does as well.

What You're Not to Read

If you want to get straight to the nitty-gritty, and extract all the vital bits as quickly as possible so you can make a start on what you need to do, you can skip the following bits and still accomplish your goal:

✔ **Text in sidebars.** These shaded boxes appear here and there throughout the book. They share anecdotes and observations, but aren't essential reading.

✔ **Anything with a Technical Stuff icon attached.** This information pumps you with a few more technical facts or background about a particular subject, but isn't essential reading if you don't want to know the why, but just the how!

Of course, when you're ready (and have the time or curiosity to spare), remember that these pieces of info are well worth dipping into.

Foolish Assumptions

Every *For Dummies* book is written with a particular reader in mind, and this one is no exception. So, I made the following basic assumptions (rightly or wrongly) about you:

- ✔ You're not a doctor so don't have the technical understanding about the PCOS condition, but you are interested in getting a basic understanding of it.

- ✔ You have the condition, and you want to know how to reduce your PCOS symptoms so that you can improve your quality of life.

- ✔ You're confused about the right dietary and exercise route to take to get you on track to reducing your symptoms.

- ✔ You're dissatisfied with quick fixes, fads, and wonder diets and treatments and need a realistic alternative that works.

- ✔ You want straight talking, understandable information. You want to know enough to help yourself to feel better, but don't need to become an expert on PCOS.

- ✔ You don't want to spend hours digging around for information but want a one stop shop that's going to cut to the chase but not mislead you.

How This Book Is Organised

The great thing about *For Dummies* books is that you don't have to read them all the way through. You can simply turn to the bit you want – a chapter, a section, even just a paragraph. The table of contents and the index help you out. This section gives you an idea of what lies ahead.

Part 1: PCOS in a Nutshell

When you're initially diagnosed with any condition, the first order of business is getting a good enough understanding so that 1) you're not terrified or panicky and 2) you can make good decisions about how to take care of your health. So in this part, I give you basic information about PCOS: what it is, what causes it, what symptoms may accompany it, what changes you can expect as you age, and – most importantly – how you can take control and manage it.

Part II: Taking Control of Your Diet

Your diet can really help to control symptoms of PCOS. This part covers following a balanced low glycaemic index (GI) diet, whether simply to control PCOS or also to lose weight. As many PCOS sufferers tend to be overweight, this part is full of helpful and practical tips to keep the weight off.

Part III: Recipes for Life

Part 3 is very practical, explaining how watching the calories and the GI gets translated into actual meals and recipes. You don't need to look at another recipe book with these chapters! As well as tips and advice, the recipes cover breakfasts (Chapter 6), lunches and starters (Chapter 7), snacks (in Chapter 8 and, yes, they are allowed!), and last but not least dinners and puds (Chapter 9). The recipes also include some indulgent ones and meals you can safely serve up at a dinner party.

Part IV: Other Helpful Stuff for PCOS

This part looks at other ways that you can help to reduce your PCOS symptoms, including the importance of physical activity. When you have PCOS you may well be tempted to try all sorts of other 'cures' that you find out about. Part 4 sorts out the good from the bad, and points out the downright ugly of these so called 'cures'. PCOS is often accompanied by psychological problems such as depression, loss of control, and stress, so this part helps you find the right balance between body, mind, and spirit. Finally, this part gives you some really down to earth advice on what to do to ensure that you maximise your chances of getting pregnant and having a beautiful bouncing baby.

Part V: The Part of Tens

This part contains five lots of ten tips, which form a quick reference guide. Most of these tips are mentioned throughout the rest of the book, but this part brings them all together as a handy reference. You can find tips on the PCOS symptoms that you can diminish by using the advice in this book; how to distinguish the good diets from the bad; good reasons for following a low-GI diet; and ten superfoods you can incorporate into your diet to help reduce your PCOS symptoms. Finally, Chapter 18 lists ten organisations that offer support and advice to people like you who have PCOS or have a close friend or relative with it.

Icons Used in This Book

Icons are a handy *For Dummies* way to catch your attention as you slide your eyes down the page. The icons come in several varieties, each with its own unique symbol and meaning.

Your understanding of the health and diet world may be riddled with myths or old wives tales. Some of them may be based on truth, but most came from another planet and don't apply to human beings living today on earth. This symbol means that the myth has been exposed for what it is!

This symbol marks the place where you can find explanations of the terms used by nutrition experts. Skip them if you like, but expanding your understanding is always good, if you have the time!

This icon draws your attention to an important point to bear in mind about dealing with PCOS.

These details add to your understanding of PCOS. You can get on in life perfectly all right without them, so skip them if you want to, but try a few first – they may give you some facts that may help you to answer the questions in obscure quiz shows!

The Tip icon does exactly what it says – cherish these little nuggets because they're there to make your life a little easier.

This icon points to certain pitfalls or things that may actually harm you. Ignore at your peril!

Where to Go from Here

Where to go from here? Wherever you like, and you certainly don't need to read from cover to cover, unless you like to follow tradition! You can dive right in anywhere in the book, because each chapter (and even each section) delivers a complete message. The table of contents is detailed enough to help you to pinpoint the area you want to know about, and you can use the index.

If you want to know more about exercising to achieve weight loss, go straight to Chapter 10. If you want a healthy but tasty recipe for dinner tonight, jump to Chapter 9.

If you're really not sure where to start, read Chapter 1, which gives you all the basic information about PCOS and helps you to decide which area you want to home in on first.

Part I
PCOS in a Nutshell

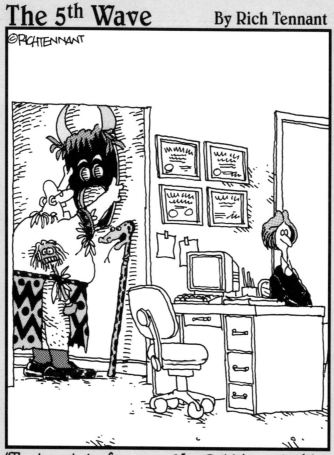

In this part . . .

This part gives you an overview of everything PCOS-related, and helps you to identify whether you have PCOS by listing all the symptoms.

In this part you get some straight facts about your condition, how it plays out in your body, how it changes when you change (such as when you get older or heavier) and how you can start to tackle it.

Chapter 1

Sensible and Straightforward Solutions for a Difficult Condition

● ●

In This Chapter

▶ Understanding PCOS and its symptoms

▶ Looking at treatment options

▶ Working out what you can do to help yourself

● ●

*T*his chapter is a great place to start to get on the right course if you suffer or suspect you suffer from PCOS, or if you have a friend, relative, or partner with the condition and you want a quick overview of the most important things you need to know about it.

This chapter gives an overview of the entire book; so in one chapter you get a feel for what PCOS really is and what its symptoms are. Most importantly you get an overview of treatments that are aimed at reducing the symptoms, mostly looking at what you can do for yourself.

Understanding PCOS

PCOS is the most common ovarian function disorder in women during the period of time before the menopause arrives. An estimated 20 per cent of women have polycystic ovaries (PCO), but despite having small cysts on their ovaries, they don't have any symptoms of PCOS. For actual PCOS, where definite symptoms are present, the incidence in women is as high as 5–10 per cent and the rate appears to be increasing.

Defining the condition

According to the American Society for Reproductive Medicine, PCOS is defined by having any two of the following signs and symptoms:

✔ Lack of ovulation for an extended period of time (which probably manifests itself as the stopping of your monthly period).

✔ High levels of androgens (male hormones).

✔ Many small cysts on the ovaries (normal ovaries have 5–6 follicles (cells), whereas polycystic ovaries have ten or more).

The hormones involved in controlling periods, and ultimately reproduction, are produced in the pituitary gland located in the brain. In PCOS two of these, called luteinising hormone (LH) and follicle stimulating hormone (FSH), are produced in proportions that are off kilter. The imbalance of these two hormones is thought to prevent the follicles in the ovary from developing properly: They tend to remain small and don't mature enough to release an egg. As a result, a string of small follicles forms on the ovary giving rise to the characteristic polycystic ovary.

Trigger factors

PCOS is often described as being a condition of hormone imbalances and probably has a genetic basis, so you may inherit it from a parent. You are more likely to develop PCOS if:

✔ You have a relative with PCOS (female relative of course!).

✔ You have a relative with type 2 diabetes (male or female).

✔ Your father went bald prematurely (yes, honest, it's true!).

Obesity is also believed to act as a trigger to PCOS in women with a genetic pre-disposition.

You Know You Have PCOS Because . . . : The Symptoms

The symptoms of PCOS vary from woman to woman and can be present in any combination. They can also change over time and so, if you have PCOS, your symptoms are likely to be different from someone else you know with PCOS.

The most common PCOS symptoms include the following:

- ✔ Weight gain, especially around the tummy.
- ✔ Increased hairiness on the face and other regions (called *hirsutism*).
- ✔ Male pattern baldness or thinning hair.
- ✔ Oily skin with acne.
- ✔ Absent or irregular menstrual cycles which leads to infertility.

For detailed information on the symptoms of PCOS, go to Chapter 2.

Weight gain

Not being able to control weight gain is often the most distressing symptom in PCOS, and unfortunately the rate of obesity in women with PCOS is 50 per cent. If you have found that you are gaining weight easily, you are likely to find that it tends to go on around your middle, a condition that your doctor or specialist calls 'central adiposity'.

The symptoms of PCOS are more severe if you gain a lot of weight; as you lose weight, the symptoms diminish. If you are an overweight woman with PCOS even a modest weight decrease of 5 per cent leads to:

- ✔ A decrease in your insulin level.
- ✔ An improvement in your menstrual cycle (or acts as a trigger for it to start again).
- ✔ Reduced testosterone levels leading to reductions in hirsutism and acne.

Emotional manifestations

If you have PCOS you are more likely to suffer from depression, anxiety, irritability, and mood swings. In fact it can seem as if you have premenstrual syndrome (PMS); the difference is that in PCOS, the symptoms don't just appear before a period.

The emotional symptoms that accompany PCOS may be due to one, or all, of the following:

- ✔ Hormone disturbances.
- ✔ A host of upsetting symptoms caused by PCOS.
- ✔ The stress of living with a long-term medical condition.

Another emotional manifestation of PCOS is the tendency toward eating disorders. A link exists between having an abnormal eating behaviour and PCOS. Binge eating and bulimia is more common than in the general population: 1 per cent of women have bulimia in the general population, whereas 6 per cent of women who have PCOS are bulimic. Go the section 'Looking after the inside' for basic info on dealing with an eating disorder; for detailed information about these disorders and PCOS, head to Chapter 2.

Insulin resistance

You may be told that you have insulin resistance if you have PCOS, but this is not something you can see, although it does lead eventually to physical conditions such as diabetes and heart disease. Insulin resistance, with the resultant high level of circulating insulin, is very common in PCOS. This condition is due to the muscles becoming resistant to the action of insulin, so that more insulin has to be pumped out to have any effect. Insulin resistance is more likely if you gain weight.

One of insulin's functions in your body is to help your cells take up glucose which is used to create energy. If you're insulin resistant, not only do you end up feeling tired and lacking in energy, but also, because your cells can't utilise the glucose in the blood, blood sugar levels rise, resulting in type 2 diabetes. Type 2 diabetes is known as a silent but deadly condition because its symptoms can go unnoticed for many years, by which time damage to the eyes and kidney may have occurred and risk factors for heart disease increased.

Insulin resistance also leads to the development of abnormal levels of fats in the blood with rising levels of harmful cholesterol increasing your chances of having heart disease or a stroke. Again you don't know you have high cholesterol unless you have a blood test.

Insulin resistance is the root of most symptoms in PCOS. When insulin resistance is present, normal amounts of insulin are insufficient to bring down blood glucose levels, which are a result of consuming carbohydrates. Your pancreas has to make even more insulin to compensate, which leads to a rise in the amount of insulin circulating through your body. High insulin levels mean that:

 ✔ Your body stores more fat resulting in weight gain.

 ✔ Your ovaries produce more testosterone which has an adverse effect on the reproductive hormones that control the formation of follicles in the ovary. The result is that your menstrual cycle may become irregular or your periods may even stop altogether.

✔ Extra testosterone causes more free testosterone to circulate in your body causing acne and hirsutism.

Metabolic syndrome (syndrome X)

You may well ask what on earth this syndrome is. Here's a quick definition: Metabolic syndrome is a cluster of conditions that often occur together, including obesity, high blood sugar, high blood pressure, and high levels of harmful blood fats, and it puts you at an increased risk of getting heart disease and type 2 diabetes.

If you have PCOS, you have an eleven fold increased risk of getting metabolic syndrome. (Fortunately, your risk of getting it decreases if you put into practice some of the advice in this book!). The diagnosis of metabolic syndrome (also known as syndrome X) is made when you have at least three of the following going on in your body:

✔ Abdominal obesity (excessive fat tissue in and around the abdomen).

✔ Abnormal blood fat levels, which includes high triglycerides, low HDL cholesterol (good cholesterol), and high LDL cholesterol (bad cholesterol). These together cause plaque build-ups in the artery walls.

✔ High blood pressure.

✔ Insulin resistance where the body can't properly use insulin and more is pumped out to compensate.

✔ An increase in certain substances in the blood which increase the likelihood of blood clots.

✔ A rise in substances in the blood (with complicated sounding names such as C reactive protein!) that cause inflammation leading to an increased risk of damage to the artery wall and an increased risk of cardiovascular disease.

PCOS through Life Stages

Unless kept in check, PCOS can have an influence on each of your reproductive stages throughout your life. PCOS may be diagnosed at different life stages; for some women it may not be diagnosed until the menopause. At different life stages, the symptoms that lead to a diagnosis of PCOS can differ. Table 1-1 lists what kind of symptoms can be expected at each life stage.

Table 1-1	PCOS and Life Stages
Life Stage	*Most Notable Symptoms*
Puberty	Early menarche (the start of your periods).
	Acne.
	Weight gain.
	Irregular periods or periods that start then stop altogether.
Adulthood	Weight gain.
	Continued acne and hirsutism.
	Irregular or absent periods.
	Inability to conceive.
	PMS type symptoms.
During pregnancy	Greater tendency towards developing high blood pressure.
	Developing gestational diabetes (diabetes that develops during pregnancy).
	Higher rate of miscarriage.
Menopause	Late menopause.
	Increased tendency to put weight on around the middle.
	Developing type 2 diabetes, high cholesterol, and high blood pressure.
Post menopause	A tendency towards weight gain, insulin resistance, metabolic syndrome, and type 2 diabetes.
	Other symptoms probably diminish.

The Three-Pronged Attack

Unfortunately no cure exists for PCOS, but you can control the symptoms so that the effect of PCOS on your body is minimal. Basically treatment involves the following:

✔ Improving insulin sensitivity. This improvement prevents the whole cascade of later problems such as developing type 2 diabetes and abnormal blood fat levels which can give rise to heart disease.

✔ Restoring normal ovulation and hence fertility.

✔ Stopping the male hormone, androgen, levels in the blood from rising.

Treatment of PCOS therefore involves the three-pronged attack of:

✔ **Diet:** using a weight control diet if necessary with low-GI advice.

✔ **Exercise:** encouraging you to be more physically active on a day-to-day basis and throughout the day.

✔ **Emotional well-being:** If you lack motivation, or are moody and/or depressed, you need to also incorporate some techniques for mood lifting and motivation.

Even if you are normal weight, research has shown that if you have PCOS, you still have a tendency to have raised blood concentrations of insulin compared to women without PCOS of the same weight. Eating a low-GI balanced diet and being physically active is therefore important, even if you don't have a weight problem.

Treatment should be tailored to you and the symptoms you are experiencing, but it should also take into consideration whether you are aiming to get pregnant or not.

If you are not imminently planning a baby, treatment needs to focus on:

✔ Correcting abnormal hormone levels.

✔ Reducing weight (or maintaining a healthy weight if you aren't overweight).

✔ Managing cosmetic concerns, such as increased hairiness where you don't want hair, and the loss of hair on your head where you do want it!

If you're hoping to get pregnant, treatment needs to focus on:

✔ Reducing weight, as a healthy diet with increased physical activity allows more efficient use of insulin and decreases blood glucose levels and may help you to ovulate more regularly.

✔ Promoting ovulation with ovulation induction medications.

Maximising your health before you conceive and normalising blood sugar and blood insulin levels also make sure that, if you do conceive, there's less risk of miscarrying or having a baby that develops problems.

Diet under the spotlight

The high insulin level commonly found in PCOS sufferers is to blame for the tendency to gain weight and the inability to lose it. That's why, when you have PCOS, your diet is of vital importance because you have to balance several factors: calorie intake (to avoid excess weight gain), carbohydrate intake (to stabilise blood sugars), and so on. Therefore, a PCOS-friendly diet helps you to:

✔ Lose weight to get to a healthy weight, or to maintain a healthy weight.

✔ Reduce insulin resistance and the risk of developing type 2 diabetes.

✔ Reduce the risk of cardiovascular disease.

✔ Ensure a balanced and nutritionally adequate dietary intake.

The following sections explain the basic components of the low-GI diet and what you need to know to lose weight (or maintain a healthy weight). For detailed information on the low-GI diet and how to lose weight successfully, head to Part II.

Know your GI (glycaemic index)

Insulin resistance (a key symptom of PCOS) results in high circulating blood levels of insulin, especially when you eat carbs that break down very rapidly resulting in glucose entering the bloodstream very rapidly (glucose is the most common breakdown product of starchy and sugary food). To avoid stimulating a high release of insulin, you want to avoid the foods that result in the biggest increases in blood glucose. That's where the glycaemic index (GI) comes in.

If you have PCOS, you need to eat meals based on low-GI foods, with medium-GI foods taken in moderation and high-GI foods eaten only occasionally. Table 1-2 lists a few examples of low-, medium- and high-GI foods (for more detailed lists, go to Chapter 4).

The glycaemic index (GI) is a method of expressing the glycaemic response of individual foods in relation to the glycaemic response of glucose. Glucose is given a GI of 100 so that other foods are given appropriate numbers relative to this. For example, spaghetti is given a GI of 41. Only carbohydrate containing foods can have a GI value, so for example meat, cheese, and some green vegetables aren't given a GI value.

Diets to avoid

Avoid diets that restrict the intake of certain groups of foods or ban them completely. Avoid diets that advocate you take certain supplements too. Such diets are likely to be unbalanced. Low-carb diets are often advocated in popular books and Web sites for PCOS. These diets aren't recommended because they:

✔ Are high in fat and so are likely to raise your cholesterol level, putting you at a higher risk of heart disease.

✔ Tend to be high in protein which may put you at a higher risk of kidney problems, especially if you already have diabetes.

✔ Cause you to produce more ketones from the breakdown of fats. As well as making you feel awful and causing your breath to smell, if you do fall pregnant, you can damage the baby with such high ketone levels in the blood.

Table 1-2	GI Ranking of Foods
Food	*GI Ranking*
Cornflakes	High
Weetabix	Medium
All Bran	Low
Porridge	Low
White Rice	High
Basmati Rice	Medium
White/Wholemeal bread	High
Mixed grain bread	Low
Pasta	Low
Potato, mashed	High
New potatoes, boiled	Medium
Sweet potato	Low
Baked beans	Low
Apples	Low
Grapes	Low

Balanced eating

Watching the GI value of food shouldn't be the be-all and end-all of eating for PCOS. Here are some other diet bits you need to keep an eye on:

- ✔ Establish a pattern of regular meals and snacks.

- ✔ Avoid low-carb diets as they don't do your overall health much good.

- ✔ Eat a varied diet to ensure that you have the complete range of vitamins and minerals that your body needs.

- ✔ Fat is twice as high in calories gram for gram as carbs or protein, so don't pile on the spreads, oils, butter, cheese, or mayo, and avoid pastry. The fat you do eat should be the unsaturated type.

- ✔ Salt and alcohol intakes should follow healthy eating and drinking guidelines (see Chapter 3 if you're not sure what the guidelines are).

- ✔ Don't forget to include some oily fish (like mackerel and sardines) in your diet every week.

- ✔ Your requirement for calcium may be higher than expected because of PCOS; so if you're concerned that you don't have much milk, milk products, or alternatives such as calcium fortified soya products, you may need to take a calcium and vitamin D supplement.

Weight loss practicalities

You can measure your weight in three ways:

- ✔ Body mass index (BMI). You need to aim for a normal Body Mass Index of between 18.5 and 25. BMI is covered in Chapter 5.

- ✔ Body fat percentage. This measurement should be around 20–30 per cent. (You can buy scales for home use that measure this for you.)

- ✔ Waist circumference. For women, a waist circumference measure over 80 centimetres (31.5 inches), regardless of your height or body type, indicates an increased risk of developing heart disease, diabetes, blood pressure, and other related diseases.

If you want to lose weight, you should be aiming for a calorie allowance of around 1500 cals a day, which should allow you to lose about half a kilogram to one kilogram (1 to 2 pounds) a week, depending on how active you are. You also need to make sure that your portion sizes are reasonable – use a smaller plate so that you can't actually serve yourself a meal that is overly large. A healthy dietary plan involves having three meals with two small snacks. For great tasting low-GI recipes, go to Part III.

Get physical

The good news about getting more active is that it offers huge benefits to symptom reduction in PCOS. The benefits extend well beyond PCOS and into many other areas from cancer prevention to lifting moods.

Benefits of exercise

The reasons to exercise if you have PCOS (and for general health) include the following:

- ✔ Helps maintain weight loss and allows you to have a few more calories while on a weight loss diet.

  The ideal combination is to lose weight by following a sensible weight control diet along with a minimum of half-an-hour physical activity a day.
- ✔ Improves the relative mount of muscle to fat and improves overall body shape.
- ✔ Improves insulin sensitivity.
- ✔ Increases the levels of good cholesterol in the blood (HDL).
- ✔ Reduces blood pressure.
- ✔ Decreases the risk of developing heart disease and diabetes.
- ✔ Improves bone density and so reduces your risk of developing osteoporosis (brittle bones).
- ✔ Improves your psychological health, such as self-confidence, well-being, and self-image.

To maximise the advantages of doing exercise you need to combine aerobic exercise (which causes you to get a bit breathless) with some resistance training (such as lifting some weights), and some stretching and flexibility work to maintain joint and muscle strain-free movement. Chapter 10 explains what you need to know.

Tips for exercising success

There's a high drop out rate among people who take up exercise. To avoid this drop off yourself, and make sure that you reap the maximum benefits from exercise, plan ahead and bear a few things in mind:

- ✔ Don't be too ambitious or you'll never keep it up!
- ✔ Plan to do exercise that fits into your lifestyle and that you enjoy doing.

- ✔ If time is a barrier, incorporate exercise into your daily routine. For example, if you normally pop to the shops most days to top up on your food shopping, think about walking or cycling there instead.

- ✔ You don't have to join an expensive gym: Do exercise you can perform from home, or just go out for a brisk walk, cycle, or jog.

- ✔ The amount of moving about you do throughout the day is as important as any formal exercise session you undertake. So think about how you can build in more activity throughout the day.

Looking after the inside

Knowing about what wonderful results can be achieved by diet and exercise is all very well, but if you are unable to take the advice due to an overload of stress, anxiety, or depression, having an encyclopaedic knowledge of PCOS is going to do you a fat lot of good. In order to be able to act on your knowledge about what you should do, you need to feel fired up, ready for action, and on a fairly emotional even keel.

An important key to getting well is to treat yourself kindly. Recognise that PCOS is a major stressor in your life and give yourself permission to work through the feelings associated with it. If you are to diminish the symptoms associated with PCOS you must also recognise the emotional effects of PCOS.

PCOS often leads to feelings of anxiety, low self-esteem, and loss of control. The emotional effects of PCOS can start in the teenage years when the symptoms such as weight problems, excess facial or body hair, and acne, start to emerge. To make matters worse, the journey to a diagnosis can be long and painful. Once a diagnosis is made, it can be a relief to know that the symptoms aren't just in your mind. But then you're left with the stress of knowing that you have to cope with a long-term condition. Empowering yourself by knowing what PCOS is about and what you can do about it so that you are in control can help to lessen the emotional frustrations.

Dealing with emotional symptoms

One of the best ways to deal with the emotional fallout of PCOS is to find support from people who understand what you are going through. Online support groups, national associations with local chapters, group meetings, and many other ways are available to get to know people who are struggling with the same problems you have. When you feel isolated you are more likely to experience depression. If the depression is serious you may need to see a counsellor.

Chapter 12 explains in more detail the effects of PCOS on your emotional well-being and offers strategies and advice on how to avoid or ameliorate the most common emotional pitfalls.

Mood and motivation

Vicious circles are common in PCOS. Getting into shape and reducing the symptoms can seem such an uphill struggle that it may seem easier just to give up and give in. But in doing this you feel more and more depressed and feel that extreme actions are required. However extreme actions just set you up for failure once more and the circle continues. To offset a complete relapse you should bear the following in mind:

- ✔ Tripping up from time-to-time is inevitable. When it happens, pick yourself back up and set yourself back on the road.
- ✔ Start things gradually.
- ✔ Make sure that the changes you make can be incorporated easily into your lifestyle and that you can keep them up long term.
- ✔ Set yourself smaller mini goals along the way and reward yourself with something other than food each time you achieve a mini goal.

Keep a food diary and an exercise diary. If keeping a diary permanently is too much, just fill it in for a week initially, and then from time-to-time when you feel your resolve is slacking. Include keeping a track of your moods too. A diary can remind you what you were doing when things were going well, but it can also help bring things to light when things aren't going so well.

Eating disorders

If you have a distorted pattern of thinking about food and behaving around food, you may have an eating disorder. If you have an eating disorder you'll also have a pre-occupation and/or obsession with food and your use (or indeed non-use) of food is likely to be out of control.

Any eating disorder requires professional help and usually cognitive behavioural therapy (CBT) is given. Acknowledging what the triggers are to this behaviour is important – they are frequently mood-based, especially feelings of low self-esteem. CBT is given alongside dietary advice aimed at restoring normal meal patterns of three reasonable meals a day plus snacks if appropriate. This restoration of regular meal patterns is to break the cycle of bingeing then purging or starving.

Trying Out Other Stuff

Paying attention to your diet, your exercise levels, and your emotional health are things that you can do yourself, with a bit of support from friends, family, and some relevant experts such as personal trainers and dieticians. However, there may be times when you feel this just isn't enough and you may have to get extra support, as outlined in the following sections.

Medication

As well as taking on board the diet, exercise, and motivational advice in this book, it may be that your doctor feels you also need some medication to help reduce your symptoms, as not doing so quickly can put you at risk of developing other diseases such as diabetes, heart disease, or possibly even endometrial cancer (cancer of the womb lining).

You should only take medication that is prescribed by your doctor or specialist especially for you.

For insulin resistance

Although not favoured by all doctors and PCOS experts, many still use metformin, an insulin sensitising drug, to treat PCOS. The drug seems to help with the following PCOS symptoms:

- ✔ Menstrual regularity and so improvements in fertility.
- ✔ Androgen level reduction leading to reduction in hirsutism and acne.
- ✔ Weight loss.

For acne and hirsutism

If you have hirsutism and/or acne, you may be prescribed a combined oral contraceptive pill containing the anti-androgen, progesterone. 'Yasmin' and 'Dianette' are two examples of pills containing progesterone. If a contraceptive pill is not required, you may just get prescribed some anti-androgenic medication such as 'Spironolactone' or cyproterone acetate.

For fertility problems

Lifestyle changes are the best way to address fertility problems, but if some help is needed, you may be prescribed a drug called 'clomid' (clomiphine citrate), often with chorionic gonadotrphin (a reproductive hormone). The two together help the follicles in the ovary to develop properly and for ovulation to occur. If you don't ovulate, no egg is released to be fertilised by the sperm.

For weight loss

If you are finding it tough to lose weight, despite having tried to do so on numerous occasions, and/or your current weight is endangering your health, your doctor may put you on one of the three anti-obesity drugs that are on the market. You need to be carefully monitored while you are on such medication, as these drugs are not without some side effects.

Supplements and herbals

When you read up about PCOS, or surf the Web on the subject, you find that a whole plethora of herbal remedies and supplements are recommended for PCOS. Go to Chapter 11 for more information about supplements and herbals.

Be wary of the advice you find. Supplements and herbal remedies can be harmful, especially if you decide to take them without the backing of a professional medically qualified practitioner. Before you take any herbal or supplement, consult your doctor.

Supplements

The following list explains what supplements you can safely take, unless advised otherwise by a doctor or dietician:

- ✔ **Calcium and vitamin D:** Take these supplements if you don't include much milk or dairy products (or their alternatives such as fortified soya products) in your diet.

- ✔ **Iron supplements:** Iron supplements may be necessary if you have heavy periods and have been found to be anaemic.

- ✔ **A multivitamin and mineral supplement:** If you know your diet has been unbalanced for a while, you may need multivitamin and mineral supplements. Only take a supplement that provides up to the recommended intake of the nutrients and choose one that includes chromium.

- ✔ **Folic acid:** If you are planning on getting pregnant, you want to make sure that you get enough folic acid. The dose advised is 400 micrograms per day.

Herbals

As far as herbals go, the really strong contender as being truly effective in PCOS is Agnus Castus. Other herbals may have an effect but so far, the evidence supporting them is still weak.

Agnus Castus is available as a dried berry extract in tablet, capsule, or liquid form. The active ingredients are compounds similar in structure to sex hormones that act on the pituitary gland in the brain to affect ovarian hormonal production, helping to normalise menstruation patterns.

Alternative therapies

Natural remedies should only be tried if you follow the advice of an experienced qualified practitioner with an interest in women's health including fertility. At present, no clinical trials have been completed on alternative therapies in this area. However, you can try some treatments that may help you to relax and which should be relatively safe, including massage and reflexology. Chapter 11 discusses the alternative therapies – both good and bad.

Chapter 2

Knowing You Have PCOS

. . . .

. . . .

*I*f you have PCOS, you have the most common hormonal and reproductive problem affecting women of child-bearing age. In recent years it has become apparent that PCOS is much more common than was previously realised.

In the past, only women with the most severe symptoms were acknowledged to have the condition that is now known as Polycystic Ovary Syndrome. (Previously the condition was known as Polycystic Ovarian Disease or Stein-Leventhal syndrome, after the two doctors who discovered it in the 1930s.) Nowadays, with much more advanced diagnostic tools being available such as ultrasound, doctors are better at recognising the condition, even if the symptoms are only mild.

This chapter spells out how you can recognise if you have PCOS by exploring the physical, emotional, and hidden symptoms of PCOS. It also looks at how you or your doctor can spot PCOS and touches on how to cope with PCOS through your life stages.

Overweight and under the Weather: Symptoms of PCOS

PCOS is associated with multiple cysts on the ovaries (sometimes described as a 'string of pearls'). These cysts are immature *follicles*, the egg-containing structures in the ovary, one of which should grow monthly to release an egg (ovulate). The cysts themselves are harmless, but PCOS is also accompanied by a host of other symptoms which are caused by certain hormones being out of balance, and this inhibits the normal growth of the egg-containing follicles. (In fact the word *syndrome* means a group of symptoms.) The following sections outline both the obvious and not-so-obvious symptoms of PCOS.

You and your PCOS are unique. You can get quite a few symptoms with PCOS, but the combination of particular symptoms probably varies from someone else's symptom profile. Some symptoms are more common than others; namely weight gain (especially around the middle), skin problems, hairiness, and a tendency towards diabetes and infertility.

Around 20–30 per cent of women have polycystic ovaries, but not all go on to develop symptoms. Once symptoms do develop, that marks the change from simply having symptom-free polycystic ovaries to polycystic ovary syndrome. The incidence of actual PCOS is probably around 5–10 per cent of women in the developed world, although it is on the up which experts claim is due to the increasing number of overweight and obese people in the population.

Physical symptoms

Several symptoms manifest themselves physically in PCOS. Because many of them affect the way you look, they can have a large impact on your psychological health too. The situation isn't all doom and gloom though – these symptoms start to lessen as you take on the advice in this book.

Period disruption

In PCOS, your period may be:

- ✔ Absent altogether – known medically as amenorrhoea.
- ✔ Irregular – known medically as oligomenorrhoea.
- ✔ Heavy – known medically as menorrhagia.
- ✔ Lasting for a long time.

As a PCOS sufferer you are more likely to have higher than normal levels of *androgens* sloshing around your body. Androgens are male hormones – the best known being testosterone – which all women produce in their ovaries. The abnormal level of these male hormones, along with other hormonal disruption, is responsible for the period problems you may be experiencing. However, you may be one of the lucky ones because about 1 in 5 women with PCOS have perfectly normal menstrual cycles.

Weight gain

You have a 50 per cent chance of being overweight with PCOS (but that also means you have a 50 per cent chance of not being overweight!). Insulin resistance and the increased levels of male hormones that occur in PCOS are believed to be the main causes of weight gain, which occurs particularly around the middle. If you observe any male friends (or maybe your partner!) who are getting a bit chubby, you often find that this is where they first put on weight. In males, weight gain around the middle is sometimes referred to as a beer belly.

The elevated levels of glucose in your blood stream, which occur, for example, after you eat a carbohydrate-containing meal, trigger the pancreas to release insulin which allows the cells in the body (such as muscle cells) to absorb the glucose. If you are *insulin resistant* (a common condition in PCOS), excessive amounts of free-floating glucose remain in the blood stream because it can't properly enter the cells. This excess amount is eventually sent to the liver and converted there to excess body fat.

Different hair growth patterns

A change in hair growth usually manifests as excessive hair growth on parts of the body that ought not to be hairy on a woman. (The term for this pattern of hair growth is *hirsutism*.) You may find that you develop hairiness on your face, chest, stomach, and back.

Unfortunately, as well as gaining more hair in places where you don't want it, with PCOS you are more likely to lose it on your head, a condition known as *alopecia*. Don't worry: You aren't going to go completely bald! What tends to happen with PCOS is that you get a gradual overall thinning of the hair, or thinning at the corners above the temple. As thinning continues the hair may go see-through so that it looks like a fine, fuzzy halo when light shines on it.

If you do suffer from alopecia, it's rarely severe and can be controlled by bringing down your male hormone levels by following the diet and exercise advice in this book (in the short-term your GP may also prescribe medication to do this). Remember that losing around 100 hairs a day is normal. Keep this in mind before you convince yourself you have alopecia.

Fatigue/exhaustion

You may find that you need more sleep than you used to and perhaps also crave a nap in the middle of the day. Even so you may still feel tired a lot of the time and have a real job waking up in the morning. This kind of tiredness is commonly associated with PCOS.

Lack of good quality sleep also means you're more prone to tiredness and exhaustion. Although some women with PCOS do go on to develop chronic fatigue, dealing with symptoms early can help avoid this happening.

The hormonal fluctuations underlying PCOS can mean that you experience difficulties in getting a full night's restful sleep. Worry and frustration associated with having PCOS may also be contributing to any rough nights you're experiencing.

With PCOS, the root cause of the feeling of tiredness and exhaustion is resistance to insulin, which makes your body turn carbohydrates you eat into fat rather than a fuel source for energy. So at the same time as gaining more and more weight, you also feel more and more tired. Also, blood sugars may dip quite low overnight if you suffer from PCOS, giving rise to fatigue the next day.

Digestive disorders

Many women with PCOS have digestive problems, especially constipation and irritable bowel syndrome (IBS). The reason why is not clear but it can be linked to the fact that you may have a lowered metabolic rate after a meal which may result in:

- Food taking longer to digest.
- Food not being digested efficiently.

Nausea

In the same way that fluctuating hormone levels may lead to nausea in pregnancy, and also during PMS, the altered hormone levels in PCOS can also give rise to nausea.

Dizziness and fainting

The dizziness and fainting associated with PCOS can be linked to the tiredness, but it does seem that sometimes blood sugar levels can drop abnormally low and can give rise to symptoms of dizziness and fainting. Again a low-GI diet helps to alleviate low blood sugars (see Chapter 4).

Hot flushes/flashes

Hot flushes or flashes are normally associated with the menopause, but they can occur in PCOS too. Hot flushes themselves don't cause any harm, but they are a nuisance. They are characterised by:

- Rapid heart beat
- Rise in temperature
- Clammy palms
- Sweating

You may get hot flushes with PCOS because of the underlying hormone disturbances.

Pain

PCOS doesn't result in the type of pelvic pain that is sometimes associated with larger ovarian cysts but you may notice some pelvic discomfort at times. This may be due to the effect of hormones on the flow of blood through the pelvic veins.

Skin changes

You may develop *skin tags* – small pieces of skin that form on the neck or armpits. You may also develop darkened skin areas on the back of the neck, in the armpits, and under the breasts. The medical term for this condition is 'acanthosis nigricans'.

Acne and oily skin

If your androgen (male hormone) levels are high, you may develop acne on your face, chest, or back. The skin's sebaceous glands are stimulated to over-produce an oily substance called sebum and this over-production gives rise to acne.

Psychological symptoms

The psychological symptoms you get with PCOS can be as a result of having an illness that can have so many physical manifestations. Even the most naturally cheery of souls can get down in the doldrums from time to time. Some experts believe that the syndrome itself can have mind-altering effects – and not the pleasant 'way out, man' type!

Depression

One of the less recognised symptoms of PCOS is depression. Depression is more likely if you have more extreme symptoms of PCOS. Although depression stems from many factors, considering PCOS as a possible cause is always a good idea if you experience other PCOS symptoms as well.

Many experts are unclear as to whether depression really is a symptom of PCOS or whether your PCOS symptoms (such as weight gain and so on) cause depression. Whichever comes first – the depression or the PCOS – a vicious cycle can develop because the depression makes you less likely to want to deal with your PCOS symptoms and so they get worse, and as the symptoms get worse, so does the depression.

If you experience even some of the following symptoms of depression, seek some help from your doctor:

✔ Feeling down, for no apparent reason, for more than a couple of days in a row, especially if you feel far more down than any possible trigger warrants.

✔ Avoiding having a social life, preferring to stay at home by yourself, and inventing excuses not to go out with friends or visit family.

✔ Experiencing crying episodes, often for no real reason.

✔ Having persistent trouble sleeping.

✔ Being overly critical of yourself.

✔ Having suicidal thoughts.

Depression can also be a side effect of drugs that you may have been given to treat your PCOS. At least 100 fairly common prescription drugs can bring about the side effect of depression. If you're feeling depressed, mention it to your doctor. If the cause is due to the drugs you are on, he or she may well be able to find alternative medications.

In some medical practices antidepressants are prescribed. These drugs don't alleviate the underlying issues but may help you to get motivated to tackle your PCOS.

Irritability, mood swings, and other psychological symptoms

In PCOS, the following symptoms sometimes appear on their own; sometimes they accompany PCOS-related depression (explained in the preceding section):

✔ Feeling stressed.

✔ Feeling anxious.

✔ Feeling out of control.

✔ Experiencing a lack of mental alertness.

✔ Experiencing a decreased sex drive.

Some of the 'mood' symptoms associated with PCOS can make it seem as if you have PMS (premenstrual syndrome, characterised by a wide array of symptoms including irritability, anxiety, and wild fluctuations in mood). Indeed the irritability and mood swings seen in both PMS and PCOS are both triggered by fluctuating hormone levels. However, in PMS the symptoms occur *only* prior to your period starting, whereas in PCOS no recognisable monthly pattern exists.

Binge eating/bulimia

Having PCOS seems to make you more prone to developing abnormal eating patterns. The most common effect is the desire to binge eat. In fact, up to 60 per cent of women with bulimia have been found to have PCOS.

The binge eating/bulimia cycle is a vicious one. You binge and then feel so guilty for bingeing that you do one of the following:

- ✔ Starve yourself until you can't hold out without food any longer.
- ✔ Try to get rid of the excess food you have eaten by making yourself sick.
- ✔ Try to get rid of the excess food you have eaten by using lots of laxatives.

What normally happens after this is that you are either so hungry or so fed-up that you binge all over again, and the cycle continues. Chapter 5 has more information on bingeing cycles. If you recognise a tendency in yourself to binge eat, you may need to seek some professional help in order to break out of this vicious cycle.

Unseen, lurking symptoms

As if the physical and mental symptoms of PCOS aren't enough to be dealing with, you may also have symptoms that lurk unseen until you have medical tests.

Fertility problems

Your PCOS may first have been diagnosed because you were trying to conceive but couldn't. When an ovary doesn't produce an egg, the result is infertility. An egg is not produced because the levels of hormones are insufficient to mature an egg in the ovary, and so it doesn't get released.

Infertility usually happens when PCOS becomes quite advanced. Around 90–95 per cent of women attending infertility clinics due to lack of ovulation have PCOS. You can help to restore your fertility by adopting the lifestyle changes outlined in this book, and in particular in Chapter 13.

Metabolic syndrome

If you have PCOS, you are at an increased risk of developing a condition known as *metabolic syndrome*. Around 45 per cent of women with PCOS are believed to have this condition in addition to the PCOS.

Metabolic syndrome is a whole mix of health problems which together lead to the development of full-blown type 2 diabetes and heart disease. You may not know you have any of these problems, but your doctor can usually pick them up in fairly routine blood tests. Here are some of the conditions associated with metabolic syndrome:

✔ Insulin resistance (refer to the later section 'Insulin resistance' for more).

✔ High cholesterol levels.

✔ Too much weight gain, and that weight developing particularly around the waist and abdomen (apple shape).

✔ High blood pressure.

✔ High levels of a protein in the blood called *C-reactive protein*, a marker protein for inflammation which can be a sign that the arteries and heart may be prone to damage.

✔ High levels of substances in the blood that make it clot more quickly. A high level means that the blood is more likely to clot and this may mean that it clots while travelling around the arteries. If a clot does get lodged in the arteries leading to the heart, this can give rise to a heart attack. If a clot gets lodged in the artery leading to the brain, it can cause a stroke.

With PCOS, you are more likely to have metabolic syndrome if

✔ You gain a lot of weight.

✔ Your periods have stopped (even though you aren't menopausal).

PCOS is a condition that can be relieved by breaking the vicious circle of weight gain which leads to worsening of symptoms and the development of new symptoms. By losing weight you can reverse the symptoms of metabolic syndrome and regain your periods. Gaining weight leads to an increasing likelihood of your periods stopping, a worsening of metabolic syndrome, and the developing of full-blown diabetes.

Insulin resistance

Having insulin resistance means that normal amounts of insulin produced by the pancreas can't adequately do the work of controlling the glucose levels in the blood so that they remain within normal parameters. The body detects that blood glucose levels aren't being adequately controlled and so pumps out more insulin in order to try and achieve some sort of blood sugar control. However, the result is that insulin levels in the blood become very high and this itself causes other symptoms commonly seen in PCOS, including:

✔ Weight gain.

✔ Increased production of male hormones, namely testosterone, by the ovaries, which in turn are responsible for such symptoms as acne, facial hair growth, and irregular periods.

✔ Abnormal blood fat levels which can lead to heart disease.

✔ Damage to blood vessel walls which can lead to heart disease or stroke.

✔ Kidneys retaining too much sodium, which in turn causes blood pressure to rise.

✔ Insulin resistance commonly resulting in the development of type 2 diabetes.

Even if you're not overweight and have PCOS, you may still have a raised level of insulin in the blood. However, eating a low-GI diet (see Chapter 4) combined with exercise can help you to bring insulin levels down, even if you're normal weight.

Endometrial cancer

The lining of the womb is known as the endometrium, and it varies in thickness throughout a normal monthly menstrual cycle. So in a normal menstrual cycle the lining builds up in preparation for the implanting of a fertilised egg. However, if the egg is not fertilised, this extra lining is shed and that's when a period happens.

Often, in PCOS, no egg is released, but the lining of the womb still builds up. However, because ovulation never happens, this lining is never shed but keeps building up. Known as endometrial hyperplasia, this condition can increase the risk of developing endometrial cancer, although even in PCOS, this cancer is not very common.

Restoring a normal menstrual cycle is therefore important, not only for restoring fertility but also so that the risk of developing endometrial cancer is reduced.

Endometriosis

Having both PCOS and endometriosis is not uncommon, but no one really knows whether the two conditions are actually linked.

Endometriosis is a condition where tissue that is similar to the lining of the womb grows at other sites of the body that are outside the womb. The most common sites are the pelvis, on the ovaries, and in the bowel. These growths also react like the womb to oestrogen and so tend to swell and become painful at the time of the month when the womb lining would be building up. They can also then bleed when a normal period is due.

If you have PCOS, you tend to have a lot of oestrogen slushing around and very little progesterone which dictates when the oestrogen should stop having its effect of building up womb tissue and trigger the monthly bleed. Being in a mode of continual build-up of womb tissue is just what you don't need if you have endometriosis, and this is likely to make the condition worse.

Other PCOS symptoms

Other, less common, symptoms can occur if you have PCOS. Most of these symptoms are a result of the disrupted hormone levels and include:

- ✔ Migraine
- ✔ Feeling perpetually hungry
- ✔ Abdominal pain

Detecting PCOS

Although PCOS is a tendency you're born with and so can be lurking throughout your life, you're statistically most likely to have it diagnosed in your early- to mid-30s, perhaps because you're having difficulty in conceiving.

Self identification

Symptoms of PCOS may be vague or they can be caused by something definite. Here are some pointers which may indicate that you need to get yourself checked out (you can read a full list symptoms in the section 'Overweight and Under the Weather: Symptoms of PCOS' at the beginning of this chapter):

- ✔ Weight gain, despite eating the same as usual.
- ✔ Periods becoming irregular or stopping altogether which coincides with weight gain.
- ✔ Excessive hair growth on the face, chest, or stomach, and thinning of scalp hair.
- ✔ A need to binge on food and developing periods of intense hunger.
- ✔ Depression, tiredness, and moodiness.

Even if your mother or sister has PCOS, and you think that you do too, don't expect to have exactly the same symptoms. Symptoms of PCOS vary between women, even within the same family. So your sister with PCOS may have periods whereas you have none at all. Also, your symptoms may change over time; expect them to get worse and expect more symptoms to develop if your weight continues to increase.

You can't really diagnose yourself with PCOS; if you think you have it, you need to get properly diagnosed by your doctor or specialist because other conditions have symptoms which are shared with PCOS. These other conditions include:

- **PMS (premenstrual syndrome)**, which occurs in many women from 2 to 14 days before the onset of menstruation and is characterised by a wide array of physical and mental symptoms.

- **Low thyroid function**, known as hypothyroidism, where the thyroid gland in the neck doesn't produce enough thyroid hormone. This condition can result in you feeling tired, perpetually cold, and you may put on weight.

- **Adrenal deficiency**, also known as Addison's disease, which is a hormone deficiency caused by damage to the outer layer of the adrenal gland and results in you feeling weak and tired.

- **Cushing's syndrome**, caused by increased production of cortisol, or by excessive use of cortisol or other steroid hormones. Weakness, acne, and weight gain are common symptoms.

- **Hyperprolactinaemia**, characterised by increased levels of the hormone prolactin in the blood. Women with this condition mainly experience disrupted or absent periods and infertility.

- **Androgen-producing tumours**, which result in the production of high levels of male hormone, particularly testosterone.

Getting a doctor's clarification

If you suspect that you have PCOS, your doctor or specialist can give you a proper diagnosis. As well as taking a medical history from you and conducting a physical examination, your doctor may look for at least two symptoms of PCOS. According to the American Society for Reproductive Medicine, PCOS is defined by the presence of any two of the following characteristics:

- Lack of ovulation for an extended period of time (which probably manifests itself as the stopping of your monthly period).

- High levels of androgens (male hormones).

- Many small cysts on the ovaries.

Your own doctor may need to send you for some tests in order to detect if any of the above are occurring. These tests may include a number of the different procedures covered in the following sections.

Scan of the ovaries

A woman's ovaries are where her eggs are stored. Each egg is stored in a capsule called a follicle. Once a month, one follicle grows to produce a mature egg, which is released at ovulation. In normal circumstances, the remaining follicle dissolves. In PCOS, the egg doesn't mature fully and remains at a size of about 2–9 millimetres diameter within a fluid-filled cyst. (A mature follicle that is ready to release an egg reaches 20 millimetres in diameter.) Over time, the ovaries fill with many cysts and this is why PCOS is described as *polycystic* which means 'many cysts'. These small cysts in the ovaries don't get larger; in fact, they eventually disappear and are replaced by new cysts.

Figure 2-1 shows how normal ovaries look compared to an ovary of someone with PCOS. In PCOS, your ovary is also slightly enlarged.

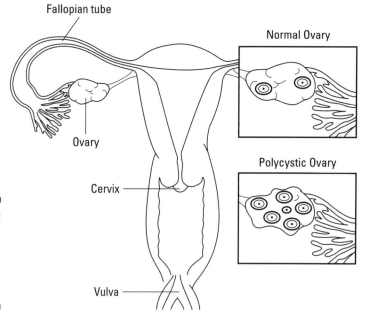

Figure 2-1: Comparing a normal ovary with a polycystic ovary.

In order to look at the ovaries, an *ultrasound* (sometimes called a *sonography*) scan is done. This procedure uses safe high-frequency sound waves and allows an image of the ovaries to be seen on a special computer. The ultrasound can detect if a woman's ovaries are enlarged (which can happen in PCOS) or if cysts are present. This sort of scan can also pick-up a thickening of the endometrium.

Glucose tolerance test (GTT) explained

If you have diabetes, or even severe insulin resistance, the body is unable to make normal use of glucose as fuel, and it accumulates in high amounts in the blood. Even in healthy people, glucose levels in the blood rise after a meal, but they soon return to normal as the glucose is used up or stored. A glucose tolerance test can distinguish between the normal pattern of clearing glucose and what happens if diabetes or severe insulin resistance (sometimes known as glucose intolerance or pre-diabetes) is present.

A GTT is performed after an overnight fast. A sample of your blood is taken and your blood glucose level measured. Then you're asked to drink a standard amount of glucose dissolved in water. Two hours later, you have another blood sample taken and the blood glucose level is measured again. The levels of glucose in the two samples are then carefully measured.

A diagnosis of diabetes is made if the level of glucose is over a set level:

- ✔ If the fasting blood sample is over 6.7 millimoles per litre (mmol/l).

- ✔ If the level of the sample taken 2 hours after the glucose drink is more than 11.1 mmol/l.

Approximately 20 to 40 per cent of women with PCOS have an abnormal glucose tolerance test.

Hormone tests

Your GP or specialist may refer you to have some blood tests done. These tests show up any disturbed levels of the hormones controlling ovulation and give an indication that PCOS may be the problem.

Hormones are substances that get released into your blood stream and circulate around the body influencing other organs. In PCOS the hormones that control ovulation are out of balance, such as progesterone (too little is produced), androgens (in PCOS the ovary tends to make too much of this male hormone), and also too much luteinising hormone (LH). LH is an important hormone throughout the cycle because it influences hormone production and acts as a trigger for ovulation. The disrupted hormone levels cause the period irregularities. Another hormone called *follicle stimulating hormone* (FSH) should be in the right proportion to LH. Doctors can measure the ratio of LH to FSH and use it as a means of monitoring the condition and whether various treatment options are working.

Testing, testing!

Your doctor may check certain other blood levels which are often out of kilter in PCOS. These tests may include the following:

- ✔ **Glucose tolerance test:** Checks whether you can cope with a certain load of sugar. If your body is not coping very well with a sugar load, this is an indication that you have, or are on the threshold of developing, type 2 diabetes.

✔ **Fasting glucose level:** If your body has not been able to bring down glucose levels to a normal value first thing in the morning before eating, this can also be a sign that you have diabetes or are borderline.

✔ **Blood cholesterol measurements:** These can include measurements of cholesterol and bad fats (called triglycerides) which circulate in the blood.

Knowing you're at risk

The exact cause of PCOS is unclear, but certain conditions do pre-dispose women to developing it. These conditions include:

✔ **Someone in your family has (or had) PCOS:** You are at increased risk if your mother or sister has the condition or your father has family members with PCOS. So there appears to be a genetic link.

Here are the stats showing that genetic tendency toward PCOS (you can read more about the link in the sidebar 'It's in the genes'):

- 35 per cent of PCOS sufferers inherit it from their mother.

- 35 per cent of PCOS sufferers inherit it from their father's side of the family.

- 50 per cent of PCOS sufferers have female relatives with PCOS on both sides of the family.

✔ **Past diagnosis of insulin resistance:** Being insulin resistant means your body can't use insulin efficiently. This leads to high circulating blood levels of insulin (called *hyperinsulinaemia*). This high level of insulin sloshing around the blood may gradually cause PCOS symptoms to get worse and worse.

It's in the genes

Researchers in the United States studied 215 mothers of women with PCOS and compared them with mothers of women who didn't have PCOS. Results showed that mothers of women with PCOS themselves had some of the symptoms of PCOS including high cholesterol levels, insulin resistance, and other metabolic abnormalities associated with PCOS. In addition, a high proportion of these mothers who had daughters with PCOS reported that they had had menstrual irregularities. Those mothers who had reported the menstrual problems had higher male hormone levels than those who hadn't reported irregularities. All this points to the fact that the mothers who had had daughters with PCOS had a much higher incidence of PCOS symptoms than mothers of non-PCOS daughters. It seemed that whether they had been diagnosed with it or not, a genetic tendency was definitely present.

Type 2 diabetes

The two types of diabetes are:

✔ Type 1

✔ Type 2

Type 1 normally occurs in childhood or in a young person. The pancreas simply stops producing insulin altogether and so injections of insulin must be given. Type 2 diabetes is normally preceded by insulin resistance so that the pancreas is still capable of producing insulin, and does so in increasing amounts, but the body is resistant to it. This can happen when someone gains too much weight. Eventually, if weight remains high or continues to increase, the body may give up producing insulin altogether, so like its type 1 cousin, insulin may be required in order to keep blood sugar levels at a controlled level.

Both type 1 and type 2 diabetes can cause similar long term damage to the body if blood sugars are not controlled sufficiently. The effects include heart disease, kidney damage, gangrene, and blindness.

PCOS through Life's Changes

Your PCOS symptoms will probably change with each stage of your life. Symptoms will get worse if you gain extra weight and may also get worse if you get stressed or ill. So are you stuck with it for life? Well, yes and no! No cure exists for PCOS, and if you make no changes to your lifestyle, you're going to get symptoms throughout your life. But you can rid yourself of symptoms by changing your lifestyle into a healthy one, whether you're 14 or 40!

Puberty

PCOS doesn't just suddenly appear; it's a disorder that is present throughout life. However, it may not manifest itself until the menstrual cycle is established, or rather should have manifested itself.

Diagnosing PCOS in young teenage girls is not a clear-cut thing, because during puberty the hormones are jumping all over the place anyway and the body goes through some fairly major changes! Weight gain, acne, and irregular periods are a common female teenage trait.

Going through adolescence is tough enough with all the changes that go on, but it can be harder still when this time heralds the start of PCOS symptoms. If the tendency to develop PCOS exists, weight gain during this time may act as a trigger to developing the condition.

The danger of weight gain during adolescence

Recent research shows that, during the transition to puberty, if weight gain occurs that leads to obesity, it is associated with an increased production of androgens – a possible forerunner to the development of PCOS and a sign that insulin resistance is occurring.

In the girls measured who had gained weight and become obese, total testosterone levels (an androgen) were over twice as high as normal weight girls. Obesity in childhood is associated with insulin resistance, raised blood pressure, and adverse changes in blood fat levels which may lead to future heart health problems. However, doctors are now realising that obesity may also be pre-disposing these girls to PCOS along with all its problems, including cosmetic problems such as hairiness, delayed or irregular periods, and later problems of infertility.

If PCOS is in the family, keep an eye on any developing symptoms. Watch particularly for rapid weight gain and periods that start suddenly and then stop for months on end.

Weight gain needs to be tackled sensitively – all teens need to avoid it, but particularly so if it is likely to set off the full-blown syndrome. However, teenagers hate being preached at and care should be taken to avoid triggering abnormal eating patterns and eating disorders.

Pregnancy

Unfortunately your PCOS can put you at increased risk of having a miscarriage (see Chapter 13), of developing gestational diabetes, and also of developing pregnancy toxaemia (also known as pre-eclampsia, where blood pressure can reach a dangerously high level for both mother and baby). Gestational diabetes is a transient diabetes that occurs in pregnant women, particularly if they are overweight at the start of pregnancy and/or gain a lot of weight during pregnancy.

Being in tip-top shape prior to getting pregnant can offset any pregnancy problems and hopefully help to reduce the risk of miscarriage. Chapter 13 has some tips on how to get into shape for pregnancy. Getting down to your target weight prior to pregnancy and avoiding excessive weight gain during pregnancy can help to offset the risk of developing gestational diabetes.

Menopause

Menopause is the time when you have your last period and fertility ends. The average age of menopause in the developed world is 51. However, the wind down to menopause can happen for a number of years before periods actually end for good, and this time period is known as the peri-menopause.

You may find it difficult to distinguish peri-menopause symptoms from PCOS symptoms because they include:

  ✔ A tendency to gain weight.

  ✔ Irregular periods which can get heavier or lighter.

  ✔ Hot flushes/flashes.

  ✔ Fluctuating hormone levels which can bring about mood changes.

Unfortunately, hitting the menopause doesn't mean that PCOS suddenly goes away. What tends to happen is that symptoms remain that predispose you to developing heart disease. These symptoms include weight gain around the middle, insulin resistance, type 2 diabetes, and distorted blood fat levels – a condition known as *dislipidaemia*. Unfortunately, evidence exists that the high androgen (male hormone) levels remain too, so that male-pattern hair growth on the face and other parts of the body also remain.

A lifetime of PCOS

Unfortunately, period (menstrual) irregularities and the metabolic symptoms such as insulin resistance and abnormal blood fat levels of PCOS seem to be inherited and persist throughout life. Unfortunately neither the removal of ovaries, nor going through the menopause, seem to get rid of the symptoms. However, you can look for a light at the end of the tunnel and that is the fact that by adopting a healthy lifestyle you can reduce most symptoms down to insignificance.

No cure as such exists for PCOS, but it can be controlled so that symptoms disappear. Treatment involves breaking the vicious cycle of obesity leading to increased insulin levels, which in itself leads to higher insulin levels and triggers worsening PCOS symptoms.

If you know you have PCOS in your family, the only way to prevent it from developing in the first place is to stay within the right weight for height ratio. This can be measured by a ratio called the body mass index (BMI). Your BMI is your weight, in kilograms, divided by your height, in metres, squared. The formula is therefore $BMI = kg/m^2$. A healthy BMI is typically between 18.5–24.9. A general guide is given in Table 2-1, and Chapter 5 has more information.

Table 2-1	BMI Weight Status
BMI	*Weight Status*
Below 18.5	Underweight
18.5–24.9	Normal
25.0–29.9	Overweight
30.0 and above	Obese

Waist circumference is another way of checking how much fat you're carrying, particularly in the danger area around the middle. You're in the danger zone (as a woman) if your waist circumference is more than 80 centimetres (31.5 inches). See Chapter 5 for more on this.

Part II
Taking Control of Your Diet

The 5th Wave   By Rich Tennant

"Oh, I have a very healthy relationship with food. It's the relationship I have with my scales that's not so good."

In this part . . .

Reading this part gives you the know-how on nutrition and diet and how following a low-GI eating plan can dramatically help your PCOS symptoms. This part helps you to choose a healthy balanced diet, containing everything that your body needs in the right proportions. This part is packed full of tips about losing weight and keeping to a healthy weight in the easiest and least stressful way.

Chapter 3

Understanding the Important
Bits about Your Diet

....

In This Chapter

▶ Looking at the benefits of eating a healthy diet for PCOS

▶ Exploring the various nutrients that make up the diet

▶ Balancing your overall diet to maximise health

....

*Y*our daily diet needs to be composed of many different foods which supply a mixture of all the nutrients you need to keep your body working efficiently. In fact, the more variety you can include in your daily food intake, the easier it is to get the full range of nutrients you need in your diet. In the case of your diet, variety really is the spice of life.

The trick is to get a mixture of all the nutrients you need and in the right proportion, known as a *balanced diet*. A balanced diet equals a healthy diet, and it's not that hard to achieve, even with PCOS. You just have to give it a little extra thought. This chapter helps you to choose a balanced diet and the most appropriate diet for you. It also helps you to realise why sticking to a healthy diet is so important in PCOS.

Benefits of Eating the PCOS Way

Eating a good diet has lots of positive effects for your health, such as reducing your chances of heart disease and cancers, or just helping you to feel your best. Along with being active, healthy eating is key to reducing the symptoms of PCOS:

> ✔ Although no actual 'cure' exists for PCOS, the right diet can help the symptoms of PCOS shrink away. Many of the symptoms are due to the fact that PCOS causes insulin to work less efficiently in your body. So higher amounts of insulin are needed to deal with sugar released from carbohydrates (sugars and starches) in your food. However, following the right diet combats this problem by lowering the level of insulin

required by your body while ensuring that the lowered amount works more efficiently.

✔ If weight is an issue, symptoms of PCOS are going to be worse. Losing excess body fat, and keeping it off in a sensible fashion, is the only way to help reverse these symptoms.

✔ Moodiness, irritability, and depression have a tendency to rear their ugly heads pretty often in PCOS. The right diet can have a positive effect on your mood.

✔ The right diet is essential if you are planning to have a beautiful bouncing baby. (Pregnancy is explored in more detail in Chapter 13.)

An increasing number of food labels carry 'Guideline Daily Amount' (GDA) nutrition information or 'Daily Values'. These figures are a guide to how much of certain nutrient you should be having each day. Most food labels also tell you how much of certain key nutrients are in a serving (or portion) of the food. By having the GDA or Daily Value alongside the amount of nutrient in the food you can compare what is in the food to your guideline amount. Many labels also do this comparison for you as a percentage figure. For example, if a food contains 10 grams of fat per portion and the GDA or Daily Value for fat is 70 grams, the percentage of your GDA, or Daily Value, provided by a portion of that food is 14 per cent.

The Oxford English Dictionary defines a nutrient as 'a substance that provides nourishment essential for life and growth'. This means that the body cannot function, repair itself, or grow without all the nutrients it needs, which include proteins, fats, and carbohydrates as well as an assortment of vitamins and minerals.

By using GDAs, you can tell more easily which foods are particularly high in certain nutrients, and the information can help you track your total intake of these nutrients over the day.

The GDAs for women shown in Table 3-1 have been developed for the average woman who wants some idea of how much of each nutrient she should be eating each day for optimum health and for weight maintenance. If you need to lose weight, take a look at Chapter 5 which gives you average GDAs developed specifically for weight loss.

Table 3-1	Guideline Daily Amounts for Women
Nutrient	*GDA*
Energy (calories)	2000
Fat (grams)	70
Saturated fat (grams)	20

Nutrient	GDA
Carbohydrate (grams)	230
Total sugars (grams)	90
Protein (grams)	45
Dietary fibre (grams)	24
Sodium (grams)	2.4
Salt (sodium chloride) (grams)	6

The following sections outline the nutrients that go to make up your daily diet. Although not strictly nutrients, you also find out about antioxidants in food which play an important health-protecting role in the body.

Fats and Oils

Don't think that fats and oils are necessarily the baddies of the diet world; experts are beginning to see how important many fats and oils are for achieving optimum health. A certain amount of fat in the diet is important for food palatability but also to provide certain vitamins and important fatty acids. The fat in your food also helps certain nutrients to be absorbed into the blood. Total fat intake should not exceed more than 35 per cent of your total energy intake (which translates into a GDA of 70 grams for women).

Fats provide about twice the amount of energy (calories), weight for weight, than carbohydrates and proteins. Because fat is so energy (calorie) dense, eating more calories than you realise is all too easy. Fat has an added 'sting' in its tail because, compared to the other nutrients that give you energy (protein and carbohydrate), fat is the least likely to make you feel full-up during a meal. Likewise after eating a fatty meal, you are more likely to start feeling hungry soon after eating, compared to a meal high in protein or carbohydrate. This situation is definitely bad news for PCOS sufferers who already have a fight on their hands to try and keep their weight off and is why high-fat diets aren't recommended if you have PCOS.

Saturated fats

Saturated fats (also known as 'saturates') should be limited in the diet to no more than 10 per cent of your total calorie intake (which translates into a GDA of 20 grams for women).

Saturates (along with trans fats covered below) are particularly harmful if eaten in excess in PCOS because:

✔ They raise the level of bad cholesterol in the blood, known as LDL (low density lipoprotein) and VLDL (very low density lipoprotein), thus increasing the risk of heart disease. In PCOS these levels tend to be raised anyway, without the added damage inflicted by consuming too much saturated and trans fats.

✔ They are associated with the development of insulin resistance and dys-lipidaemia (abnormal blood fat levels). If you have PCOS, you already have a tendency to develop insulin resistance and so lowering your intake of saturated fats helps to reduce this tendency.

✔ They are associated with raised blood pressure levels, which is a risk factor for stroke and heart disease.

Saturates tend to be hard at room temperature and are mostly found in:

✔ Animal products such as dairy products and meat.

✔ Some vegetable oils such as coconut oil and palm oil.

✔ Hard margarine, ghee (clarified butter), and cooking fat.

✔ 'Hidden' fats in cakes, biscuits and puddings.

In order to help reduce PCOS symptoms keep saturates to a minimum by eating less animal fat, full-fat dairy products, pies, and pasties.

Cholesterol levels in women with PCOS

PCOS increases your risk of getting heart disease, which is partly due to:

✔ **A rise in bad cholesterol levels.** Bad cholesterol is measured by the level of 'low density lipoprotein' (LDL) and 'very low density lipoprotein' (VLDL) in the blood. These substances tend to cause a build up of 'plaque' in the artery walls, which causes arteries to get furred-up and which can eventually lead to a heart attack or stroke.

✔ **A fall in good cholesterol levels.** This fall is measured by the level of 'high density lipoprotein' (HDL) in the blood. HDL helps to remove cholesterol from the blood stream so that it doesn't get a chance to cause a furring up of the arteries.

Normally women up to the menopause tend to have relatively higher HDL levels than men. However, having PCOS causes you to have less of the HDL and more of the LDL cholesterol, so women with PCOS lose the normal protection from heart disease conferred by being a woman.

Trans fats

Trans fats should be restricted in the diet to no more than around 4 grams a day. Trans fats are used by the food industry to harden-up vegetable oils which would otherwise be too soft to use in particular products. However, the food industry is now beginning to move away from using trans fats because of the health implications.

Trans fats are thought to be even more harmful than saturates because as well as raising harmful cholesterol levels in the blood, LDL, and HDL, they also lower the levels of the good cholesterol, HDL. HDL is protective because it removes harmful cholesterol from your blood, stopping it from building up in the arteries. Therefore, staying away from foods containing trans fats is particularly important for women with PCOS.

Trans fats can be particularly high in foods that contain hardened vegetable oils which are labelled as containing partially hydrogenated fats. Trans fats are most commonly found in:

- Some pizza bases, pies, and pastries.
- Some biscuits and cakes.
- Some margarines and spreads. However, most of the more expensive brands have now cut the trans levels of their products to negligible amounts.

To help reduce PCOS symptoms avoid foods that are labelled with partially hydrogenated fats/oils. These may include pies, pastries, cakes, biscuits, and pizza bases.

Poly and mono fats

Also known as unsaturated fats or simply as 'unsaturates', poly and mono fats tend to be liquid at room temperature and are found in vegetable oils such as sunflower, corn, soya, and olive oils, in soft margarines, and in nuts, seeds, and oily fish. Polys and mono fats help to lower cholesterol levels.

Some experts fear that increasing poly levels in the diet too much may cause more harm than good. These experts believe that polys can be oxidised in the body (made into a highly reactive body-damaging substance). The damage imposed by these reactive substances makes you more prone to heart disease and cancers. Make sure that your intake doesn't exceed 20 grams per day of polyunsaturated (poly) fats, 30 grams per day of monounsaturated (mono) fats.

Cholesterol

Cholesterol is a fat-like substance found in the body cells of humans and animals and has many important functions in the body, such as the production of essential hormones and the proper function of the brain. However, when the level carried in some blood fractions exceeds certain levels, it becomes dangerous because excess cholesterol is then deposited in artery walls and can lead to heart disease or stroke. Interestingly though, cholesterol blood levels are more affected by the amount of saturated and trans fat levels in your diet than by the amount of cholesterol in your diet.

Ideally, cholesterol levels in the blood should be below 5.2 millimoles per litre (mmol/l). Get your GP to check out your cholesterol level if you have PCOS. Your GP can advise you if you need to do anything specifically to bring the level down if it is deemed too high.

However, providing you are getting enough antioxidants in your diet, such as vitamin E, this oxidation process shouldn't be an issue. Because of this slight risk, Government experts have recommended that the 10 per cent of your total calorie intake for polys should not be exceeded. Currently in the UK people are consuming about 6 per cent of their total calorie intake as polys, well within the Government top recommended level.

Monos are a safe bet when it comes to fats. They do contain the same amount of calories as other fats but, as well as protecting against heart disease, they are also believed to offer protection against certain cancers, such as breast cancer and colon cancer.

Diets rich in monos (monounsaturated fats) are also believed to help with weight loss. Research has shown that including a fist-full of unsalted nuts such as peanuts (which are high in monos) every day in the diet can help you control your food intake during the rest of the day and so help you to stay slim.

To help reduce PCOS symptoms eat most of your fats as monos, such as using olive oil in cooking or in salad dressings and dips. (Hence, the recipes in this book predominantly use olive oil). Many nuts and seeds are good sources of monounsaturated fats, as is avocado. Oils extracted from these are also good to use in dressings and sauces, but they do not take to being heated as well as olive oil, and often have a very distinct flavour. These include (with the richest source at the top):

- ✔ Hazelnuts
- ✔ Almonds

- ✔ Brazil nuts
- ✔ Cashews
- ✔ Avocado
- ✔ Sesame seeds
- ✔ Pumpkin seeds

Other oils: The essential fatty acids

The body needs two particular polys (polyunsaturated fats) for health, an because your body can't manufacture them and you have to get them from your diet, they are referred to as essential fatty acids (EFAs). These two EFAs are:

- ✔ **Linoleic acid**, which is a type of omega-6 oil.
- ✔ **Alpha linolenic acid**, which is a type of omega-3 oil.

These essential fats are very important in the body because they:

- ✔ Serve as the building blocks for other important fatty acids that are needed by your body to work efficiently.
- ✔ Play a major role in the development of every single cell in the body.
- ✔ Have vital physiological functions such as regulating blood pressure and immune responses.
- ✔ May help to prevent blood clots that lead to heart attacks or strokes.

Because of their role in promoting a healthy heart, getting an adequate supply of these essential fatty acids is particularly important if you suffer from PCOS.

Omega-6 fatty acids

Omega-6 fatty acids are found largely in fats of plant origin. Sources include:

- ✔ Sunflower, corn, soya bean, and sesame oils and margarines or spreads containing a good proportion of these oils
- ✔ Wheat germ
- ✔ Sunflower and sesame seeds
- ✔ Nuts

Omega-3 fatty acids

Omega-3 oils are particularly important if you have PCOS as they can help alleviate several conditions associated with having PCOS. For example, omega-3 oils:

- ✔ May help to alleviate depression.
- ✔ May help protect against heart disease in a number of ways. For example, they can prevent blood clots from forming and stop the heart developing an irregular rhythm.
- ✔ Can lower blood pressure.
- ✔ May help to prevent the development of insulin resistance and so may prevent you from developing type 2 diabetes.
- ✔ Can lower the level of fats called triglycerides in the blood, high levels of which are a risk factor for heart disease.

Omega-3 fatty acids are also found in fats of plant origins and in oily fish. Sources include:

- ✔ Nuts and seeds (in particular linseed).
- ✔ Flax, soya, and walnut oil and margarines or spreads containing a good proportion of these oils.
- ✔ Oily fish such as mackerel, herrings, salmon, sardines, fresh tuna, and trout.
- ✔ Dark green leafy vegetables.
- ✔ Sweet potatoes.
- ✔ Omega-3 enriched eggs.
- ✔ Meat from grass-fed animals.

The modern diet usually provides more than adequate amounts of omega-6 oils, but less of the omega-3s, and so many experts now believe that for maximum health benefits, you need to consciously try to get more omega-3 rich foods in the diet, such as nuts and seeds.

In addition, experts also recommend that your diet contain some omega-3 oils in the form of fish oil (either by eating oily fish or taking a supplement). Omega-3 oils from plant sources tend to be processed quite slowly into the substances needed by the body to function properly, but fish oil provides the body with oils that have already started to be processed into these essential substances. Fish oil sources of omega-3 are thought to be particularly important for proper immune function, for heart health, and they also have anti-inflammatory properties.

Oily fish: How much is too much?

The levels of certain harmful toxic residues found in oily fish can build up in the body. These chemicals include dioxins, polychlorinated biphenyls (PCBs), and mercury compounds. Because of these toxic residues Government experts advise that pregnant and lactating women, or those considering becoming pregnant, should eat no more than two portions of oily fish a week, whereas men and boys and other women can have four portions a week quite safely. The real danger is to the unborn baby, and that levels may build up to a toxic level in women who may fall pregnant. In addition, pregnant and lactating women need to avoid eating marlin, swordfish, and shark and restrict the amount of tuna eaten to four medium-size cans or two tuna steaks per week because of the mercury exposure.

Two common types of omega oil are found in fish and provided in fish oil supplements: Eicosapentanoic acid (EPA) and Docosahexanoic acid (DHA). But don't get freaked by their names as they're usually referred to by their acronyms!

For general health benefits, and to help reduce PCOS symptoms, eat two portions of fish a week, one of which should be oily. Oily fish include kippers, fresh tuna, mackerel, canned pilchard, trout, salmon, sardines, and herring.

The Right Carbs Are Your Friends

After fats, public enemy number two has been the poor old carbohydrate (carbs) found in foods such as bread, potatoes, breakfast cereals, pasta, and rice. But don't forget that sugar and sugary foods such as jam, honey, white sugar, and treacle are carbs too.

Carbs are broken down in the body to glucose which is the body's main fuel supply. In fact the brain can only run on glucose, it can't burn fat or protein to keep functioning. The other thing about carbohydrate-rich foods is that they are often a good source of fibre (at least the good carbs are) and essential vitamins and minerals.

As a PCOS sufferer, you need the same amount of carbohydrate as recommended for the rest of the population. In other words, carbs should supply about 50 per cent or more of your calorie needs with sugars providing a maximum of around 20 per cent (which translates into a GDA of 230 grams and 90 grams respectively).

So, now's the time to sort the good carbs from the bad – as far as PCOS is concerned. This exercise is vitally important because eating the good carbs can help you to get your health back on track, but the bad carbs can make it worse.

Here's what you need to know: Whether a carb is good or bad depends on how quickly it is broken down in the body into glucose. The slower the breakdown, the better the carb. If you suffer from PCOS, the body has a tendency to be unable to cope with a sudden rapid influx of glucose into the blood stream, which is what happens if carbohydrates are broken down rapidly by your digestive system.

The *glycaemic index*, more commonly known as the GI, is a measure of how high the level of glucose peaks in the bloodstream within two hours of eating a carbohydrate-containing food. The higher the peak achieved in that 2 hour period, the higher the GI (and the worse the carb).

GI is measured on a scale of 0 to 100:

- ✔ A carb food with a GI of less than 50 is a *low-GI* food.
- ✔ A carb food with a GI of between 50 and 65 is a *medium-GI* food.
- ✔ A carb food with a GI of more than 65 is a *high-GI* food.

Some supermarkets have started to label the GI level of their carb-containing foods, so always check your labels.

Only foods with significant levels of carbs can have a GI score. So if you see a GI value for a food such as meat or cheese, just ignore the score because it contains very little carb and so is unlikely to raise blood sugar levels. However, fruit and vegetables can contain quite a lot of sugar and/or starch, and so they do have a GI value.

Good carbs

Good carbs are those that are broken down slowly in the body, so the body's blood sugars don't swing from high to low. In some people with PCOS, a tendency exists for the rapid rise in blood sugars, brought about by certain carbs, to be followed by blood sugars crashing to a low point, which can result in feelings of anxiety, shakiness, and severe hunger. Some people have such a severe reaction that they can faint. If these symptoms sound familiar to you, you need to concentrate on eating good carbs and avoid the not-so-good carbs. Good carbs give you a more sustained release of energy, and stop you feeling hungry too soon after a meal because they're broken down more slowly.

Good carbs are those with a low GI (glycaemic index) and include the following foods:

- ✔ Granary/grain bread
- ✔ Soya and linseed bread
- ✔ Fruit bread
- ✔ Pasta
- ✔ Beans
- ✔ Oats
- ✔ Basmati rice, especially brown
- ✔ Noodles
- ✔ Apples
- ✔ Sweet potato
- ✔ Lentils

You may find that you're advised to keep your carb intake low in order to offset the effect of insulin resistance and resultant high insulin levels which tend to occur in PCOS. However, more evidence is accumulating to show that this advice is misguided. The evidence shows that diets containing plenty of carbs that are low GI and high in fibre help the body to deal with glucose efficiently. These diets may help to prevent the onset of insulin resistance (when the insulin released into the bloodstream from the pancreas is not working efficiently) and the more extreme type 2 diabetes (both common conditions in PCOS if care is not taken with the diet). So avoiding carbs in the belief that they may lead to a worsening of insulin resistance appears not to be a good idea, providing you mostly stick to the good low-GI carbs.

A carb can have a low GI, but this doesn't automatically make it a good carb as it may still be a carb food that is high in saturated fat, calories, or salt. So to be a good all-rounder a carb needs to be:

- ✔ Low in saturated fat.
- ✔ Low in calories if you're watching your weight.
- ✔ Low in salt.
- ✔ High in fibre.
- ✔ A rich source of other nutrients.

All the foods in the good carb list earlier in this section are good all-rounder carbs.

Carbs and exercise

Two of the most important things you can do to overcome your symptoms of PCOS is to eat the right diet and do some physical activity. These two factors also affect each other. Recent evidence has emerged to show that if you restrict carbs in your diet, you experience more tiredness when you try to exercise. Carbohydrates provide a ready supply of glucose, the fuel required for exercise. However, having just a burst of energy and then running out of fuel is no good. For this reason, athletes follow a high carb but low-GI diet which provides them with a sustained supply of glucose.

Not so good carbs

The good carbs alter ego is the not-so-virtuous carb. These guys are not necessarily bad or even lacking in nutrients – they simply don't help with tackling the problems caused by PCOS. The reason is that these not-so-good-carbs cause blood sugar levels to rise very quickly after consumption and they give rise to a high peak in glucose levels. In other words they are high-GI carbs.

Not-so-good carbs include:

- Mashed or baked potatoes (new boiled potatoes have a lower GI)
- Water melon
- Pumpkin
- Ripe bananas
- White or brown bread
- Cornflakes
- Rice cakes

 You don't have to avoid these high-GI foods completely because many of them contain lots of nutrients and don't do you harm if eaten occasionally. However, to help your PCOS, try to substitute the high carb options for low carb ones when you can.

 The advice on carbs is dead simple – where possible in a meal you need to try and swap the not-so-good carbs for the good carbs or, in other words, swap the high-GI foods for lower GI options. Table 3-2 offers some healthy and tasty substitution ideas.

Table 3-2	Substituting Not-So-Good Carbs for Good Carbs	
Meal Occasion	*Instead Of:*	*Have:*
Breakfast	Cornflakes	Muesli
	Instant porridge oats	Unprocessed oats made into porridge
	White toast	Granary toast
Lunch	Jacket potato with filling	Sweet potato (baked) with filling
	White filled baguette	Pitta bread filled with hummus
	Canned spaghetti in tomato sauce on toast	Beans on toast
	Brown bread sandwiches	Wholegrain bread sandwiches
Dinner	Curry with white rice	Curry with basmati rice
	Shepherds pie	Spaghetti Bolognese
	Stir-fry with instant rice	Stir-fry with noodles
	Meat, veg, and mashed potato	Meat, veg, and baby new potatoes
Desserts	Bread and butter pudding made with white bread	Bread and butter pudding made with fruit loaf
	Fruit crumble made with white flour	Fruit crumble made with oat topping
Snacks	Muffins/cakes/biscuits	Cakes, biscuits or muffins made with fruit, oats and wholegrains
	White bread and jam	Fruit loaf with ricotta
	White crackers and cheese	Wholegrain crispbread with avocado or hummus dip

A word about sugary foods

Sugary foods are also carbs and have a bad reputation. However, foods such as honey and molasses, which are another form of sugar, have a slightly better reputation. The truth is that some forms of sugars have a high GI, for example glucose, but others have a low GI, such as fructose. So not all sugary and sweet foods or forms of pure sugar cause a rapid rise in blood sugar levels.

Wholegrains and Fibre

Wholegrains are defined as grain foods where all parts of the grain (such as the germ, endosperm, and bran layer) are intact and retained. Examples included wholegrain wheat and wholegrain (brown) rice.

Fibre, on the other hand, is defined as food substances found in cereals, fruits, and vegetables that are not digested but help the function of the intestines.

Fibre is usually found on the outside of plants, and was thought to be unnecessary to the body, and so milling used to strip this part away from plant. For example, the outer bran layer in the grain of wheat was stripped off to make white flour. However, over the last few decades research has shown that having fibre in the diet is very important – even if it is just to prevent constipation!

Holy wholegrains

Diets that are rich in wholegrain foods have been shown to offer a number of health benefits.

One large study found that women who ate 2.7 servings of wholegrain foods a day were 30 per cent less likely to suffer from coronary heart disease. Regular consumption of wholegrains also appears to lower the risk of certain types of cancer, stroke, and type 2 diabetes. These findings have been backed-up by other research which shows that a link exists between the consumption of wholegrains and insulin resistance; eating more wholegrain foods seems to give you a decreased likelihood of developing insulin resistance. Wholegrains are also believed to help you to keep your weight down and increase your body's sensitivity to insulin.

The sum of all parts: Why wholegrains are so darn good

The health benefits associated with eating wholegrain foods are thought to be due to their unique mix of properties, which seem to act together to exert a greater health benefit from the whole package than would be achieved from the sum of the individual components. The mix includes the following components:

✔ Fibre.

✔ Mostly low-GI carbohydrate.

✔ Some protein.

✔ A wide range of vitamins and minerals including vitamin E, a wide range of B vitamins, iron, magnesium, zinc, and selenium.

✔ Phytochemicals (plant chemicals) that act as antioxidants.

Foods in which 51 per cent or more of the ingredients consist of wholegrains are described as wholegrain foods. Wholemeal bread, brown rice, and now many breakfast cereals are wholegrain.

The GDA for wholegrains is 3 servings of grains a day, which comes to a total of 48 grams daily.

Some rough (age) facts

Fibre doesn't exactly conjure up an appetising image for many people and usually people think of bran when the word *fibre* is mentioned. But fibre plays a number of important jobs in the body and it's particularly helpful for PCOS sufferers for a number of reasons:

- ✔ If you are trying to lose weight, fibre can help you feel full as it bulks food out without providing calories.
- ✔ Fibre can help to lower the GI of a food. Soluble fibre in particular forms a sticky gel when it absorbs fluid and this gel can slow down the rate at which sugar is released into the bloodstream.

More and more benefits of fibre are being realised. From being considered as something that was unnecessary in the diet, fibre has come a long way! Here are some of its other benefits:

- ✔ **Constipation:** Fibre helps to keep the bowels healthy and functioning regularly.
- ✔ **Cholesterol levels:** Research has shown that a high intake of fibre, especially soluble fibre, can help lower cholesterol levels.
- ✔ **Cancer:** Fibre has a protective effect against colorectal cancer. Studies carried out in countries that had a high intake of fruit, vegetables, and cereals were found to have a low incidence of chronic bowel diseases, including cancer.

Fibre is a mixture of the non-digestible carbohydrate part of a plant that passes unabsorbed through our body such as fruit, stems, leaves, and seeds. Fibre naturally occurs in a wide range of foods and these can easily be incorporated into your diet. Fibre-containing foods are usually also rich in vitamins and minerals and so are good to include in a balanced and varied diet.

Getting enough of the rough stuff

The Guideline Daily Amount for fibre is 24 grams. But please note that this is a minimum recommendation! Table 3-3 shows some sources of fibre and the amount they contain.

Table 3-3	Sources of Fibre in Your Diet	
Food Source	*Portion Size*	*Amount of Fibre (grams)*
All-bran	6 tablespoons	13
Unsweetened muesli	3 tablespoons	4.5
Porridge	1 bowl	2
Granary bread	1 slice	2
Wholewheat pasta, cooked	230 grams	11
Brown rice, cooked	180 grams	2
Avocado	½ small	4.5
Dried apricots	6	4
Apple	1	2.5
Baked beans	1 small can (200 grams)	10
Frozen peas, cooked	3 tablespoons (90 grams)	6
Sunflower seeds	1 tablespoon	1.5
Roasted peanuts	50 grams bag	4

Getting more fibre into your diet can be quite easy. Here are a few suggestions to get you going (oh no, another pun!):

✔ Aim for at least 5 portions of fruit and vegetables per day.

✔ Have a wholegrain breakfast cereal – you can add fresh or dried fruit to this to increase the fibre content further.

✔ Eat granary bread or rolls instead of white.

✔ Use brown or wholegrain rice instead of white.

✔ Use wholewheat pasta instead of white or green.

✔ Use a wholemeal flour or a mixture of white and wholemeal flour when baking.

✔ Add lentils, beans, or pulses to stews, soups, and casseroles.

Increase the amount of fibre in your diet slowly otherwise you may suffer from abdominal discomfort. Also ensure that you're taking in enough fluids (see the later section 'Getting enough fluid').

Consuming 'too much' fibre is unlikely, but just in case you decide to overdo a good thing, studies have shown that in individuals who have excess raw wheat bran, absorption of certain minerals is prevented.

Soluble and insoluble fibre

Two main types of fibre are present in our diet: soluble and insoluble. All plants contain both types of fibre but can be higher in one type than the other.

- ✔ **Insoluble fibre:** Insoluble fibre passes through the body mostly unchanged but absorbs water and consequently swells, which has the effect of adding bulk to the stool and helps to prevent constipation. Sources of insoluble fibre include:
  - Wholegrain wheat
  - Rye
- ✔ **Soluble fibre:** Unlike insoluble fibre, soluble fibre is broken down once it reaches the large bowel. The natural gut bacteria feed and multiply on this broken down fibre resulting in softer, bulkier stools. Good sources of soluble fibre include:
  - Oats
  - Barley
  - Pulses
  - Beans
  - Apples
  - Berries

Protein Power

Everyone needs protein in the diet, but even if you are a bodybuilder you don't need a lot. Proteins are the body's building blocks, and the body's protein is continually being turned over, which means more protein needs to be eaten to replace it. The body can also use protein as an energy source. Like all sources of calories (protein, fat, and carbohydrate), an excess intake of calories from protein gets stored as fat. However, of all the so called 'macronutrients' (protein, fat, and carbohydrate), protein is the most likely to help you feel full-up. So some protein in a meal can help you feel satisfied with what you have eaten and less likely to reach for the biscuit tin straight after your meal!

The GDA for protein is 45 grams. Dieticians recommend that you include a good source of protein in two of your meals. But, as you can see from Table 3-4, getting enough protein in your diet is really easy.

Table 3-4	Sources of Protein (Single Servings)	
Good Sources (15 grams or more per portion)	*Fair Sources(9–14 grams per portion)*	*Poorer Sources (8 grams or less per portion)*
Sirloin steak (100 grams) provides 35 grams of protein	Baked beans (225 grams) provides 12 grams of protein	Soya milk (0.28 litres) provides 8 grams of protein
Tuna, canned, (100 grams) provides 33 grams of protein	Plain yoghurt (I pot/ 125 grams) provides 12 grams of protein	Muesli (60 grams) provides 8 grams of protein
Chicken, meat only, (100 grams) provides 31 grams of protein	Lentils (120 grams) provides 9 grams of protein	Egg, boiled, provides 7 grams of protein
Turkey breast, meat only, (100 grams) provides 24 grams of protein	Cow's milk (0.28 litres) provides 9 grams of protein	Peanuts (30 grams) provides 7 grams of protein
Chick peas, cooked, (200 grams) provides 16 grams of protein	Tofu (100 grams) provides 9 grams of protein	Bread (2 slices) provides 7 grams
		Hard cheese (30 grams) provides 7 grams
		Porridge, bowl, (400 grams) provides 6 grams

Proteins are made up of smaller units called amino acids. About 20 different amino acids exist, eight of which must be present in the diet. These eight are the essential amino acids, called 'essential' because your body can't manufacture them itself – they have to come from your diet.

Protein can be derived from plant and animal sources. However, unlike animal proteins, plant proteins may not contain all the essential amino acids in the necessary proportions.

If you suffer from high blood pressure you may want to note that people who eat more vegetable proteins (such as from beans, peas, and lentils) are more likely to maintain a normal blood pressure than those who eat less. You may want to try some of the bean and lentil recipes in the recipe section in Chapter 9. Vegetable protein is also associated with soluble fibre.

Vitamins, Minerals, and Other Bits and Bobs

I've talked about the nutrients that provide calories to the body – namely protein, fat, and carbohydrate – but a plethora of nutrients provide no calories and are required only in relatively smaller amounts: the vitamins and minerals essential to the working of the body.

Increasingly scientists are also discovering that other substances in our food, not known as nutrients, can also play an important protective role in the body. These substances include those in tea and red wine that help protect you from cancers and heart disease.

The big deal on vitamins and minerals

Vitamins and minerals are essential to the body – you can't survive long without any of them. A balanced diet provides you with all the vitamins and minerals you need, but there may be times when supplementation is required and some of the most common causes are listed in Table 3-5.

Table 3-5	When You May Need a Supplement
Micronutrient Which May Need Supplementing	*Reasons for Requiring Supplementation*
Multivitamin and mineral supplement	If diet has been poor for over 2 weeks for whatever reason, perhaps due to illness.
Multivitamin and mineral supplement	If you have been on a low calorie diet for more than a month and it provided you with less than 1600 calories per day.

(continued)

Table 3-5 *(continued)*

Micronutrient Which May Need Supplementing	*Reasons for Requiring Supplementation*
Folic acid	A dose of 400 micrograms (mcg) should be taken if you are planning to get pregnant and for the first 12 weeks of pregnancy.
Iron	If you have been suffering with heavy periods for more than 3 months. It may be best to see the doctor to get advice on the best type of iron and the quantity to take.
Vitamin C	If you are a smoker you require extra of this antioxidant vitamin. Ideally however you should give up this weed!
Calcium and vitamin D	If you do not eat any dairy products or calcium containing alternatives. It may be advisable to also seek dietary advice from a dietician.
Calcium and vitamin D	If you are at risk of getting osteoporosis or have borderline osteoporosis. Again, seek some medical advice on the best form of calcium to take and how much, and also seek dietary advice.
B vitamins	If you have been consuming high levels of alcohol for more than three months.

Except for folic acid, doses larger than the recommended intake should not be taken unless prescribed by your doctor.

Chapter 11 of this book describes some vitamins and minerals that may play a particular role in helping with PCOS. *Nutrition For Dummies*, UK Edition, by Nigel Denby, Sue Baic, and Carol Ann Rinzler (Wiley) offers a more thorough discussion of all the different vitamins and minerals.

Antioxidants

Antioxidant is the name given to a group of several substances found in food and drink. At the molecular and cellular levels, antioxidants serve to stop havoc happening as a result of 'free-radical' damage. A *free radical* is a highly reactive chemical that can damage important cellular molecules such as DNA or lipids (fats found in the membrane surrounding a cell) or other parts of the cell. An antioxidant simply renders the free radical harmless by de-activating the free reactive electrons.

They don't really know enough about supplements

The situation is actually quite frightening. You see vitamins and minerals for sale in healthfood shops, supermarkets, health clubs, and chemists and hundreds of millions of people worldwide take them regularly. Half of American adults take a multivitamin and in the USA alone this makes a tidy $20 million for their manufacturers. But scientists don't really know if these vitamins are doing you any good, or if they may be doing harm; scant information on their benefits and safety is available.

Scientists are not even sure if multivits can compensate for a bad diet as it seems to be that those people who already eat healthily are the ones taking the supplements!

However, what scientists are united over is that a balanced and varied diet should provide you with all your normal requirements of vitamins and minerals.

The most common *free-radical* found in the human body is oxygen, which is essential to life but highly reactive and highly destructive unless kept under control by antioxidants. Free radicals are the natural by-products of the essential processes that occur in your body. They are also created by exposure to various environmental factors, tobacco smoke and radiation, for instance. If oxygen and other free radicals were allowed to let-rip in the body, humans would develop cancer and heart disease very quickly.

Women with PCOS are thought to be more prone to damage caused by free radicals thus increasing their likelihood of developing cardiovascular disease. So, ensuring that your diet is rich in antioxidant nutrients is particularly important.

Antioxidants don't have to be nutrients but the ones that are nutrients include:

- ✔ Vitamin C.
- ✔ Vitamin E.
- ✔ Vitamin A.
- ✔ Beta carotene and other carotenoids (pigments that add colour to many fruits and vegetables such as the orange colour in peppers and carrots).
- ✔ Selenium (a mineral).

Together as antioxidants, these substances are thought to be effective in helping to prevent cancer, heart disease, and strokes.

Different parts of plants are now believed to contain a variety of antioxidants that aren't minerals or vitamins, including:

- Grape skin (anthocyanins)
- Garlic (allium sulphur compounds)
- Blueberries (anthocyanins)
- Tea, especially green tea (flavonoids)
- Apples (flavonoids)
- Tomatoes (lycopene)
- Chocolate (flavonoids)
- Red wine (flavonoids)
- Soya beans and products made from them (isoflavonoids)
- Olive oil (phenols)

Don't be tempted to take antioxidant supplements in the belief that they're going to help you overcome free-radical damage. Research has shown that taking supplements of some antioxidants, such as vitamin E, actually increases your likelihood of heart disease. Research also shows that smokers who take beta carotene as an antioxidant actually go on to develop higher rates of lung cancer than those who don't take the supplement.

A little of what you fancy does you good!

Did you know that chocolate can be good for you providing you don't eat too much? Cocoa contains a flavonol called catechin. Flavonols are a group of antioxidant substances found in some foods, which are believed to lower the risk of heart disease and insulin resistance: good news for PCOS sufferers. However, you should only be having a few squares of dark chocolate (preferably with at least 70 per cent cocoa solids) a day – no more than 25 grams. Chocolate is high in fat and sugar so although the fat in chocolate is not believed to raise harmful cholesterol levels, the heady fat and sugar combination delivers quite a high calorie kick. Therefore, a little can be great for you but too much can be dangerous!

Flavonols may also help to reduce the incidence of other diseases too, including cancer, dementia, blood pressure, and strokes.

Other flavonol-rich food and drinks include red wine, tea, and blueberries.

Eating a varied and balanced diet gives you all the antioxidants you need. Eat a variety of different coloured fruits and vegetables to get a good mixture of antioxidants because many antioxidants are found in the part of fruit and veg that gives them the colour.

Alcohol and Other Bevies

Keeping hydrated is important for everyone, but especially if you have PCOS because you can mistake thirst for hunger and eat more – not a good idea! Tea and coffee can hydrate and also provide some antioxidants.

Getting enough fluid

Fluid is essential to life. Remember, you are made up of 80 per cent water so allowing yourself to get dehydrated is not good for you and can cause the following symptoms:

- Headache
- Lack of concentration
- Tiredness
- Dizziness or light headedness
- Burning sensation in your stomach

To tell if you're dehydrated, check your wee! It should be odourless and relatively clear. If it's a golden or deep colour with a strong odour, you're dehydrated and need more water.

At normal temperature, with little or no exercise, you need around 2.5 litres (10½ cups) of fluid per day, whereas in hot conditions and with heavy exercise you need a lot more. During exercise you need to replace water losses as much as possible by drinking at every opportunity.

As well as water, tea, fruit juice, and soft drinks can provide fluid. Coffee and alcoholic drinks can also provide fluid but some people find that these can act as a diuretic and so may not be ideal for replacing fluid.

Drinking quite a few calories without noticing is all too easy. Experts are now beginning to believe that the calories in the fluid you drink may override any appetite control you have. This means that you can down a glass of orange juice (about 100 calories) without registering that you've drunk the equivalent of about 3 oranges.

Having a tipple

Alcohol is something to be enjoyed and most of the time drinking doesn't cause any problems. But drinking too much or at the wrong time can be harmful. The important thing is to know where the benefits end and the risks begin. Medical experts advise that women should drink no more than 2–3 units of alcohol per day (see the sidebar 'A unit of alcohol' to find out how much a unit is). These daily benchmarks apply whether you drink every day, once or twice a week, or only occasionally.

Of course, some occasions exist when it makes sense to drink less than the daily benchmarks, or not to drink at all. For example, women who are trying to become pregnant or are at any stage of pregnancy, shouldn't drink more than 1 or 2 units of alcohol once or twice a week, and should avoid episodes of intoxication.

Benefits of alcohol to PCOS sufferers

More and more evidence is accumulating that alcohol acts as a protector against cardiovascular disease. However, the protection seems to be mainly for older women (of around menopause age) and men. Also, drinking more than about 3 units a day increases your risk of cardiovascular disease. PCOS carries with it an increased risk of developing cardiovascular disease so it would be nice to know whether alcohol can offer you any protection. The problem is that no one really knows yet. Even why alcohol can be protective isn't fully understood, but part of the answer probably lies in the following facts:

- Many alcoholic drinks are particularly rich in antioxidants.
- Alcohol raises the level of good cholesterol in the blood, known as HDL (see the sidebar 'Cholesterol levels in women with PCOS' earlier in this chapter for more information). A high level of HDL is associated with reduced heart disease. Women usually have higher levels than men, but only up to the menopause. As a consequence women tend to suffer less heart disease than men up until the menopause. The protection conferred by alcohol in older women may be due to the fact that alcohol raises this good cholesterol level.

In addition to the possibility of cardio-protection, alcohol is also a great stress reducer – but relying on it too much for this purpose is a slippery slope to alcoholism!

Risks of alcohol to PCOS sufferers

So what are the downsides of drinking alcohol for PCOS sufferers in particular? Alcohol can:

✔ **Increase appetite**, which is fine if your appetite needs stimulating, but that's not normally a problem associated with PCOS.

✔ **Contain quite a few calories without even making you feel full up.** A glass of dry white wine (175 millilitres) provides about 115 calories, whereas half a pint of larger provides about 100 calories.

✔ **Lower your reserve.** So if you are determined to keep the calories down, but you have a glass or two of wine, that reserve may well crumble when faced with some tasty looking desserts!

✔ **Interfere with certain medicines.** If your doctor prescribes you drugs for your PCOS, always check that drinking alcohol with them is safe.

The low-down on caffeine

Caffeine is found in food and drinks such as chocolate, cola, tea, cocoa, and energy drinks. Drinks containing caffeine taste nice (otherwise why would you bother with them?) and they stimulate alertness. So a cup of coffee can be just what you need at certain slump times, such as:

✔ Keeping your attention going during that post-lunch dip.

✔ On a long car journey to keep your concentration levels up.

✔ When you feel lousy with a cold, caffeine can perk you up (in fact caffeine is often used in cold remedies).

However, the downside of all this is that, if you're a regular coffee drinker and you suddenly stop, you can end up feeling fuzzy-headed, and possibly with a headache. Another effect of all this stimulation is that turning it off is not always easy. If caffeine is still giving you a zing at bed time, you may find it hard to drop off to sleep!

TIP

A unit of alcohol

A unit of alcohol is 10 millilitres of pure alcohol. Counting units of alcohol can help you to keep track of the amount you're drinking. The list below shows the number of units of alcohol in common drinks:

✔ A pint of ordinary strength lager: 2 units

✔ A pint of strong lager: 3 units

✔ A pint of bitter: 2 units

✔ A pint of ordinary strength cider: 2 units

✔ A 175 millilitre glass of red or white wine: around 2 units

✔ A 25 millilitre measure of spirits: 1 unit

Keep in mind that lagers and ciders sold in bottles are usually stronger than those sold on draught. The labels of some bottled drinks tell you how many units of alcohol are in the bottle.

Caffeine has been accused of having a number of harmful effects on the body including high blood pressure and raised cholesterol levels, of particular concern to PCOS sufferers.

However, providing you're sensible about it, having PCOS doesn't mean that you have to avoid all caffeine-containing drinks completely. Four to five cups of normal strength coffee or five to six cups of normal strength tea a day is pretty safe, even if you have PCOS.

Salt: Getting the Measure

Experts now agree that you shouldn't have more than about 6 grams of salt a day. The problem is that, if you are Ms Average, you're probably having about a third more than this – somewhere in the region of 9 grams a day. This intake can happen without consciously adding a lot of salt to your food. About 75 per cent of your salt intake may be hidden by being included in processed foods such as ready meals and from eating out.

Eating more than 6 grams a day over a period of time may lead to an increased risk of developing high blood pressure. High blood pressure puts you at an increased risk of having a stroke or a heart attack. Having PCOS itself already ups your risk of these problems, so you need to try and watch your salt intake in the following ways:

- ✔ Try to cut down on the amount of salt and salty ingredients you use in cooking: If your food is cooked well – using herbs and spices and fresh good quality ingredients – you don't need to add salt to the recipe or at the table.

- ✔ When you buy processed foods such as ready meals, soups, and sauces, check out the amount of salt on the label. Food manufacturers have been reducing salt in the food they make on a gradual basis and also telling you how much salt is in the food.

Putting It All Together

You now know a little bit more about all the different nutrients in your diet but the key to healthy eating is knowing how to put the whole diet together: In other words, knowing how many and how much of different foods you should have. When you get this balance right, it is called a *balanced diet*. No one food can be held up as being 'good' or 'bad' – what really matters is how you put them all together and balance them out over the course of a day (or even several days).

Looking at the label for salt

Food labels are now a mine of information, but you do need to know how to interpret them. In the UK, legally salt has to be labelled as sodium but the label often gives you the salt equivalent. The US tends to stick to labelling sodium only. Salt is actually a substance called sodium chloride and once in the body, the sodium and chloride elements separate. The sodium part of salt is thought to have the harmful effect if taken in excess.

The GDA for salt of 6 grams is actually equivalent to about 2.5 grams of sodium (or 2,500 milligrams).

This is because 1 gram of sodium is equivalent to 2.5 grams of salt. So if the label only tells you the amount of sodium, you can work out the amount of salt by multiplying by 2.5.

Some labels also tell you what percentage of your GDA is in a portion of the food. Therefore, if a pizza slice contains 3 grams of salt, that's 50 per cent of your GDA for salt (and therefore it's giving you quite a lot of your salt limit for the day).

In order to help you to visualise the proportion and types of foods that are needed to make up a healthy balanced diet, nutritionists have developed a pictorial model called The Balance of Good Health, shown in Figure 3-1.

Fruit and vegetables

Bread, other cereals and potatoes

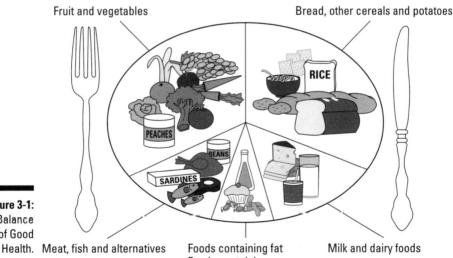

Figure 3-1:
The Balance of Good Health.

Meat, fish and alternatives

Foods containing fat
Foods containing sugar

Milk and dairy foods

Chapter 4

Eating the Low-GI Way: The Right Way for PCOS

This chapter explains the principles of eating the low-GI way – the cornerstone to controlling PCOS symptoms. And the low-GI diet is a great way to eat healthily, so the whole family can follow this diet too. On the face of it, there seems no logic as to why some foods are high GI and others low. This chapter gives some explanations for what dictates whether a food is a low or high GI, before going on to explain the different effects that low- and high-GI food has on the body, especially if you have PCOS. However, this chapter also shows that following a low-GI diet is not the be-all or end-all of what you need to be thinking about from the point of view of your diet. You also discover that following the basic principles here doesn't mean that certain foods are ruled out of your diet all together or forever!

The Basics about Low-GI Diets

A low Glycaemic Index (GI) diet is one where the carbohydrates (carbs) you consume break down slowly and/or slowly release glucose into your blood stream so that your blood sugar levels remain stable. Evidence suggests that a low-GI diet may also help you to eat less because you feel less hungry between or before meals. PCOS often comes with some insulin resistance or even diabetes, which are helped by keeping blood sugar levels stable. PCOS sufferers also have a tendency to feel quite hungry and gain weight easily, so a low-GI diet is ideal for curtailing this problem.

Some research which backs the GI way

More and more research is now coming out to support the following of a low-GI diet. It seems that the low-GI way to eat is not just great for those with PCOS, but also for the general population. This is particularly the case when more and more people are carrying around too much weight, developing high blood pressure, generating high cholesterol levels, and suffering other health problems. Following is a list of what some recent research has shown with regard to the general health gains achieved by following a low-GI diet:

✔ Low-GI diets help people lose and control weight: Research has shown that moderate reductions in GI make losing weight easier, particularly for women. This may be because low-GI foods may help keep away hunger pangs for longer due to their 'slow-release' characteristic.

✔ Low-GI diets increase the body's sensitivity to insulin.

✔ Low-GI carbs improve diabetes control.

✔ Low-GI carbs may be able to reduce the risk of heart disease: Research shows that a high carb diet based around low-GI foods is overall the most effective for heart health. Research also shows that low-GI wholegrain foods (such as traditional porridge oats) provide heart health benefits over and above those of high-GI wholegrains (such as wholewheat flakes).

✔ Low-GI carbs reduce blood cholesterol levels and other harmful blood fats without lowering the body's good fat level – high-density lipoprotein (HDL).

✔ Low-GI diets may help to reduce the risk of getting certain cancers such as colorectal and breast cancer.

✔ Low-GI carbs can help prolong physical endurance (which is why sportsmen and women eat a low-GI diet before an event).

The GI concept is a fairly recent one that started in the early 1970s when scientists began to look at how different carbohydrates affect the blood sugar in different ways. Then in 1981 a Canadian doctor, David Jenkins, and his team expanded this work further; they saw that some carbs send blood sugar levels shooting up wildly almost straight after consumption, whereas other carbs cause hardly a blip in blood sugar levels. The research into the effect that fast or slow blood sugar rises have on humans who are healthy, and humans who have impaired blood sugar controls, still continues.

The low-GI diet is not just another dieting fad; it is backed by science. In the next sections you find out how it can be the sensible way to eat for life, and not just if you have PCOS.

Although the glycaemic index concept is an important one if you have PCOS, it shouldn't be used alone. The GI should be incorporated into healthy eating guidelines that are covered in Chapter 3 and later in this chapter.

GI and your blood sugar

Eating carbs affects your blood sugar levels in different ways. Quick nutrition lesson: Food is broken down in your gut into smaller elements, and these elements are absorbed into the blood stream. (Lucky for you, you only need to know how your body digests carbs, as only foods containing carbs – which includes sugars – affect your eventual blood sugar level.)

Your body can only absorb carbs when they are broken down into

- ✔ Glucose
- ✔ Fructose (found in high levels in fruit)
- ✔ Galactose (derived from milk)

Even relatively simple sugar products such as sucrose (table sugar) are broken down by the body to glucose and fructose.

The rate of breakdown and release of glucose into the blood stream has the most influence on the GI of a food.

GI watching for PCOS

The graphs shown in Figure 4-1 demonstrate what happens in your blood stream when you consume a food or drink with a high GI compared to one with a low GI. You see that the glucose drink in the first graph with a high GI of 100 requires so little breaking down by the body that the sugar from it gets rapidly absorbed, almost all at once, by the gut and gets to rush quickly into the blood stream, thus causing a rapid and sudden rise in blood sugar levels. The second graph shows blood glucose levels after eating spaghetti, with a GI of 41.

Digest this!

As soon as you eat a food containing some carbohydrate, digestive enzymes in the saliva in your mouth start to break down the carbs in your food into simpler sugars. Starch, for example, is made up of long chains of glucose molecules. So when starch is broken down, starting in the mouth, you get a release of free glucose. The breakdown process continues throughout the rest of the gut, with digestive enzymes getting released along the way, which gradually fully break down the more complicated food compounds. The chewing process in the mouth and churning process in the stomach (along with the mixing with stomach acid) also aid this breakdown of food.

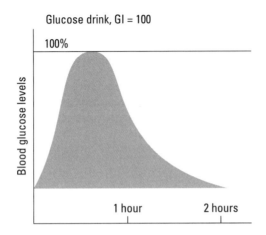

Glucose drink, GI = 100

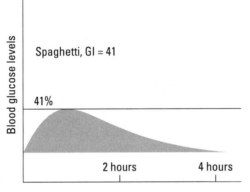

Figure 4-1:
Comparing
blood sugar
(glucose)
levels after
consuming
a high-GI
food and a
low-GI food.

Spaghetti, GI = 41

A sudden rise in blood sugar isn't terribly good news even when you don't have PCOS, but if you do, the harmful effect gets exaggerated:

✔ **Your blood sugar (glucose level) may stay elevated for extended periods of time.** When you suffer from PCOS, the body finds it difficult to bring down a high level of blood sugar and so it stays high for a long period of time, particularly if you have developed full-blown diabetes or have insulin resistance. With diabetes your body is unable to produce enough insulin to bring down the high glucose level, whereas in insulin resistance, insulin is produced but is unable to do its job of bringing down blood sugar levels very effectively. Over time, having high blood sugar levels can give rise to several complications including heart disease, kidney failure, and damage to the eyes.

✔ **Your blood sugar may drop to a level where you start to notice yourself getting a little dysfunctional.** In some cases, when your body can still pump out insulin effectively, the body responds to high blood sugar levels by pumping out too much insulin. PCOS sufferers seem particularly susceptible to this happening. So in some PCOS sufferers, a food that causes blood sugars to rise suddenly can cause a rebound effect where a high blood sugar level is followed by blood sugar levels plummeting down too low. This sudden drop leads to feelings of shakiness, severe hunger, anxiety, and even fainting.

✔ **Your body overproduces insulin.** Most of the symptoms of PCOS are due to excessive levels of insulin being produced. This is because insulin is just not effective at normal levels due to the condition known as 'insulin resistance'. Easing the symptoms of PCOS revolves around trying to reduce these excessive insulin levels. High-GI foods promote excess insulin secretion, which may increase the risk for diabetes, cardiovascular disease, some types of cancer, and generally make the symptoms of PCOS worse.

✔ **You may become hungrier faster.** When the glucose from a meal is dumped all at once into your blood stream, you're filled up for a while but there's nothing sustainable about it; after your glucose levels return to normal (or even lower than normal), you may start to feel the need to eat again. One of your body's triggers for hunger is your blood sugar level. A slow and sustained release of blood sugar that you get with a low-GI diet keeps blood sugar levels on an even keel, and levels tend not to drop to hunger point for 3–4 hours, compared to only a couple of hours with a high-GI diet.

The insulin and blood sugar link

Insulin is a clever little hormone because it allows glucose to enter certain cells of the body, such as the muscles, which need ready fuel to produce energy. If the sugar is not required immediately, insulin helps sugar to enter the liver, where it gets stored as glycogen, which acts as a reserve when you need energy quickly. Any excess glucose that is still lurking when immediate energy needs are satisfied and when glycogen stores are topped up, gets converted into fat, and again, insulin facilitates this process.

Of course, if the body is unable to produce enough insulin, such as in diabetes, your body has no way of stopping blood sugar levels shooting very high and staying high for a long time. These high levels can lead to all kinds of damage to the body in the long term and even in the short term can lead to a coma and even death. For this reason people with more severe type 2 diabetes or those with type 1 diabetes (where the body cannot produce any insulin) have to have insulin shots or injections to deal with the rises in blood sugar that occur after meals.

The good news about a low-GI diet in this context is that if you are a diabetic requiring insulin shots, you probably don't need to take so much insulin if you follow a low-GI diet.

Achieving blood sugar control

The key to achieving blood sugar control is to eat foods that have low GI rather than foods with high GI. The GI value of foods are classed accordingly:

- ✔ Low GI is a GI value of 55 or less
- ✔ Medium GI is a GI value between 56 and 69
- ✔ High GI is a GI value of 70 or more

Spaghetti and other low-GI foods don't cause a rapid rise and fall in blood sugar levels. Because your gut can't easily break down the sugar in low-GI food, it stays locked in for longer than the sugar in a high-GI food, such as a sugary drink. With low-GI foods, the sugar is slowly extracted from the food and so only gets to trickle into the blood stream as opposed to being dumped all at once. When you have PCOS, your body deals better with a steady trickle of sugar into the blood stream rather than a rush so that you avoid high and low swings, which can play such havoc in your body.

Low GI and PCOS

Because blood sugar levels don't shoot up, but stay on an even keel on a low-GI diet, your body doesn't need to pump out lots of insulin to try to lower blood sugar levels. Therefore, levels of insulin in your blood stay low, providing that you generally continue to eat low GI. This habit can help you to lose weight more easily (after all, insulin promotes weight gain) and help to relieve many of your other symptoms of PCOS.

Testing food for its GI

Testing food for its GI value is an expensive and involved process and is only done in specialised research centres. So, not every single food with a GI value (that is, it contains carbohydrate) has been tested; much to the frustration of avid low-GI followers! Here are the steps involved to determine the GI of a food:

- ✔ Testing requires 10 or more healthy subjects.

- ✔ The subjects consume a portion of the test food containing 50 grams of carbohydrate, and testers measure its effect on blood glucose levels over the next two-hour period.

- ✔ On another occasion, the subjects consume a 50 gram portion of glucose (the reference food) and the testers measure its effect on blood glucose levels over the next two-hour period.

- ✔ The GI is determined by dividing the area under the curve of the test food by the area under the curve of the reference food. In the example shown in Figure 4-1, glucose is given a GI value of 100, whereas if the 2-hour area under the blood sugar curve of the spaghetti were measured, it would be found to be 41 per cent of that of the glucose. So spaghetti is given a GI of 41.

- ✔ The final GI value is the average GI value of all 10 subjects.

Low GI and diabetes

If you have PCOS and have developed diabetes that requires insulin shots, a low-GI diet can help you achieve the following:

✔ Better blood sugar control in the short and long term

✔ Less insulin required to control your blood sugar

✔ Weight loss

✔ Lower risk of developing heart disease and other complications of diabetes

Spotting a low-GI carb

At first, spotting a low-GI carb from a high one may not seem that obvious. You may also be unsure at first about whether a food has a GI or not. Well read on to find out!

Not all food has a GI value, because not all food has any significant carbohydrate content that is likely to have an effect on blood sugar levels. So foods that are pure meat, fish, or cheese contain no carbs to speak of, and so can't be given a GI value. Table 4-1 illustrates examples of foods that do and don't have GI values.

You can quickly get to know which carbs are low GI or not, but they are hard to identify in the raw without understanding a few rules about what makes a food low GI. Bottom line to remember: Some foods take longer to break down and release their sugar content into the blood stream than others.

Table 4-1	Sample GI Values
Food	*GI Value*
Croissant	67
Cola	58
White baguette	95
Chocolate puffed wheat cereal	77
Sweetcorn	53
Apple	38
Chickpeas, boiled	28
Peanuts	14

(continued)

Table 4-1 *(continued)*	
Food	**GI Value**
Carrots	47
Cabbage	No GI value
Runner/French beans	No GI value
Courgettes/zucchini	No GI value
Cheese	No GI value
Brazil nuts	No GI value
Any plain meat	No GI value

In order to have a GI value, you have to eat the amount of food that provides 50 grams of carbohydrate. Some foods are so low in carbs that eating an amount that provides 50 grams of carbs is impossible. Therefore, some vegetables (especially green veg) and nuts may not be given a GI value.

The type of starch in food

Starch is a storage form of glucose found in plant foods. Starch is composed of hundreds or thousands of glucose molecules that are strung together in chains.

Two main kinds of starch are present in plant foods – amylopectin and amylose. When these starches are digested, their glucose molecules are liberated and absorbed, causing a rise in blood sugar. However, because of the differences in their chemical structures, these two starches have very different effects on blood sugar.

- **Amylopectin** has a structure that resembles the branches of a tree and so is easily attacked by digestive enzymes. Starchy foods that contain a high proportion of amylopectin – like baking potatoes and sticky short-grain rice – are quickly digested and produce rapid rises in blood sugar levels.

- **Amylose**, on the other hand, consists of a long, straight chain of tightly packed glucose molecules that resists digestion. Foods high in amylose – such as new potatoes and basmati rice – are absorbed more slowly and have lower glycaemic indexes.

Cooking method

Cooking can increase the GI ranking of a food. During cooking and baking, the starches in foods like grains, pasta, breads, and muffins absorb water. This causes the starch granules to swell and rupture, a process known as *gelatinisation*. Gelatinised starch is readily attacked by digestive enzymes and very quickly digested and absorbed. Bread has a high GI partly because the starch in the finely ground flour used to make bread is easily gelatinised. And soft, overcooked pasta has a higher GI than firm, al dente pasta because the overcooked pasta absorbs more water during cooking.

Degree of food processing

Highly processed foods are digested faster and usually have a higher GI index. New technologies for processing grains – such as explosion puffing, extruding, and flaking – have been developed which tend to start to break down the starch in that grain and raise its GI value. For instance, instant oat cereal has a higher GI than whole porridge oats.

Fibrous coat

An intact fibrous coat, such as that on grains and legumes, acts as a physical barrier to digestive enzymes and so slows down the digestive process, hence lowering a food's GI.

A food's fat content

Foods with a higher fat content have a lower GI rating. A high fat content means that food has to stay in the stomach longer and so the whole digestive process is slowed down. However you shouldn't use this as an excuse to eat fatty meals or you're going to end up gaining more weight and increase your risk of developing heart disease and certain cancers. The advantage gained by slightly lowering the GI of a food or a meal by upping fat intake definitely does not outweigh the health gains from keeping fat intake down!

A food's fibre content

High fibre content in a food tends to slow down the rate at which the starch in the food can be broken down. The two types of fibre are: *soluble* (found in oats, beans, fruit, and veg) and *insoluble* (found in cereal fibre such as bran). The soluble fibre lowers the GI best.

Beans and pulses have a low GI because their starch content is wrapped in a fibrous shell which the digestive enzymes take a while to get through. Research has shown that in addition to its effect on GI, a high-fibre meal seems to have a knock-on benefit to the next meal, causing a more even blood sugar control compared to a meal that had the same GI but lower fibre content.

The acid content of a food

Acid present in a food slows down your digestion of it. The naturally occurring acids in fruits, as well as the acids in fermented foods such as yoghurt, buttermilk, and sourdough bread, slow the rate of digestion and contribute to the low GI of these foods. Likewise, adding just 4 teaspoons of vinegar or lemon juice to a meal can lower the GI of the meal by about 30 per cent. For this reason, using vinegar and lemon juice to flavour foods can be a way to lower the GI of your diet.

The type of sugar present

You may be surprised to discover that, with the exception of glucose (GI = 100), most sugars have low to moderate glycaemic indexes. Fructose, the sugar that occurs naturally in fruits, is very slowly absorbed, giving it a GI of only 23. Lactose, the sugar naturally present in milk and dairy products, has a GI of 46. This is one reason why most fruits and dairy products have such low glycaemic indexes. Sucrose (white table sugar), a combination of equal parts fructose and glucose, has a GI of 65. The fact that sucrose is part fructose is one reason why many sweets have a moderate GI.

Finding resources for GI values

Below is a list of some of the Web sites that allow free access to GI values:

✔ www.glycemicindex.com: This site comes highly recommended for being clear, thorough, and reliable. The site calls itself 'The Official Web site of the Glycemic Index and GI Database' and is run by the University of Sydney. As well has having an extensive database of GI values, it also has other information about GI, the GI diet, and the most up-to-date research on GI.

✔ www.mendosa.com/gilists.htm: This site is a searchable table which includes 750 foods. The entries represent a true international effort of testing around the world. However at the time of writing this table had not been revised since September 2002.

✔ www.gilisting.com: This site has an online glycaemic index database and some diet tips.

✔ www.bupa.co.uk/health_ information/html/healthy_ living/lifestyle/exercise/ diet_exercise/gi_table.html: This table is located on the BUPA (private healthcare) site. It provides quite an extensive list of the GI of foods divided into 3 separate tables for low, medium, and high GIs.

✔ www.weightlossresources.co. uk/diet/gi_diet.htm: This site has the values of commonly eaten foods but not an extensive list. The Web site is called weight loss resources and it does contain some credible advice on how low GI can be used to help with weight loss.

✔ www.shaklee.com/pws/library/ products/wm_gi_gl_tables.pdf: This site has quite an extensive list as a pdf file (you can search it using the Adobe Acrobat search tool) and contains an example of a GI breakfast meal make-over!

If you have no computer, or dislike using one, you can buy the following:

✔ *Complete Guide to GI Values Pocket Guide* by Prof. Jennie Brand-Miller, Kaye Foster-Powell, and Dr Susanna Hold (Hodder Headline).

✔ *The New Glucose Revolution Shoppers' Guide to GI Values: The Authoritative Source of Glycemic Index Values for More Than 500 Foods* by Jennie Brand-Miller (Marlow and Co. UK).

✔ *The Low GI Shopper's Guide to GI Values* by Prof. Jennie Brand-Miller and Kaye Foster-Powell (Hodder and Stoughton).

If you were to make a banana cake without sugar, the ripe bananas and flour in the cake mean it would have a GI overall of 55. However, adding sugar to the cake in the form of sucrose brings down the average GI of the cake to 47!

However, just because sugar in the form of white table sugar or fructose doesn't have a high GI doesn't mean that you can add it liberally to everything. Pure sugar provides calories and no other real nutrients. That is why sugar is said to provide empty calories – it helps pile on the pounds without providing any other nutritional value. Far better to save those calories for something nutritious!

Meal Planning the Low-GI Way

Armed with the basics, you now need to get down to the nitty-gritty; how do you throw a low-GI meal together?

When you have a meal you need to remember two things in order to ensure that your meal is low GI:

1. You need to base your meal on a carbohydrate food.

2. You need to make sure that the carb you are basing it on is low GI.

To help you along the way, Table 4-2 gives examples of some low-GI starches you may want to base each meal occasion on. Chapters 6 to 9 have more details of how to throw some meals together based on low-GI principles.

Table 4-2	Meals and Their Carbs
Meal	*Suitable Low-GI Carb*
Breakfast	Oat-based breakfast cereal
	Barley-based breakfast cereals
	Cereal high in bran
	Cereal with plenty of dried fruit/nuts/seeds
	Granary or multigrain toast

(continued)

Table 4-2 (continued)

Meal	Suitable Low-GI Carb
Lunch	Oatcakes
	Crispbread with multigrain/seeds
	Jacket sweet potato
	Wholegrain or stoneground flour bread
	Rye or sourdough bread
	Pasta
	Cooked cold potato, for example, as potato salad or reheated
Dinner	Basmati or Doongara or Japanese koshihikari rice
	Legumes: peas, beans, or lentils
	Noodles
	Pasta
	Sweet potatoes
	New potatoes, boiled
	Have a side salad with your meal which has a vinegar dressing of some sort or just add some balsamic vinegar

Constructing a meal

Many of your meals are going to be based on one starchy component; for example in a traditional meal of meat, two veg, and potato, the potato is the starchy component. So for meals made of just one carb-containing food, if that food has a low GI, the overall meal is low GI. However if the meal is made up of more than one starchy food, the GI of that meal is the weighted average contribution of each carb; *weighted* meaning that the carb that is providing the greatest quantity exerts its GI effect more.

This weighting means that you can balance out a high-GI carb in a meal with a lower one, and so end up with a meal that is a medium GI. An example is a baked potato with baked beans. Baked potatoes have a high GI whereas baked beans have a low GI. If you eat them together, you end up with a medium GI meal (providing you're using more than just a small amount of beans!)

Adding plenty of veg or a salad also lowers the overall GI of a meal.

Three-a-day plus snacks

Make sure that you eat breakfast, lunch, and evening meal. In addition, avoid getting too hungry between meals. If you get a craving, grab a small low-GI snack, which can include fresh fruit or low-fat yoghurt. The following sample meals give you an idea of what your daily intake may look like.

Breakfast

Porridge served with semi-skimmed milk and some fruit.

Cup of tea with semi-skimmed milk.

Mid morning

Apple.

Lunch

Two slices granary bread made into a tuna sandwich with low-fat mayonnaise and some sweetcorn.

Cucumber sticks.

One low-fat yoghurt.

Mid afternoon

Two slices of malt loaf spread with a little reduced-fat spread.

Evening meal

Spaghetti bolognese made with lean mince or Quorn.

Side salad with low-fat vinaigrette dressing.

Sugar-free jelly with some canned mandarin slices in natural juice.

Bedtime

Low calorie hot chocolate drink.

Two oatcakes with some low-fat spread and reduced-sugar jam.

A note on limiting carb intakes

Although not eating starch or carbs in general may help to keep blood sugar levels down, this is not the answer.

A low carb diet means that the majority of your calories come from fat and protein. This kind of diet brings a risk of heart disease, increasing your blood pressure and possibly leading to an impairment in kidney function. The latter is particularly the case if you have diabetes or insulin resistance and high blood pressure.

Such a diet also means that you produce a lot of *ketones*, which are substances produced in elevated amounts when you're trying to metabolise a lot of fat in your diet as opposed to carbohydrate. Ketones can make you feel slightly nauseous and also make your breath smell nasty! If you are trying to conceive on a ketone-producing diet, you should be aware that ketones in the mother's blood stream have been found to be toxic to an unborn child.

Other Advice for Healthy Eating

No one likes rules and rigidity, especially to do with food. However, you do need to bear a few things in mind when following a low-GI diet.

In observing a low-GI diet, three simple guidelines apply:

1. When you plan to have a carbohydrate containing food in your diet, you need to make sure that it's a low-GI one.

2. If finding a low-GI food is difficult, or if you just fancy a change occasionally, go for a medium-GI food.

3. For a special occasion, or if nothing else is really available to eat, or if you have gone to friends for a meal, the odd high-GI food is not going to hurt too much!

These simple rules are the basics. The following sections give you some other guidance in order to make sure that your diet is both balanced and low GI.

A few friendly suggestions

To keep your diet healthy *and* low GI, follow these tips:

✔ For drinks, have sugar-free squash, diet fizzy drinks, tea or coffee (in moderation), or a low-cal hot chocolate drink. If you do need to sweeten your hot drink, use artificial sweeteners if you don't mind the taste, as doing so saves on empty calories. Also avoid drinking more than 1–2 units of alcohol a day and mostly stick to dry wines or spirits with diet mixers.

✔ Aim for a minimum of five portions of fruit and vegetable daily which should be predominantly fresh or frozen.

✔ Avoid adding salt to foods and reduce the consumption of high-salt foods.

✔ Don't eat too much protein foods such as meat, fish, eggs, poultry, and cheese. Two servings of these a day is fine. If you are a vegetarian, use Quorn, soya or peas, beans, and lentils as protein alternatives. In fact, these foods are nutritious and low in fat, and so are great to eat even if you are not veggie.

✔ Keep your fat intake down (avoid frying your food) and swap saturated fats (such as butter, lard, ordinary cakes, biscuits, and pastries) to poly or monounsaturated fats and oils. Avoid trans fats (found in oils that have undergone some hydrogenation).

✔ Try to have three servings of dairy foods a day to ensure that you get sufficient calcium. A serving is one small pot of yoghurt, ⅓ pint (200 millilitres) of milk, or 1 ounce (25 grams cheese).

✔ Get plenty of fibre in your diet as it may give an added boost to blood sugar control over and above the effect of GI alone.

✔ If you need to lose weight, watch your portion sizes and how often you eat, even if you're eating low-GI foods.

✔ Allow yourself one treat a day such as a small scoop of ice cream, or one of the bakery items from Chapter 8 which are also low GI.

✔ Don't take nutritional supplements or follow alternative therapies without guidance from a health worker who is professionally qualified, such as a doctor or dietician.

Portion size does matter

Just because you're eating mostly low-GI foods, and following the basic principles outlined above, doesn't guarantee weight loss. You may still be eating a lot of food or eating food too often. At the end of the day, no amount of low-GI eating is going to help you keep your energy intake down if you end up eating large portions and eating food too frequently. If the total amount of calories you consume exceed what your body needs, the excess calories just get stored as fat.

When may you need a high-GI food?

You may have heard about world-class footballers taking masses of certain rather sweet but low-fat foods with them to have after a gruelling match. If you're a fairly serious class athlete, sports player, or runner, during the course of whatever activity you are doing, your body uses up all its reserves of energy. This reserve would have been stored as glycogen, which is basically just a nice compact form of glucose that's fairly easy to get hold of when needed. The majority of glycogen is stored in the liver and some in muscle tissue.

However, a big match, a long run, or any jolly energetic activity conducted for an hour or so, is going to use up this glycogen store. For an athlete, restoring this store as soon as possible is essential, as you never know when you may need it again, and you can be prone to bouts of exhaustion without it.

The quickest way to restore this store is to get some glucose delivered into the blood stream pronto. And what is the best way of doing that? Well, eating some high-GI food as quickly after the match as possible. But you don't want something fatty as that slows down the digestion and adds a lot of calories.

Foods such as ripe banana and honey white bread sandwiches are great, or some commercial energy drinks.

It may be helpful to keep an eye on how much food you serve up for yourself. If you like to fill your plate with food, just use a smaller plate.

Weigh out how much of these carb foods you normally serve yourself and then compare it to the normal portion sizes in Table 4-3. For a week, try and weigh out your carb foods so that you only serve yourself a normal portion size. You'll soon get used to seeing how much a portion size looks on your plate. If you feel yourself slipping into giving yourself larger portions again, go back to weighing your carbs for a few days again.

Table 4-3	Normal Portion Sizes for Low- to Medium-GI Foods
Carb	*Normal Portion/Serving Size*
All bran	1 small bowl, 40g, 1½oz
Porridge, made with water	1 small bowl, 160g, 6oz
Muesli	1 small bowl, 50g, 2oz
Basmati rice, uncooked	4 tablespoon (tblsp), 60g, 2oz
Noodles, cooked	4 tblsp, 230g, 9oz
Macaroni, cooked	4 tblsp, 230g, 9oz
Spaghetti	4 tblsp, 220g, 9oz

Carb	Normal Portion/Serving Size
Pitta bread	1 large, 75g, 3oz
Rye bread	1 slice, 25g, 1oz
Boiled potato	2 medium, 175g, 7oz
Sweet potato	1 medium, 130g, 5oz
Baked beans	1 small tin, 205g, 8oz
Butter beans	4 tblsp, 120g, 5oz
Chick peas	4 tblsp, 140g, 6oz
Red lentils	4 tblsp, 160g, 6oz
Peanuts	1 small handful, 50g, 2oz
Apple juice	1 glass, 160ml, 6fl oz
Orange juice	1 glass, 160ml, 6fl oz

The food industry and GI

The food industry has not been blind to all the GI excitement going on. In Australia everyone knows about GI and many manufacturers and retailers label their foods with the GI value. This has been happening to a lesser extent in the US and UK, although the biggest retail chain in the UK has been putting the GI value on their foods for a while now. However, to be fair, the UK and US recognise that the real proven advantage of a low-GI diet is for diabetics and those with metabolic syndrome, insulin resistance, and PCOS. However, with growing obesity, that is likely to be an increasing number of consumers. Signs indicate that the low-GI diet may be great for people without any disease too, but this evidence has dragged behind the evidence for its benefits in the aforementioned conditions.

If a food does carry a low-GI label, this doesn't guarantee it is healthy!

The other way that the food industry has been responding to the low-GI way of eating is through research and development: producing foods that are low GI. An example of this is in one of our biggest staples in the West – bread. Breads can now be manipulated in the following ways to bring down the GI value:

- By adding different low-GI grains and/or seeds.
- By enclosing the grain kernels so they break down slower.
- By using sour dough fermentation.
- By adding acid.
- By using cereals especially bred to have higher levels of the starch which breaks down slowly.
- By upping the fibre level.

You can now find plenty of choice of low-GI breads on the market.

Going off the rails

Sticking to a low-GI regime is going to help you to feel better in the long run because it helps control your PCOS symptoms. However, you can eat some high-GI foods once in a while without causing irreversible damage! If you get the chance you can limit the effect of eating a high-GI food in the following way:

- ✔ In the same meal try and have a low-GI food such as yoghurt, some milk, or some low-GI beans as an accompaniment.

- ✔ Have plenty of veg or salad with your meal.

- ✔ If you are intending to have a pudding, make that a low-GI one, such as one that is fruit-based.

- ✔ Have something acidic with your food such as vinegar or lemon juice.

- ✔ Make sure that your next meal or snack is a low-GI one.

Sorting the GI from the GL

You may also have heard of the low GL diet and wondered what it's all about? This diet is basically another way of trying to ensure that what you eat doesn't send your blood sugars shooting up too quickly. But it does involve another layer of complication and explanation, which is unnecessary; just counting the GI is fine. However, because many people do talk about the Glycaemic Load, or GL, of a food, it is only fair to give you some sort of explanation.

As explained elsewhere in this chapter, the glycaemic index (GI) is a numerical system of measuring how much of a rise in circulating blood sugar a carbohydrate triggers – the higher the GI number, the greater the blood sugar response. So a low-GI food causes a small rise, whereas a high-GI food triggers a dramatic spike. The Glycaemic Load (GL) is a relatively new way to assess the impact of carbohydrate consumption that takes the glycaemic index into account, but also takes into account the amount of the food – the quality and quantity of carbohydrate – that you consume. To work out the GL you have to know how much carbohydrate is in a serving of a particular food.

Glycaemic Load is calculated this way:

$$GL = GI \div 100 \times \text{amount of carbs}$$

A GL of 20 or more is high, a GL of 11 to 19 inclusive is medium, and a GL of 10 or less is low.

The drawback of the GL system is that low-GL foods are likely to be low GI simply because they are low carb. What this means is that if you were to try and follow a low-GL diet alone, it may not be the healthiest way to eat because it may be high in fat and protein and low in carbs.

The key to getting the best blood glucose response is to eat more low-GI carbohydrate, not to eat less carbohydrate. GL doesn't distinguish slow carb from low carb; you need the carbs, but the slow release kind, not the ones that rush in!

Fortunately you don't need to go to the extent of working out the GL of your food, which just adds another layer of complexity you don't need. Take a look at *The GL Diet For Dummies* if you want to know more.

The GI effect of low-GI meals tends to build up. In other words, if you have a low-GI breakfast, it tends to have a lasting effect through to lunch and even dinner. Even if you have a high-GI lunch, the effect on your blood sugars isn't going to be as bad as if you had no breakfast or a high-GI breakfast. Although not as pronounced as a low-GI breakfast, other meals may be able to have a knock-on effect to the next meal as well.

Like any diet, don't let one meal or day's failure knock you back. After any relapse, just start fresh again as if you had never failed!

Not all low-GI foods are equally good!

Just because a food has a low GI, doesn't necessarily make it the healthiest choice. Table 4-4 lists some low-GI foods which may not be the wisest choice due to the fact that they may be high in fat, or salt, or both. The right-hand column offers some advice as to whether these foods should be limited to once a day, once a week, or once a month.

If the table says you can have a product once a day, week, or month, don't have this and all the other products listed once a day, week, or month. You can have one treat OR another!

Table 4-4		Low-GI Foods to Limit
Food	*GI*	*Recommended Frequency of Consumption*
Banana cake	47	Once a week.
Chocolate cake with chocolate icing (frosting)	38	Once a month.
Sponge cake	46	Once a week.
Apple muffins	44	Once a week. If you make your own low-fat version, you can have as your daily treat.
Chocolate brownie	23	Once a week.
Rich tea biscuit	55	Once a day.
Ice cream, premium, vanilla	38	Once a week. You can make your own with low-fat milk and fruit and have this as your desert or your daily treat.

(continued)

Table 4-4 *(continued)*

Food	GI	Recommended Frequency of Consumption
Custard with sugar	43	Once a week. If you make your own with low-fat milk, you can have once a day as part of a dessert.
Frozen yoghurt	33	Once a day as a dessert.
Full-fat yoghurt	36	Once a week. A low-fat yoghurt that is sugar free is allowed daily.
Milk shake/flavoured milk	35	If this is made with sugar and full-fat milk, only have once a month, but if made with reduced-fat milk and sweeteners, it can be drunk once a day.
Corn chips	42	Once a week.
Potato crisps	54	Once a week.
Salted peanuts	14	Once a week. A small handful allowed daily if unsalted.
Peanut M & Ms	33	Once a week.
White chocolate	44	Once a week.
Plain or milk chocolate	43	Once a week.
Hazelnut chocolate spread	33	Once a month.
Vegetable pizza, take away	49	Once a month. If you make your own with a low-fat base and topping (see recipe in Chapter 7 and 9), you can have it once in the day as your meal.

Chapter 5

Shedding the Extra Load

*N*o doubt about it: PCOS is associated with being overweight. More than half of patients with PCOS are obese. Recent research has also shown that if you are overweight, your chances of having PCOS are around five times higher than if you are normal weight.

This chapter goes into detail on how to lose weight if you have PCOS and how to overcome certain obstacles that come your way. If you have PCOS, you're likely to need to watch your weight quite carefully, if not actually reduce it by a certain amount. You discover in this chapter how the low-GI diet needs to be maintained, but tailored to weight loss as well. This chapter also looks at coping with hunger and cravings, which are particularly common if you live with PCOS.

Deciding How Much to Lose

You may have already been set a goal weight to reach by your dietician or doctor. If you have a lot of weight to lose, aim for a target of around 3 kilograms at a time. You may want to set your own target, and below are outlined the most scientific and sensible approaches for setting targets.

Body mass index

The healthy weight range is based on a measurement known as the Body Mass Index (BMI), determined from your weight and height. You can do the maths (have a calculator ready!) by following these three simple steps for working out your BMI:

1. Measure your height in metres and multiply the figure by itself.

2. Measure your weight in kilograms.

3. Divide your weight by the answer to Step 1.

   For example, suppose you're 1.6 metres tall and weigh 65 kilograms. The calculation is:

   $1.6 \times 1.6 = 2.56$. BMI is 65 divided by 2.56 = 25.39.

Then read the classification for your results in Table 5-1.

Table 5-1	Recommended BMI Chart
BMI	**Classification**
BMI less than 18.5	Underweight
BMI 18.5–25	Ideal
BMI 25–30	Overweight
BMI 30–40	Obese – need to lose weight
BMI greater than 40	Very obese – need to lose weight

The BMI measurement may be inaccurate if you are an athlete or very muscled (muscle weighs more than fat), because it can push you into a higher BMI category despite having a healthy level of body fat. The measurement is also not accurate for women who are pregnant or breast-feeding, or people who are frail. Health professionals are now also realising that some people can have an ideal BMI but still be at risk of developing obesity type symptoms because they are carrying too much weight around the middle area. Women with PCOS may fall into this category; your BMI may be 25 or less, but you may still develop insulin resistance because of the excess weight you carry around your tummy. So your BMI may not be the ideal measure for you if you have PCOS.

The BMI Calculator is only one guide about your overall health. Waist measurement, body fat level, blood pressure, cholesterol, physical activity, not smoking, and the healthiness of your diet are also important. You need to get the whole picture.

Waist circumference

The measurement of waist circumference provides information about the distribution of body fat and is a measure of risk for conditions such as diabetes. Experts now know that people who carry their excess fat centrally (around the tummy area) are more likely to suffer the consequences of being overweight.

The correct position for measuring waist circumference is midway between the upper hipbone and the lower rib. Place the tape measure around the abdomen at the level of this midway point, breathe out, and take a reading when the tape is snug but doesn't push down the skin. In practice if you are very overweight, it may be difficult for you to accurately find those bony landmarks; in which case placing the tape at the level of the belly button is recommended.

For women, a waist circumference measure of over 80 centimetres (31.5 inches) indicates an increased risk of developing heart disease, diabetes, blood pressure, and other related diseases.

If you have PCOS, waist circumference may be a better indicator of risk than BMI. However, not only is there a physical difficulty in measuring waist circumference if you are very obese but also, if you have a BMI over 35, waist circumference has little added predictive power of disease risk. However, if you have a BMI in the region of 25–35, incorporating a measurement of your waist circumference provides additional information about the likelihood of you developing further PCOS symptoms. It also can be used as an additional measure of progress with weight loss, especially as physical activity regimes can help you lose weight around the danger middle area without you necessarily losing any or much weight.

Being waist aware

Diabetes UK are running a campaign where they urge individuals to take a two-minute test to see if they are at risk of developing diabetes. Many people are unaware that they have diabetes and some have it for up to 12 years before getting a diagnosis, at which point serious damage to the eyes, kidneys, or circulation may have occurred. The Diabetes UK Web site (www.diabetes.org.uk/Measure_Up_-_are_you_at_risk_of_diabetes/) has a short questionnaire you can fill in which lets you know how at risk you are. One of the main risk factors of developing diabetes is having a waist circumference of over 80 centimetres (31.5 inches) (for women), so Diabetes UK is urging everyone to be waist aware!

Apples and pears

If you have too much weight around your middle, you may be described by some health professionals as having an 'apple' shape and told that you have an increased risk of developing heart disease and diabetes. When men gain weight, they often gain it round the middle, which is often referred to as a 'beer belly'. When women gain weight they don't tend to put it on around the middle as much as men, unless, that is, you have PCOS. Normally women are offered some protection against heart disease by not developing an apple shape like men. Unfortunately this protection can be lost if you

have PCOS. Women after the menopause also tend to put weight on in this area, and again this increases their risk of developing diabetes and heart disease.

However, if you tend to gain weight around your hips, you are referred to as being a 'pear' shape. This tends to be a less risky place to gain weight as far as heart disease and related health risks are concerned. Someone with an apple shape faces greater health risks than someone who has a pear shape, even if they are both overweight to the same degree.

Before You Begin to Slim

You are probably already aware that it tends to be harder to lose weight if you have PCOS. No one is exactly sure why but it may be a combination of:

- ✔ Generally having a lowered metabolic rate so that you just burn your fat up that much slower.

- ✔ Always feeling hungry and more prone to food cravings so that cutting down on your food intake is harder for you.

- ✔ The higher circulating insulin levels may mean that you have a greater tendency to store excess fuel as fat, rather than burning it up.

First rule: Lose weight slowly

Slow weight loss is better than rapid weight loss if you have PCOS, unless of course you have been told to lose weight urgently by your doctor. Therefore half a kilogram to one kilogram (1 to 2 pounds) a week is ideal. This weight loss is achievable for you, even if you struggle to diet. Weight lost slowly is also less likely to be re-gained and you are less likely to go into that yo-yo situation where you lose a bit, regain it, lose it again, and so on. Yo-yo dieting is thought to be harmful and can lead to the re-gained weight more likely to be fat, so that after a few repeating cycles you have a lower muscle mass and a higher fat mass than someone of the same weight as you who never dieted.

Second rule: Pick the best of the diet bunch

Rather than working out your own diet and checking that all the sums add up for the calorie values (and that your fat and sugars levels aren't out of balance too), you may want to pick a slimming diet 'off the shelf' or see an appropriate health professional such as a dietician and get some guidance from them. With any diet plan you choose, check that it's balanced and states how many calories it provides.

Commercial slimming organisations tend to be quite sensible these days but tell them you have PCOS and want to follow a low-GI approach. Many of them are familiar with this concept and should be able to offer some positive advice.

You can now get dietary advice by joining a Web-based organisation – some even offer low-GI diets specifically. You do have to pay to join, but they are often cheaper than joining a slimming club. You may not get the social support unless you join with a friend or the site has a members' chat-room. Again, before joining check out that the advice is sensible and follows the guidance that is given in this book.

Here are some basic guidelines to follow to make sure that you don't pick a dud diet:

- ✔ Avoid diets that claim huge weight losses in a short space of time.
- ✔ If you plan to follow a diet for longer than a month then around 1500 calories is a good level of intake. For shorter time periods, when you have less than 6 kilograms to lose, you can drop to 1300 calories, but you certainly shouldn't go below 1200 calories.
- ✔ Avoid diets that tell you to avoid certain foods or groups of food.
- ✔ Avoid diets that only advocate a narrow range of foods.
- ✔ Make sure that the diet isn't a low carbohydrate diet.
- ✔ Check whether the diet plan is also adaptable to a low-GI way of eating.

Although some procedures and drugs make you appear to have lost weight, these are only temporary solutions due to water loss. After a day or so, providing you are drinking normally, the weight goes back on because you haven't lost fat. The following techniques make you lose water, but don't provide a real loss in fat mass:

- ✔ Body wraps
- ✔ Saunas or steam rooms
- ✔ Diuretic pills, including 'natural' herbal diuretics

You may also see claims that certain natural chemicals can make you lose weight including:

- ✔ Caffeine and other stimulants
- ✔ Green tea extract
- ✔ Conjugated Linoleic Acid, a type of fat naturally present in small amounts in dairy foods and that you can buy as a supplement

Some evidence suggests that these substances can speed up metabolism, but the evidence is not yet conclusive, and the extra calories you burn off by consuming these substances is minimal. Stimulants such as caffeine are not well tolerated by everyone and can lead to high blood pressure.

Following a Low-GI and Weight Loss Diet

The theory behind weight loss is very simple:

- ✔ If energy in equals energy out, weight remains stable.
- ✔ If energy in is greater than energy out, weight gain occurs.
- ✔ If energy in is less than energy out, weight loss occurs.

That's the theory, but in practice it's a little more complicated because trying to reduce your energy in (by cutting down on the food you eat) and increase your energy out (by doing more exercise) tends to induce complaints from your body! The task becomes even trickier if you have PCOS. Ideally, you need to think about low-GI requirements as well as calorie requirements.

You don't have to lose a lot of weight to start to see the benefits in terms of your PCOS symptoms. If you're overweight, even losing 5 per cent of your body weight leads to the following beneficial changes:

- ✔ A decrease in insulin resistance leading to a beneficial lowering of circulating insulin levels.
- ✔ An improvement in the regularity of your periods, or if they have been absent they may well return with even this small weight loss.
- ✔ A lowering of testosterone level leading to the reduction of unwanted facial hair (hirsutism) and acne.
- ✔ More general health benefits such as lowering your cholesterol levels, and reducing your risk of developing diabetes and heart disease.

Combining low GI and low calories

For maximum health benefit, and particularly if you have weight to lose, a low-GI diet alone just doesn't cut it! Check out Chapter 4 for more information on the GI diet.

Basically all you need to do is to make sure that the starchy foods in the diet are low-GI starches. You may also need to avoid certain foods that, although low in calories, aren't low GI. Don't forget that certain low-GI foods may also not be low in calories. Table 5-2 lists low calorie, high-GI foods and low-GI, high calorie foods to avoid, if possible.

Table 5-2	Low- and High-GI foods to avoid
Low/Moderate Calorie but High-GI Foods	*Low-GI but High Calorie Foods*
Cornflakes	Full cream milk
Puffed wheat	Chocolate
Puffed rice	Fruit cake
White rice	Sponge cake
Rice cakes	Ice cream
White flour crackers	Creamy sauces
Bagel	Greek/wholemilk yoghurt
French bread	Tortilla/corn chips
Baked potato	
Meringue	
Sorbet	

When you have PCOS you have a tendency to feel very hungry, quite often. Some of this hunger may be due to fluctuating glucose levels. A low-GI diet can help to stabilise hunger by reducing blood sugar fluctuations. Having a regular meal pattern also helps to avoid extreme hunger and this pattern may involve having some small low-GI snacks between meals too.

Several research studies show that a low-GI diet can lead to weight loss and increased feelings of satiety. However, some other studies have failed to prove this, so to a certain extent, the jury is still out. The reason for following a low-GI diet when you have PCOS is to bring circulating insulin levels down and hence alleviate some of the symptoms. The fact that a low-GI diet may help with weight loss is an added bonus!

Knowing what you need: GDA

GDA stands for Guideline Daily Amounts and is explored in more detail in Chapter 3. The GDA tells you how much of certain nutrients you are guided to eat every day for a balanced and healthy diet. These figures are for women who have no excess weight to lose, so if you consumed the GDA for energy in a day, which is 2,000 calories, you would probably not lose or gain weight (unless of course you were very active or very slothful indeed in which case you may lose or gain weight respectively on 2,000 calories).

If you have a lot of weight to lose, you may be able to lose it by only cutting down by a couple of hundred calories on this 2,000 GDA figure. However, a good general rule is to cut your calorie intake by about 500 calories. Table 5-3 shows what the set GDAs are for weight maintenance and for weight loss.

Table 5-3	Weight Maintenance and Weight Loss GDA	
Nutrient	*Weight Maintenance GDA*	*Weight Loss GDA*
Calories	2,000	1,500
Total fat (grams)	70	50
Saturated fat (grams)	20	15
Total sugars (grams)	90	70

Armed with a calorie counter guide and by looking at the nutritional label, you can see whether a food is likely to fit into your overall calorie controlled diet. For example, if you fancy a ready meal but it says it provides 600 calories, 40 grams total fat, and the full total of your GDA for saturated fat, you may want to think twice: Is it so desirable that you want to blow nearly half your calorie allowance for the day on it plus over half your total fat and all your saturated fat limit?

The recipes in this book have been nutritionally analysed so that you can easily slot them into your calorie-controlled plan.

A typical 1,500 calorie controlled plan

A basic calorie-controlled diet should be based on healthy eating advice as advocated in Chapter 3.

To give you a taster of how you can eat well on a calorie-controlled diet, following are two different daily meal plans for a healthy low GI, 1,500-calories-a-day approach. The first plan gives quite specific guidance whereas the second is less precise and enables you to ring the changes. You may be surprised by how much food is in it, but don't forget that it's not just about the ingredients, but about the way you prepare and cook the food.

Plan 1

Breakfast

BLT (bacon, lettuce, and tomato) sandwich and fruit: 2 slices granary bread filled with 2 grilled rashers lean back bacon, lettuce, tomato, and 2 teaspoons reduced-calorie mayonnaise. Plus 1 satsuma.

Lunch

Ploughman's lunch: Serve a 10-centimetre piece French granary bread with 50 grams reduced-fat Cheddar cheese, 2 pickled onions, 1 tablespoon sweet pickle, and salad.

Dinner

Sweet potato, lentil, and cauliflower curry: Spray a non-stick pan with a spray oil. Heat and gently fry 2 tablespoons split red lentils, ½ sliced small onion, 1 teaspoon curry powder (or to taste), and 1 bay leaf for a few minutes. Add enough water to cover and 1 small can chopped tomatoes. Bring to boil and simmer for 20 minutes. Remove the bay leaf and add 1 chopped sweet potato and cauliflower florets. Cook until the sauce has thickened and serve with 6 tablespoons cooked brown rice.

Snack

1 slice granary toast topped with 2 teaspoons peanut butter and 1 teaspoon jam.

Daily milk allowance

275 millilitres/½ pint skimmed milk.

Plan 2

Breakfast

Bowl of low-GI breakfast cereal and semi-skimmed milk or fortified soya milk.

Piece of fruit or glass of fruit juice.

Mid morning

Fresh fruit.

Lunch

Sandwich made with 2 slices granary bread, cold meat, cheese or egg, tomato/salad.

Pot of fruit-flavoured low-fat yoghurt.

Mid afternoon

Slice of malt loaf or two oatcakes.

Evening meal

Meat/Fish/Chicken/veggie dish using recipes in Chapter 9. Vegetables or salad. Sweet potatoes/basmati rice/pasta.

Getting the right portion sizes

When following a 1,500 plan, in order for it to be balanced and stay within your calorie limit, use the recommended number of portions mentioned in Table 5-4.

Table 5-4 Recommended Portions of Food on a 1,500 Calorie Diet	
Food	*Daily Portions*
Breads, cereals, potatoes, rice, pasta	6
Meat, fish, eggs, pulses, and nuts	2
Milk and dairy foods	3
Vegetables	At least 3
Fruit	3
Oils, dressings, and spreads	3
Extras, such as snacks, alcohol	1

Guide to portion sizes

So that you know roughly what one portion equates to, use the following guidelines.

Breads, potatoes, cereals, rice, pasta

- Small bowl (about 3 heaped tablespoons) breakfast cereal or porridge
- 1 medium slice of bread or mini pitta or small tortilla
- Half a medium pitta, tortilla, wrap, or roll
- 3 crispbreads or 2 oatcakes
- 2 new or 1 medium potato (including sweet potato)
- 3 heaped tablespoons/half a cup cooked pasta, noodles or 25 grams/ 1 ounce uncooked
- 2 heaped tablespoons/⅓ cup cooked rice or barley or 25 grams/1 ounce uncooked
- 1 small slice malt loaf or half a fruit scone

Meat, chicken, fish, eggs, pulses, seeds, and nuts

- 75–100 grams/3–4 ounces cooked lean meat or oily fish (uncooked weights are about a quarter heavier)
- 150 grams/6ounces white fish, seafood, or Quorn
- 150 grams/6 ounces meat-based tomato type sauce such as Bolognese or chilli
- 2 eggs (but avoid more than 6 a week if your cholesterol is high)
- 5 tablespoons cooked beans, lentils, baked beans, or tofu
- 35 grams (just under 1½ ounces) nuts, seeds or nut butter or 75 grams/ 3 ounces reduced fat hummus

Milk and dairy foods

- 300 millilitres/½ pint skimmed or 200 millilitres/⅓ pint semi-skimmed milk or fortified Soya milk
- Small pot low-fat yoghurt, fromage frais (flavoured or plain), or soya desert
- 25 grams/1 ounce cheese
- 50 grams/2 ounces half-fat soft cheese
- 2 heaped tablespoons or small pot cottage cheese

Vegetables

- 3 heaped tablespoons any type, fresh, frozen or canned
- Bowl of salad

Fruit

- ✔ 1 medium piece of fruit such as apple, orange pear
- ✔ 1 cupful berries or grapes
- ✔ 2 small fruit such as satsumas or plums
- ✔ 1 large slice large fruit such as melon or pineapple
- ✔ 3 tablespoons canned or stewed fruit in juice
- ✔ 150 millilitres/6 fluid ounces glass of unsweetened fruit juice
- ✔ 1 tablespoon dried fruit

Oils, dressings, and spreads

- ✔ 1 teaspoon oil, spread, margarine, or mayonnaise
- ✔ 2 teaspoons low-fat spread or salad dressing
- ✔ 1 tablespoon single or sour cream or half-fat crème frâiche
- ✔ 2 tablespoons fat-free dressing

Extras (these are around 100 cals each)

- ✔ Two fruit servings
- ✔ One dairy serving such as small pot low-fat yoghurt
- ✔ 1 slice of low-GI bread with low-fat spread and yeast extract
- ✔ 2 low-GI crispbreads with 50 grams/2 ounces tuna or thinly spread peanut butter or half-fat soft cheese
- ✔ 25 grams/1 ounce nuts and raisins
- ✔ 1 mini fruit bun or small cereal bar or mini chocolate bar
- ✔ Small bag of savoury snacks such as reduced fat crisps that don't exceed 100 calories
- ✔ Small glass of wine or half a pint of beer or cider or 25 millilitres spirit with a low-cal mixer

Free stuff

Don't forget to have at least 6 to 8 drinks throughout the day. You can have the following drinks and not need to count them as part of your diet:

- ✔ Water, including still or sparkling mineral water and flavoured low calorie still or sparkling waters
- ✔ Sugar-free squash/cordials
- ✔ Sugar-free jelly

✔ Diet soft and carbonated drinks

✔ Herb teas

✔ Tea and coffee

✔ Bovril or yeast extract drinks, but limit to one a day because they are quite salty

Here's some stuff that you don't have to count which you can use to spice up your food:

✔ Lemon or lime juice or vinegars

✔ Herbs and spice

✔ A few capers or olives

✔ Stock cube

✔ Soy or teriyaki sauce (but not too much because these are quite salty)

✔ Hot pepper sauce, such as Tabasco or Worcestershire sauce

✔ Mustard

✔ Tomato purée

✔ A splash of wine

Pacing yourself

Although you need to decide how you spread these portions around in a day, Table 5-5 offers a suggested approach.

Table 5-5	Spread of Portions for Each Meal			
Food	**Breakfast**	**Lunch**	**Main Meal**	**Snacks**
Breads, cereals, potatoes, rice, pasta	1	2	2	1
Meat, fish, eggs, pulses, and nuts		1	1	
Milk and dairy foods	1	1		1
Vegetables		1	3	
Fruit	1		1	1
Oils, dressings, and spreads	1	1	1	
Extras, such as snacks, alcohol				1

Ready meals

If you're out and about and want to grab a quick sandwich for lunch, or a ready-made salad, go for one that's around 300 calories. If you don't have time to cook in the evening and you want to just heat up a ready meal, just choose one that's around 400 calories but don't forget to serve it with plenty of extra veggies or a bowl of salad.

Food Addiction and Cravings

Craving for starchy foods, such as bread, and sweet foods is common if you have PCOS but nobody really knows why. One theory is that it is a similar craving that women with PMS get and is linked with changes in mood.

Overcoming cravings

You can try a few things such as the following to stop yourself craving certain foods:

- Don't let yourself get starving hungry because this often triggers a craving.
- Keep your blood sugar level on an even keel by following a low-GI diet.
- Don't skip meals. Allow yourself a small between-meals snack if you are likely to get too hungry before your next meal thus avoiding downward swings in blood sugar levels that can trigger a craving.
- Don't totally deny yourself foods that you really crave and love; if it's chocolate, have it after you have had a proper meal and just have a little bit of some really good quality stuff.
- Doing some exercise every day can often help to normalise hunger and eating patterns.
- Don't diet or restrict your eating too strictly because this is a common trigger for cravings. The body can't stay in such a state of denial for too long!

Wanting a binge

Bingeing is a form of eating disorder; an eating disorder is a distorted pattern of thinking about food and behaviour towards food. If you tend to binge on a regular basis you may well have a pre-occupation or an obsession with food. You probably feel out of control as far as food is concerned. Women with

PCOS are prone to binge and to have bulimia, which is where you binge, feel guilty, and therefore try to purge yourself of what you have eaten and then tend to repeat the cycle again.

The binge cycle typically takes the following steps in PCOS:

1. Feeling low in energy/mood/self-esteem.
2. Feeling you need to eat 'comfort foods' such as bread or chocolate.
3. Gaining a short-term feeling of comfort.
4. Increase in blood sugar levels.
5. Increase in insulin levels.
6. Hormone imbalance.
7. Which leads back to the feeling that you have low energy, low mood, and/or a reduced self-esteem, and so the cycle repeats itself.

The cycle has to be broken because the outcome of this repeated cycle is the following:

✔ Weight gain

✔ Bloating

✔ Further hormonal imbalances

✔ Increasingly low self-esteem

✔ Inappropriate compensatory practices such as missing meals

So why are you more likely to have a binge eating disorder compared to someone without PCOS (6 per cent of women with PCOS have bulimia compared to 1 per cent without PCOS)?

✔ PCOS is a collection of disorders, which include menstrual problems, an above average weight, anxieties about fertility, and increased facial hair; these factors are not something that make you feel particularly good about yourself. These symptoms can set up a situation where a normal relationship with food is not possible and bingeing becomes the way in which you deal with the emotional stress.

✔ The fluctuating insulin levels that occur in PCOS and their subsequent effect on blood sugar levels can result in a feeling that you need to binge. After bingeing you may feel that you have to compensate somehow so you attempt to starve yourself. The problem is that this sort of behaviour, where bingeing is followed by starvation, can actually make insulin resistance worse.

Evidence is emerging that the desire to binge and the lack of a subsequent feeling of being satiated, which is commonly seen in PCOS, is due to hormone levels that are out of kilter. The body depends on these hormones to be at normal levels so that food intake can be kept on an even keel.

Some evidence suggests that cravings for sweet food and a desire to binge on them is related to testosterone levels (which tend to be higher in women with PCOS). Testosterone may drive down the level of a hormone, called *cholecystokinin*, which controls appetite. A lowered level of this hormone may predispose you to having an increased tendency to binge and gain weight, compared to women with a higher level. Further evidence exists that appetite regulation is impaired in women with PCOS due to another appetite hormone, called *ghrelin*, being disrupted. Normally ghrelin levels increase sharply before a meal and this stimulates hunger and drives food intake. As consumption of a meal progresses, the level of ghrelin falls and this helps the feeling of becoming satiated. However, in PCOS this decline in ghrelin levels doesn't happen, or happens to a lesser extent, so that the trigger to stop eating is reduced.

If you suspect you truly have an eating disorder and/or that your bingeing behaviour is out of control, you need some professional help from your GP who can refer you to a specialist if necessary. You may be asked to see a dietician and possibly concurrently the help of a psychotherapist.

Dieting Do's and Don'ts

No one has a sure-fire successful formula for dieting because the reasons people become obese may be very different and the way that they respond to weight loss may be very different too. However, this section offers a few tricks of the trade, which can help you along the path to your goal weight.

Keeping a diary

The diet diary is an essential tool for weight loss. It puts you in control and shows where things may be going wrong and enables you to do some detective work on where and why you may be failing. Table 5-6 shows such a diary.

Table 5-6		A Diet Diary			
Time	*Place*	*Food Eaten*	*Quantity*	*Mood*	*Hungry: Y/N*
0730	Walking around kitchen	Granary bread Orange juice	1 med. slice 1 cup	Tired, stressed (late for work)	N

To get the most benefit from a diet diary, heed these bits of advice:

- ✔ **Keep your diary with you at all times, and religiously write everything down as soon as you eat anything.** Even the simple act of knowing you have to write it all down can be enough to make you think twice about eating something you know you shouldn't. With the best of intentions, you probably won't remember everything you've had all day if you jot it down in the evening, thus negating the usefulness of keeping the diary in the first place.

- ✔ **Try to spend some time analysing your diary at the end of every week to see whether any patterns emerge.** If you think you have had a good week and have lost weight, look back to see what you actually did to cause that weight loss. If you don't lose weight one week, go back through the diary to see whether you can spot where you went awry.

- ✔ **Keep up the diary for a period of time.** If you think that you are slipping back into old habits you can look back on the good week to remind yourself what you did.

Keep the diary for at least week and use it to build up a picture of how you eat. Then if you find the weight loss isn't going well, go back to keeping a food diary again and see if you can spot what's happening.

Recording your weight and body fat

Weight recording can be done in conjunction with your food diary. You can then match-up your intake with what's happening to your weight and hence get a real feeling of cause and effect.

You only need to weigh yourself once a week because weight can fluctuate quite a lot on a daily basis. Try to do it at the same time of day and with the same type of clothes. You can even do it naked if you prefer!

Consider investing in scales that measure your body fat percentage. These scales are more expensive than ordinary scales but give you a fuller picture of what's going on in your body while you lose weight. If you are also embarking on an exercise programme, you may find that you lose proportionally more body fat than you do weight. This is because some of your body fat is not simply being burned up, but is being used to make more muscle, and muscle weighs more than fat. Furthermore, if you work out, you may look more toned and slimmer than a woman of the same weight as you who doesn't work out.

Table 5-7 can help you to identify where you are healthwise with regard to your body fat percentage. You can see that as you get older, you're allowed a little more leeway with regards to how much body fat you can carry and still be in the healthy range!

Table 5-7	Recommended Body Fat Percentages for Women			
Age	**Underfat %**	**Healthy %**	**Overfat %**	**Obese %**
16–17	<16	16–30	31–34	34>
18	<17	17–31	32–31	31>
19	<19	19–32	33–37	37>
20–39	<21	21–33	34–38	38>
40–59	<23	23–34	35–40	40>

Arranging (rather than filling) your plate

When following a diet you need to eat less energy-dense food (foods that provide a lot of calories in a small amount of the food) and try to fill up on food that you can eat a lot of but that doesn't supply so many calories. Table 5-8 lists the energy density of common foods.

Table 5-8	Energy Density of Foods
Energy Density	**Food**
High	Butter, oil, cheese, fatty meat, nuts, pastry, batter, full fat dumplings, cake, biscuits, alcohol
Medium	Lean meat, poached or grilled fish, pasta, fruit juice, breakfast cereals, bread, rice
Low	Vegetables, fruit, beans, lentils

The foods with a high energy density provide lots of calories, so only eat a little of these in a day. High energy dense foods are usually high in fat: Fatty foods are high energy dense because fat has twice as many calories weight for weight compared to protein and carbs. The low energy dense foods, such as vegetables and pulses, should make up the largest part of your diet as they provide lots of vitamins and minerals but not many calories. These foods are low energy dense because they contain very little fat but usually contain quite a lot of water, which is of course calorie free.

When considering your dinner plate, plan to cover it with your dinner in the following healthy proportions (see Figure 5-1):

✔ About half of your plate can be made up of vegetables and/or pulses (peas, beans, and lentils), which are low energy dense and fill you up without many calories.

✔ About a quarter can come from starchy food such as pasta or rice, which are medium energy dense and provide the low-GI carbs, help you feel full, and provide fibre and other nutrients.

Figure 5-1: How to apportion a balanced low-GI plate.

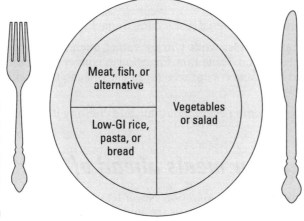

Meat, fish, or alternative

Low-GI rice, pasta, or bread

Vegetables or salad

✔ The last quarter can be the protein part of the meal, which is medium energy dense.

✔ You can add a very small amount of high energy dense foods to your plate, such as cheese, but with caution because they bump up your calories without you even noticing.

If you like to fill your plate, or pile it high, and you have largish diner plates, simply swap to a smaller plate so that even by filling your plate with food, you automatically get less!

Savouring every bite

In order for your body to register that it has had a meal and to feel satisfied with that, take time to fully appreciate a meal, or indeed even a snack. Try to be aware of every morsel that goes in your mouth: You may begin to realise that you don't really want to be eating that particular food or at that particular time. You may also be more aware of when you are feeling full and may be able to put your knife and fork down without having to finish everything on your plate.

You may find that when you have permitted yourself to properly appreciate your food, you don't need to eat as much of it. Here are some tips on how to appreciate your food more:

✔ Make an occasion of every mealtime. Light the candles, add a vase of flowers, and use the good china!

✔ Make sure you're eating food that's really tasty and nutritious; don't passively put any old rubbish in your mouth!

✔ Never eat standing up or walking around. Ideally sit at a table when you're eating.

✔ Use a proper plate (even if just having a snack) and proper utensils.

✔ Don't do anything else while you are eating, such as reading or watching television. Exception: Engaging in conversation with your family and friends is encouraged (after all, you can't talk with your mouth full)!

✔ Eat slowly, savouring every mouthful, and chewing it thoroughly.

Planning your meals ahead of time

Preparation, preparation, preparation! Never let yourself stumble up to a mealtime without knowing what you are going to have and not have the ingredients or food at hand!

Plan out your week's menu and shop for that. You can do this on a daily basis if you have the opportunity to shop daily. You then know exactly what ingredients you need and don't need to buy extras, which you may also get tempted to eat. Each morning check what you're going to have for each meal. Then if a meal needs some pre-preparation, such as soaking beans or defrosting something, make sure you do that instead of leaving it until the actual mealtime.

If you don't pre-plan, and you're ravenously hungry, you're going to be tempted to go for the first thing that comes to hand (a packet of crisps or a lump of cheese), or even send-out for a quick delivery pizza!

Using healthy cooking methods

How healthy and how low calorie your meal ends up being depends as much on the method you use to cook something as the ingredients you use.

Healthy cooking methods don't need to be involved and drawn-out; in fact they can be hassle free. Here are some tips on how to prepare food the healthy way if you want to lose weight:

- ✔ Steam or microwave your vegetables so that they retain more nutrients and you don't add extra fat to them.

- ✔ Poach, boil, or scramble your eggs; don't fry them. Scrambled eggs can be made in the microwave using a little milk and black pepper whisked up with them. Only cook until just before they are set because they carry on cooking after you remove them from the microwave.

- ✔ Grill or dry bake meat and pour away the fat.

- ✔ When cooking fairly fatty meat such as bacon or sausages, grill and then place on some kitchen roll to blot away the remaining melted fat.

- ✔ When frying mince, pour away any fat that appears.

- ✔ When making a casserole or stew using meat with some fat on it, let it go cold, take off the solidified fat that appears on top, and then re-heat.

- ✔ Don't use meat juices If you are making gravy because this is quite fatty.

- ✔ Make your own salad dressing with just a little oil, herbs, lemon juice, and balsamic vinegar, to ensure that it's much lower in calories than shop-bought dressing.

- ✔ Par boil Mediterranean vegetables and potatoes and roast in a little olive oil in the oven; you can also add minced garlic, pepper, and herbs.

The benefit of eating breakfast for weight control

If you think skipping breakfast is going to help you lose weight, think again! Studies show that breakfast, especially a cereal-based breakfast, is associated with better weight control.

An ongoing study of people who have maintained weight loss of at least 15 kilograms for more than a year shows that eating breakfast keeps people slimmer (National Weight Control Registry). Breakfast eaters tend to eat fewer calories, less saturated fat and cholesterol, and have better overall nutritional status than breakfast skippers. A Nielsen's National Eating Trends Survey showed that women who ate cereal on a regular basis weighed about 9 pounds less than those who ate cereal rarely or not at all.

When you skip breakfast, your metabolic rate tends to slow down and your blood sugar drops. As a result, you become hungry and have less energy. Indeed, children who skip breakfast aren't as able to concentrate on their lessons as children who have a cereal breakfast. Without breakfast you tend to want to snack in the morning, often on high-fat sweets, or to eat extra servings or bigger portions at lunch or dinner. However, when you eat breakfast, your body feels nourished and satisfied, making you less likely to overeat the rest of the day.

Eating breakfast every day may reduce the risk for obesity and insulin resistance by as much as 35 to 50 per cent, especially if it is a low-GI breakfast (see Chapter 6 for brekkie ideas).

Energy and cereal bars have exploded in popularity. Although they are convenient and may satisfy your hunger, read the label. Even though they contain a variety of vitamins and other added nutrients, they often contain very little fibre and are loaded with as many calories as a chocolate bar!

Top secrets from people who have kept their weight off

These tips may not have come from the stars (after all they are only human and are forever making a mess of their lives, so what do they know!), but they have come from researching successful dieters who managed to keep their weight off.

- ✔ An hour's physical activity a day helps to maintain weight loss; but if you can't manage this much, try to do at least half an hour a day.

- ✔ Weigh yourself on a regular basis and if the weight seems to be creeping up again, take things in hand immediately before things get worse.

- ✔ Continue to plan ahead with regard to your meals so that you know what you're going to eat at the next meal and you have the ingredients at hand.

- ✔ Continue to follow your low-fat diet with your carbs coming from low-GI sources where possible.

✔ Have regular meals and snacks (if necessary) and don't skip meals.

✔ Always have breakfast because this start-up meal helps to normalise your eating patterns for the rest of the day.

The National Weight Control Registry studies people who have managed to successfully maintain weight loss; they found that of those who were successful in maintaining their weight loss, only 9 per cent managed to do so without doing some regular exercise.

When the Going Gets Tough

A couple of factors may tend to throw you off your diet: not losing any weight and giving in to temptation and falling off the wagon. But help is available for both these diet failure factors, as the following sections explain.

You're not losing it

The scales at the end of the week may not always register a weight loss. Always keep a food diary when you've gone two weeks without losing weight because this record may help pinpoint what's happening.

You're self-delusional

At the start of the diet you're typically fired up and watching your food intake carefully. But after a while you may start to get complacent and let some old habits creep back in, even though you may have convinced yourself that you are still on the diet. If your weight loss has slowed down or stopped, you need to check with your food diary whether you're really still eating as healthily as you tell yourself you are.

You're already there

The reason that you're no longer losing weight, or the losses have slowed right down, may be that you've shed enough. Use the following three checks to see where you are, and if you come out normal for two out of three of them then you're okay.

✔ Your Body Mass Index (BMI) is 25 or less.

✔ Your waist circumference is 80 centimetres (31.5 inches) or less.

✔ Your body-fat percentage is 33 per cent or less (if you are aged 20–39).

You have gone too far

If you cut back too drastically on your calorie intake, or exercise too intensively, you can actually hamper your weight loss. This reaction is because the body thinks it's in a state of emergency; either in a state of starvation or in a state when extreme endurance is required. Both of these factors can tend to make the body hang on and store as much of the calories it is given as possible and stubbornly cling to its fat reserves. Watch out for these key signs, which indicate that you're not giving your body nearly enough fuel:

- Frequent, sharp hunger pangs
- Mood swings
- Strongly fluctuating energy levels
- Dizziness
- Constant thoughts about food

Check your food diary; you need to take in around 1500 calories a day and not skip meals. Also check that you're having sufficient servings of each of the food groups listed in Table 5-5.

Your metabolism is sluggish

Unfortunately, the slimmer you are, the lower your metabolic rate tends to be because it takes more energy to run a larger body than a smaller one. So, as you lose weight your metabolism falls too.

The easiest and most effective way of speeding up your metabolism is to increase the amount of exercise you do. Be sure to include weight-bearing exercise because increasing your muscle mass ups your metabolic rate. Eating little and often rather than consuming just a few large meals may also help to boost your metabolism.

You're losing inches instead

Because muscle weighs more than fat, if you are close to your ideal weight and you embark on a programme of exercise along with healthy eating, you may find that your body shape changes more than the needle on your scales. You are losing inches and gaining muscle and that may result in a drop in your dress size. You can measure the change by measuring your waist circumference or by measuring your body fat percentage. As far as your PCOS symptoms are concerned, this type of change is positive because it means that you're losing fat; at the end of the day, fat loss is what helps lessen your PCOS symptoms. As well as monitoring weight loss you may want to keep a record of a few vital statistics, such as waist measurements. When these reduce you get as much of a positive boost as any weight reduction.

You need to get moving

Exercise is important in the treatment of PCOS, but if you do enough of it, it also promotes weight loss. If you're not active, your calorie requirement to achieve weight loss may need to be less than 1,500. Maintaining a calorie intake as low as this is extremely difficult, and you may also find it hard to get all the nutrients that your body needs at this level of food intake. So if you're inactive, you may be sticking to the 1,500 but just finding that the weight is not shifting.

You need to do a minimum of 30 minutes a day of some sort of physical activity that gets you slightly out of breath. It doesn't have to be a formal exercise session and it doesn't have to be all done in one go; three 10-minute sessions work equally well. Exercise that qualifies for this 'slightly out of breath' level includes brisk walking, gardening (especially cutting the lawn), swimming at a moderate pace, and cycling with not too many hills!

Just because you've done your 30 minutes physical activity for the day, don't think you can rest on your laurels and be a couch potato for the rest of the day. That half-hour exercise is not really a lot when you think it's only half-an-hour out of a 24-hour day, and eight of those hours are spent in bed! So you need to think about how you can get physically active in your day-to-day life too; for example, find excuses to run up and down stairs when you can and avoid lifts, or ditch the remote control so that you have to stand up and walk when working the television or music system. If you work at a desk, get up once in a while to consult with a coworker face-to-face rather than sending an e-mail to the person down the hall.

You need more sleep

You may think that lying asleep in your bed not doing anything wouldn't help you to burn up more calories. But in fact the reverse is true. Recent studies show that people who sleep less have a greater increase in body mass and waist circumference over time. Indeed, a lack of sleep has been shown to be associated with an almost two-fold increase in obesity levels for both children and adults. Apparently everyone is getting less and less sleep, and so thinking about how much you get is worthwhile because almost a quarter of the adult population are believed to be sleep-deprived. Symptoms of sleep deprivation include:

- ✔ Exhaustion, fatigue, and lack of physical energy.
- ✔ Feelings of pessimism, sadness, stress, and anger.
- ✔ Insufficient rest adversely affects the frontal cortex's ability to control speech, access memory, and solve problems.

Lack of sleep may lead to obesity because of an increase in appetite that is in turn due to the hormonal changes driven by sleep deprivation. Lack of sleep can also make you more stressed, and when you're stressed you produce more of the hormone *cortisol*. Cortisol is believed to lead to a greater tendency for weight to be deposited around your middle, the danger zone!

Lack of sleep is thought to trigger an excessive production of the hormone ghrelin, which causes, amongst other things, an increase in appetite. Sleep deprivation is also believed to trigger other chronic conditions such as diabetes, high blood pressure, and early signs of aging. However more research is needed to find out exactly how lack of sleep leads to these conditions and to obesity.

To relapse is human

As well as just getting fed up with the slow or absent rate of weight loss, the other common reason for giving up on a diet completely is just by falling off the wagon and then not being able to motivate yourself back onto it again. Don't forget that from time to time you are likely to trip up and fail. This lapse doesn't mean that you shouldn't keep trying to reach your successful pinnacle! You need to keep taking more steps forwards than you take backwards! Remember that getting too negative about your occasional failures doesn't push you forward and is more likely to keep you back. If a failure happens, acknowledge it and try to work out why it happened, but then pick yourself back up and get back on the path to success as soon as you can.

Part III
Recipes for Life

The 5th Wave   By Rich Tennant

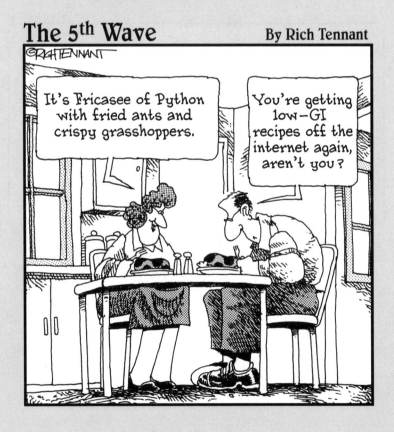

In this part . . .

This is the fun part: You get to make some really lovely meals. These recipes aren't just for you, oh no, your friends and family will love them too. You don't have to feel that you're on a diet with these gems, and they're easy to make. This part also includes some more indulgent recipes for when you're entertaining, and some yummy snacks. Oh, I nearly forgot, they're healthy and follow the low-GI plan too.

Chapter 6

Breakfast Like a King

In This Chapter

▶ Convincing you that breakfast really is an important meal

▶ Showing you how easy throwing a healthy breakfast together can be

▶ Tempting you with some delicious low-GI breakfast recipes

*Y*our mother wasn't lying when she told you that breakfast is the most important meal of the day. Breakfast is especially important for those with PCOS. By starting your day with a healthy low-GI meal, you'll find keeping your weight under control easier. Whether you take breakfast on the run or at a more leisurely pace, this chapter offers tasty recipes that are easy to prepare. Thrown in are a few PCOS-friendly recipes that dare to be indulgent. Enjoy.

Breakfast – Why Bother?

Breakfast literally means the breaking of a fast. Didn't know you fast? Well you do every day, between the last meal you eat at night and the first meal you eat the next day. If you have your evening meal at 6 p.m. and you skip breakfast, choosing instead to wait for the usual office morning round of bacon butties or pastries at elevenses, you've been fasting for 17 hours! Going without food is normal overnight, but once you're up and about, your body doesn't respond well to running on empty.

Going without food for a long period of time, especially if you're also active, may cause your body to become very efficient at surviving on very little. Your body then begins to store food rather than burn it up. With PCOS making you more likely to put on weight, encouraging the storage of fuel calories is just what you don't want to be doing.

Breakfast is also important for lots of other reasons:

- ✔ Eating breakfast helps to control glucose levels for the rest of the day, especially if the breakfast was a low-GI one.

- ✔ Eating breakfast may help you concentrate better during the morning.

- ✔ People who eat breakfast tend to have better overall nutrient intakes, in particular important vitamins and minerals such as vitamin C and iron.

- ✔ Going without food for a long period of time is associated with raised levels of cholesterol. Indeed cholesterol levels seem to improve when regular meals and snacks are consumed (providing of course this doesn't lead to an increase in calorie consumption).

- ✔ Eating breakfast helps you to control your overall calorie intake during the rest of the day and helps your body to stop the craving for unsuitable snacks between meals.

So, skipping breakfast due to lack of time, not feeling hungry, or whatever reason is not a great way of cutting out extra calories. You reap havoc later on if you do skip this vital meal. So ignite that morning boiler flame and get some good food inside you!

Tips for a Healthy Breakfast

As Chapter 4 explains, the GI (glycaemic index) of a food is an important factor in healthy diet, especially for those with PCOS. Eating a low-GI breakfast can help to stop your blood glucose fluctuating up and down for the rest of the day, even if you don't necessarily have a low-GI lunch or dinner (although a more even blood sugar control is achieved if you base each meal on low-GI foods). Following a few helpful tips can help you to get into an easy routine of knowing what the best thing to have for breakfast is, and how to achieve your breakfast goal without too much stress and strain.

Bringing down your breakfast's GI

Traditionally based on cereals or bread, breakfast tends to be a fairly starchy meal, meaning that it can also be very high GI if you're not careful.

The simple rule is to make sure that your breakfast carbs are low GI. Table 6-1 lists some typical breakfast items with their GI content, ranking them as low, medium, or high GI. Go for the low-GI foods when you can, but a medium GI-based breakfast is okay now and then too. High GI-based breakfasts are for treats or when going low GI simply isn't convenient. (For instructions on how to figure out the overall GI of a meal, refer to Chapter 4.).

As well as the GI of a food, you also need to eat food that fits into a balanced diet. If you're watching your weight, you need to keep an eye on calories, your portion sizes, and the amount of fat in your food (particularly saturated fat), and keep the salt intake down too.

Table 6-1	GI Values for Some Common Breakfast Foods	
Breakfast Item	**GI Score**	**GI Ranking**
Yoghurt, low-fat diet	14	Low
Grapefruit	25	Low
Milk, semi-skimmed	30	Low
Yoghurt, flavoured low fat	33	Low
Apple juice	41	Low
Banana, not fully ripe	42	Low
Bran cereal	42	Low
Muesli, toasted	43	Low
Bread, mixed grain	45	Low
Orange juice	46	Low
Pineapple juice, unsweetened	46	Low
Bread, fruit loaf white	47	Low
Baked beans	48	Low
Porridge	49	Low
Rye bread	50	Low
Bran flakes with sultana cereal	52	Low
Sourdough bread	52	Low
Stoneground wholemeal bread	53	Low
Rice flake type cereal	54	Low
Mango	55	Low
Sultanas	56	Medium
Muesli, untoasted	56	Medium
Muesli bar	61	Medium

(continued)

Table 6-1 *(continued)*

Breakfast Item	GI Score	GI Ranking
Raisins	64	Medium
Puffed wheat type cereal	65	Medium
One-minute oats	67	Medium
Crumpets	69	Medium
White bread	70	High
Bagel	72	High
Wheat biscuit type cereal	75	High
Rice-cakes	82	High
Cornflakes	84	High

The type of starch you choose is also important in keeping your breakfast low GI. Smart substitutions satisfy your taste buds and can be healthy. For example, if you prefer bread or toast for breakfast, choose seeded or multi-grain bread. Rye and sourdough bread is also good. Instead of butter or regular jam, use low-fat spread, low-fat cream cheese, reduced sugar or sugar-free marmalade or jam, or peanut butter (be careful with the peanut butter, which is quite high in fat). A nice alternative to pastries and croissants, which are both high GI and high fat, are fruit breads, teacakes, or any low-fat fruited tea bread/loaf or a low-fat muffin (some recipes for these can be found in Chapter 8).

Foods that aren't sugary or starchy don't affect your blood sugar levels and therefore are neutral as far as GI is concerned. This includes foods such as eggs, cheese, and meats. However, in order to keep your weight under control and to stop the level of harmful blood fats from rising, try to have non-GI foods that are low in fat, or at least low in saturated and trans fats (see Chapter 3). So a fry-up breakfast composed of bacon, eggs, and so on may not have a GI value, but eaten more than occasionally doesn't do you much good!

Only foods containing a significant amount of carbohydrate (carbs) can have a GI value.

Sugar is sweet . . . sometimes

Some of these breakfast recipes require a bit of sweetening. If the majority of your ingredients in a dish are low GI, the addition of some sugar, honey, or maple syrup doesn't significantly push up the overall GI of the meal. You may be surprised by the fact that not all sugars have a high GI. Table 6-2 shows the GI values of sugars and syrups.

TIP

Adding sugar increases the calories in your food so only add just enough to give taste. A sugary taste is a bit like a salty taste in that you can change your sensitivity to them and so eventually prefer the taste of foods that are less salty and less sweet.

Table 6-2	GI Values of Sugars and Syrups
Food	*GI Value*
Glucose (used as the standard against which other carb foods are compared, usually as glucose powder dissolved in water)	100
Honey	73
Sucrose (white table sugar)	65
Reduced sugar apricot jam	55
Maple syrup	54
Strawberry jam	51

Stocking your breakfast cupboard

The ingredients listed here are useful to have around in your cupboard and fridge and you need them for the recipes in this chapter:

- Rolled oats
- Eggs, omega-3 enriched if possible
- Low-fat yoghurt (live/probiotic if possible)
- Low-fat cream cheese
- Fresh fruit (bananas, mango, berries, apples)
- Milk, semi-skimmed or soya milk
- Runny honey
- Apricot jam
- Maple syrup
- Dried fruit
- Mixed nuts (unsalted) and seeds

Yoghurts alive!

Live yoghurts are yoghurts that have live 'good' bacteria present in them. 'Good' bacteria is beneficial to health, unlike so-called 'bad' bacteria, which can cause food poisoning. These can be present during the production of the yoghurt because yoghurt is a fermented product. However, with the pasteurisation of yoghurt the bacteria may get destroyed. Alternatively live bacteria can be added to the yoghurt. These live, 'good' bacteria are known as probiotics and they are believed to serve several important functions in the body such as helping to:

✔ Alleviate IBS (irritable bowel syndrome)

✔ Protect against food poisoning

✔ Protect against allergies and intolerances

✔ Protect against thrush

✔ Protect against bowel cancers

✔ Boost general immunity

Eating your 'live' or probiotic yoghurt may be giving you some added benefits. To get the full benefit you need to get a dose of probiotics every day because the bacteria can't hang around your gut for very long and so need to be replaced daily.

Oh, What a Beautiful Morning! Simple and Quick Breakfasts

To be healthy, breakfast doesn't have to be drab. Scrambled eggs, bacon, pancakes, smoothies, ham crisps . . . believe it or not, low-GI breakfasts can include these delectables. The recipes in this section are not only guaranteed to be low GI, they're also low calorie and have been 'controlled' for fat, salt, and saturated fat (in other words, I've kept the levels as low as possible). But the health benefits aren't the only good things about these recipes; they're also great tasting.

Oh-so-smooth smoothies

The ultimate fast breakfast is something you can drink in a glass. *Smoothies* are a delicious mix of yoghurt and fruit and sometimes ice that you can whip up in a blender. Smoothies are a great start to the day if you are pushed for time because they are low GI and very nutritious.

Smoothies may not keep you satisfied for long. If you choose a smoothie for breakfast, be prepared to think about a low-GI top-up two to three hours later. You can find good snack ideas and recipes in Chapter 8.

Berry Smoothie

Berries are rich in antioxidants and vitamins such as vitamin C. They have a low GI and combined with the yoghurt, milk, and a banana that isn't too ripe, this smoothie has a very low GI which is not significantly raised by the addition of a little honey (if needed for taste).

Preparation time: *10 minutes*

Serves: *1*

225 grams (9 ounces) strawberries or a mixture of berry fruits

1 banana, use one that's just ripe

150g (6 ounces/1¼ cups) plain live yoghurt

200 millilitres (¼ pint/¾ cup) semi-skimmed (low-fat) milk

1 tablespoon honey

1 Wash all the fruit then hull any strawberries and trim any other berries. Drain and dry thoroughly and transfer to a food processor or blender.

2 Add the peeled banana, yoghurt, milk, and honey and process until smooth.

3 Pour into a glass and chill for a few minutes before serving.

Tip: *You can add some ice before blending and this helps to chill the mixture.*

Per serving: *Calories 431 (From Fat 82); Fat 9g (Saturated 5g); Cholesterol 30mg; Sodium 188mg; Carbohydrate 79g (Dietary Fibre 8g); Protein 15g. Approx. Salt (g) 0.5.*

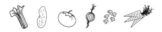

Coffee Banana Smoothie

As well as being a reasonably filling breakfast smoothie, this recipe can get you going in the morning with its shot of coffee. Feel free to use decaff coffee if you don't want the stimulant!

Preparation time: *10 minutes*

Serves: *2*

2 heaped teaspoons instant coffee granules

500 millilitres/2 cups semi-skimmed milk

1 large banana

4 ice cubes

Ground cinnamon (optional)

1 Put the milk, coffee powder, banana, and ice in a blender and blend until smooth.

2 Pour into 2 tall glasses and serve immediately; sprinkle with cinnamon if desired.

Vary It! *If you have an espresso coffee maker you can use a double espresso in this recipe instead of the instant coffee granules.*

Per serving: *Calories 173 (From Fat 28); Fat 3g (Saturated 2g); Cholesterol 10mg; Sodium 133mg; Carbohydrate 29g (Dietary Fibre 2g); Protein 9g. Approx. Salt (g) 0.3*

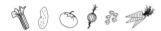

Mango and Peach Smoothie

Once you have the essential elements – milk and/or juice, a banana, and something to sweeten such as a little honey – you can whizz up almost any fruit to make a smoothie. This one uses some summer fruit: a mango and some peaches or nectarines. But experiment yourself with other variations.

Preparation time: *10 minutes*

Serves: *4*

1 large ripe mango..

1 banana (not too ripe)

2 ripe peaches or nectarines

200 millilitres (½ pint/¾ cup) milk (use soya milk if preferred)

200 millilitres (½ pint/¾ cup) orange juice

3 tablespoons plain yoghurt

2 tablespoons runny honey

1 Peel the mango and peaches or nectarines and remove and discard the stones.

2 Roughly chop the flesh of both fruits.

3 Place the fruit in a food processor or blender with the milk, orange juice, honey, and yoghurt.

4 Process until smooth then pour into glasses.

Tip: *If you use live/probiotic yoghurt, this recipe can give you an added advantage of promoting gut health.*

Per serving: *Calories 175 (From Fat 22); Fat 3g (Saturated 1g); Cholesterol 9mg; Sodium 33mg; Carbohydrate 38g (Dietary Fibre 3g); Protein 4g. Approx. Salt (g) 0.1.*

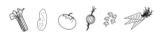

Pease porridge hot . . . : Cereals

A low-GI cereal such as muesli or porridge can be a very quick, very tasty meal. Serving cereal or porridge with low-fat milk, soya milk, or even apple juice helps keep this meal in a bowl low GI. You can make up your own cereals and add some nuts, seeds, and dried fruit.

Porridge with Berry Purée

No apologies for having so many oat-based cereals: Oats are a great breakfast food because their low-GI value helps to keep you feeling full through the morning. They are also a good source of soluble fibre, which can help to lower your cholesterol level.

Preparation time: 10 minutes

Cooking time: 10 minutes

Serves: 4

175 grams (6 ounces/2 cups) rolled oats

750 millilitres (1¼ pints/3¼ cups) skimmed milk or water

2 level tablespoons soft brown sugar

100 grams (3 ounces) strawberries, hulled

100 grams (3 ounces) raspberries

100 millilitres (4 fluid ounces) orange juice

1 Place the oats, milk or water, and sugar in a large saucepan and bring to the boil. Reduce the heat, and simmer for about 10 minutes until the oats are softened and the mixture is as runny or thick as you prefer it.

2 Meanwhile, place berries and orange juice in a food processor or blender and process until smooth.

3 Press the berry mixture through a fine sieve to remove seeds.

4 Serve the berry purée over the porridge.

Tip: If you get a glut of berry fruits, you can make up a larger quantity of the purée and freeze it in portions. You can then add it to cereals or porridge at a later stage or even pour it over ice cream as a dessert.

Per serving: Calories 293 (From Fat 31); Fat 3g (Saturated 1g); Cholesterol 4mg; Sodium 106mg; Carbohydrate 53g (Dietary Fibre 7g); Protein 14g. Approx. Salt (g) 0.3.

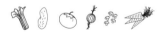

Caribbean Porridge

An unusual slant to plain old porridge which successfully brings together the Scottish and the Caribbean!

Preparation time: *10 minutes*

Cooking time: *10 minutes*

Serves: *2 to 3*

80 grams (3 ounces/½ cup) porridge oats

50 grams (2 ounces/½ cup) desiccated (dried) coconut

200 millilitres (½ pint/1 cup) semi-skimmed milk

375 millilitres (¾ pint/1½ cups) coconut milk

3 tablespoons maple syrup

1 large papaya

1 Mix the oats and desiccated coconut together in a saucepan. Stir in the milk and coconut milk and place the pan over medium heat. Bring the mixture to the boil, stirring all the time, and then reduce the heat to minimum and continue to cook, stirring, for 5 to 10 minutes until the porridge reaches the consistency you prefer.

2 Peel the papaya, cut it in half, and scoop out the seeds.

3 Transfer the fruit to a food processor or blender and purée.

4 When the porridge is cooked, stir in the maple syrup and then swirl in the papaya purée to serve.

Vary It! *If papaya is a little too exotic for you, use a mashed banana instead. You can use soya milk instead of the semi-skimmed milk if you prefer.*

Per serving: *Calories 345 (From Fat 125); Fat 14g (Saturated 10g); Cholesterol 3mg; Sodium 107mg; Carbohydrate 50g (Dietary Fibre 7g); Protein 9g. Approx. Salt (g) 0.3.*

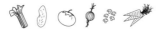

Vanilla Granola Breakfast Trifle

Although not strictly a trifle, that is the best way to describe this layered oat-based breakfast. This recipe provides you with a good helping of carbs, protein, some good fats, and plenty of vitamins and minerals, such as B vitamins and calcium.

Preparation time: *15 minutes, plus 10 minutes standing time*

Cooking time: *30 minutes*

Serves: *4*

200 grams (8 ounces/1½ cups) oatmeal or porridge oats

50 grams (2 ounces/½ cup) slivered or sliced almonds/brazils

25 grams (1 ounce/¼ cup) demerara (raw cane) or soft light brown sugar

Small pinch ground cinnamon

2 teaspoons sunflower oil

2 teaspoons runny honey

1 teaspoon vanilla extract

100 grams (4 ounces/½ cup) low-fat plain Greek yoghurt

3 tablespoons blueberry or blackcurrant conserve (fruit spread)

2 tablespoons dried cranberries or cherries

1 Preheat the oven to 150°C/300°F/Gas Mark 2. Line a large baking tray with greaseproof (parchment) paper.

2 Mix the oats, almonds, sugar, salt, and cinnamon together in a large bowl.

3 Stir the oil and honey together in a small saucepan and heat over medium-high heat, stirring, until quite hot. Remove from the heat and stir in the vanilla extract. Pour into the bowl with the oat mixture and stir well until all the dry ingredients are thoroughly coated.

4 Spread the mixture on the lined baking sheet and bake in the centre of the oven for 30 minutes.

5 Remove from oven, and leave to cool on the tray for 10 minutes, and then pour into a bowl to cool completely – don't leave it any longer or it sticks to the greaseproof paper.

6 To assemble the dish, pour a couple of spoonfuls of cooled granola into the bottom of a tall glass. Add a tablespoon of the fruit conserve and then a couple of tablespoons of yoghurt. Add another layer of the granola and then more fruit conserve and yoghurt. Repeat to fill three more glasses. Top each one with a tablespoon of dried cranberries or cherries.

Per serving: *Calories 386 (From Fat 118); Fat 13g (Saturated 2g); Cholesterol 3mg; Sodium 19mg; Carbohydrate 57g (Dietary Fibre 7g); Protein 13g. Approx. Salt (g) 0.0.*

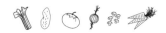

Apple Muesli

This recipe is packed with superfoods. The secret of this recipe is the blending of the flavours and the mix of crunchy and smooth textures. The overnight soaking allows the oat flakes to soften and take up the flavours from the apple juice. The oats and apple juice make this a low-GI dish.

Preparation time: *10 minutes plus overnight soaking*

Serves: *6 to 8*

200 grams rolled oats (8 ounces/2 cups)

350 millilitres apple juice (14 ounces/1½ cups)

1 red apple

125 grams/½ cup natural low-fat yoghurt (live yoghurt is good)

A mixture of fruits in season (berries work well in the summer)

Runny honey to drizzle

Handful of toasted almonds to serve

1 Place oats in a bowl and cover with enough apple juice to moisten them. Cover the bowl and chill overnight in the fridge, or for at least an hour.

2 Coarsely grate the apple (including the skin) and stir into the oats. Stir in enough yoghurt to achieve a mixture that's not too sloppy but not overly stiff. Add more apple juice at this stage too if the mixture is too stiff.

3 Serve the muesli in individual bowls topped with the fruit of your choice, a drizzle of honey, and a sprinkling of toasted almonds.

Tip: *This recipe can keep for three days in the fridge, but don't add the fresh fruit or nuts until just before serving because these need to be crunchy.*

Vary It! *You can use milk to soak the oats if you prefer and the fresh fruit can be substituted partly or wholly with dried fruit.*

Per serving: *Calories 169 (From Fat 19); Fat 2g (Saturated 1g); Cholesterol 1mg; Sodium 14mg; Carbohydrate 34g (Dietary Fibre 5g); Protein 5g. Approx. Salt (g) 0.0. Analysed with 2 tablespoons honey and 2 cups raspberries.*

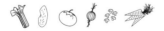

Breakfasts to Relax and Enjoy

Weekends and holidays are the ideal time to try out dishes that take a little more preparation and inspire a little more awe. Believe it or not, you can eat healthily and enjoy egg-based dishes, pancakes (yes, they can be low GI), and hot-from-the oven muffins. Using fine ingredients such as smoked salmon, Greek yoghurt, and fresh fruits and veg, you can cook up low-fat, low-GI breakfast dishes that *anyone* wants to sit around and savour.

Don't forget that the fresher the ingredients, especially fruit and veg, the better the taste is and the more nutrients are present.

Egg dishes

Eggs have had a bad press lately due to both their salmonella carrying risk and the fact that they are high in cholesterol. But eggs are versatile, tasty, and very nutrious while also being fairly low in fat. Eggs with the UK Lion mark are guaranteed to be salmonella free, and even if you suffer from high cholesterol, doctors still say you can have one egg a day.

Baked Eggs and Mushrooms in Ham Crisps

This recipe is a healthy variation on bacon and eggs. This dish is quite filling and works well as a brunch recipe.

Preparation time: *20 minutes*

Cooking time: *10 minutes*

Serves: *4*

1 teaspoon sunflower oil for greasing

4 large mushrooms, very finely sliced

2 tablespoons low-fat Greek yoghurt

Freshly ground black pepper

8 slices very finely sliced Parma ham or pancetta

4 eggs (omega-3 enriched if possible)

Granary/multigrain toast, to serve

1 Preheat the oven to 200°C/400°F/Gas Mark 6. Using the oil, lightly grease four cups of a Yorkshire pudding tin (muffin pan).

2 Place a cast-iron skillet or heavy-based frying pan over medium heat. When the pan is hot, dry fry the mushrooms for about 10 minutes until they darken, release their juices, and then reabsorb them. Allow them to cool slightly, and then mix with the Greek yoghurt.

3 Place two slices of ham in each of the four greased cavities, pressing them to make a well. Allow the ham to come up the sides of the cup.

4 Fill each ham-lined cup with the mushroom mixture.

5 Break one egg on to each of the four mushroom mixtures, taking care not to allow the white of the egg to run over the edges of the tin.

6 Bake in the middle of the oven for 10 minutes until the whites of the eggs are set but the yokes are runny.

7 Remove from oven and carefully ease each Ham Crisp out of the tin. Serve at once with some multigrain toast.

Per serving: *Calories 158 (From Fat 91); Fat 10g (Saturated 3g); Cholesterol 239mg; Sodium 613mg; Carbohydrate 2g (Dietary Fibre 0g); Protein 15g. Approx. Salt (g) 1.5. Toast not included.*

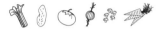

Ham and Eggs on Sourdough Bread

Sourdough bread has a lower GI than ordinary white or brown bread, and so trying to get hold of it, to make this slightly more glamorous version of poached egg on toast, is worthwhile.

Preparation time: *10 minutes*

Serves: *4*

One small loaf of sourdough bread	*A few drops of balsamic vinegar*
Olive oil to drizzle	*4 slices good quality ham*
Ground black pepper	*4 eggs*

1 Drizzle the four slices of bread with some olive oil and grill for a few minutes under a hot grill on both sides.

2 In the meantime poach the eggs (using your own preferred method).

3 Place a slice of ham on each slice of bread and top with the well-drained poached egg.

4 Top with a splash of balsamic vinegar and some ground black pepper.

Vary It! *A slice of lean grilled bacon can be used instead of the ham.*

Per serving: *Calories 341 (From Fat 125); Fat 14g (Saturated 4g); Cholesterol 239mg; Sodium 999mg; Carbohydrate 239g (Dietary Fibre 2g); Protein 20g. Analysed with 1 tablespoon oil. Approx. Salt (g) 2.5.*

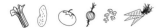

Creamy Scrambled Eggs
with Smoked Salmon

This recipe is a luxury breakfast and can be saved for special occasions. Try to get hold of the omega-3 eggs for their extra nutritional benefit. The salmon also contains omega-3 so you get a good dose of this important essential fatty acid in this recipe, which doesn't have a GI rating because on its own it contains no carbs. Team it up with some granary toast for a low-GI complete breakfast, maybe downed with some orange juice, or bucks fizz if the occasion is very special.

Preparation time: *10 minutes*

Cooking time: *5 minutes*

Serves: *4*

100 grams (4 ounces) smoked salmon

100 grams (4 ounces/½ cup) low-fat cream cheese

8 eggs

½ red onion, finely chopped

½ teaspoon chopped fresh dill, or a pinch of dry dill

1 teaspoon of butter

4 slices granary toast

1 Break up the smoked salmon into small pieces. Cut the cream cheese into small pieces. Break the eggs into a large bowl and whisk until well blended. Stir the salmon, cream cheese, red onion, and dill into the eggs.

2 Melt the butter in a cast-iron skillet or large non-stick frying pan over medium heat until the butter is foaming; don't allow it to brown.

3 Pour in the eggs and turn down the heat to low. Cook, stirring constantly, for 5 minutes until the mixture is lightly scrambled.

4 Remove the pan from the heat and serve at once with granary toast.

Per serving: *Calories 321 (From Fat 159); Fat 18g (Saturated 7g); Cholesterol 447mg; Sodium 849mg; Carbohydrate 18g (Dietary Fibre 2g); Protein 23g. Approx. Salt (g) 2.1.*

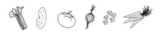

Scrambled Eggs with Spanish-style Hash

This recipe makes a great winter breakfast because the chilli really warms you up from the inside! The sweet potato really works well here and combines well with all the other ingredients, giving the recipe a great taste and a low GI.

Preparation time: *20 minutes*

Cooking time: *15 minutes*

Serves: *4.*

2 tablespoons cold pressed/virgin olive oil

1 large sweet potato, peeled, chopped, and par boiled for 5 to 7 minutes

100 grams (4 ounces) mushrooms, sliced

1 red chilli, seeded and finely sliced

8 large eggs

Fresh chives, finely snipped

Ground black pepper to season

1 Heat oil in a large frying pan. Add potatoes and fry for 5 to 7 minutes, and then add the mushrooms and fry for a further 5 to 7 minutes until tender.

2 Add more oil and toss in the chilli. Cook for a minute or two.

3 Lightly beat the eggs in a bowl and pour into the pan. Stir as the eggs begin to cook. Just before the eggs are completely cooked, remove from the heat and stir in the chives and the ground pepper.

4 Divide between warmed plates and serve.

Per serving: *Calories 363 (From Fat 156); Fat 17g (Saturated 4g); Cholesterol 425mg; Sodium 145mg; Carbohydrate 36g (Dietary Fibre 3g); Protein 16g. Approx. Salt (g) 0.4.*

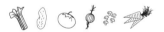

Pancakes!

Pancakes aren't a traditional breakfast dish in the UK, but Brits should take a leaf from the American recipe cookbooks. Pancakes are delicious and can give you all your food groups in one dish – fruit, milk, protein, and carbs. Pancakes are low GI and so keep you going until lunchtime. What better way to set yourself up for the day?

Apple and Raisin Oven Pancakes

This recipe is for an unusual pancake because you bake it rather than fry it, so you don't have to worry about getting the tossing right! An ideal filling start to the colder autumn mornings when cooking apples are in season.

Preparation time: 10 minutes

Cooking time: 15 minutes plus 15 minutes

Serves: 6

1 large baking apple – cored and thinly sliced	2 tablespoons apple juice
⅓ cup golden raisins	4 large eggs
2 tablespoons brown sugar	⅔ cup semi-skimmed milk
½ teaspoon ground cinnamon	⅔ cup plain wholemeal flour
2 teaspoons lemon juice	2 tablespoons low-fat margarine, melted

1 Preheat oven to 180°C/350°F/Gas Mark 4.

2 Grease a 9-inch (25-centimetre) non-stick pie plate.

3 Sprinkle the apple, raisins, brown sugar, lemon and apple juice, and cinnamon on the bottom of the pie plate.

4 Bake uncovered 10 to 15 minutes or until apple begins to soften. Remove from oven and increase temperature to 230°C/450°F/Gas Mark 8.

5 Whisk eggs, milk, flour, and margarine in a medium bowl until blended. Pour batter over apple mixture.

6 Bake for 15 minutes or until golden brown.

Tip: The batter improves if you can leave it to stand for half an hour before using. You can even make up the batter the night before and keep it in the fridge until next morning.

Per serving: *Calories 193 (From Fat 61); Fat 7g (Saturated 2g); Cholesterol 143mg; Sodium 100mg; Carbohydrate 28g (Dietary Fibre 3g); Protein 7g. Approx. Salt (g) 0.3.*

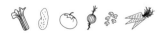

Banana Walnut Pancakes

These pancakes are very filling so worth having if you wake up starving. They are also very nutritious, providing plenty of protein from the eggs and nuts and lots of minerals.

Preparation time: *10 minutes*

Cooking time: *15 minutes*

Serves: *4*

1 medium banana (not too ripe) – mashed	*1 cup semi-skimmed milk*	*2 teaspoons brown sugar*
½ cup plain white flour	*½ cup finely chopped walnuts*	*1 teaspoon baking powder*
½ cup plain wholemeal flour	*1 large egg, beaten*	*½ teaspoon vanilla extract*
	2 tablespoons sunflower oil	*Maple syrup to serve*

1 In a large bowl, sift together both of the flours, sugar, and baking powder.

2 In a separate medium bowl, mix together milk, egg, oil, and vanilla.

3 Add wet ingredients to dry ingredients and mix well.

4 Stir in banana until just mixed. Fold in walnuts.

5 Pour in ¼ cup amounts of the mixture onto a heated (medium-high), greased griddle or large fry pan.

6 Turn the pancake when the visible side starts to show a lot of bubbles. Turn and cook other side until golden brown.

7 Serve with a little maple syrup.

Per serving: Calories 347 (From Fat 172); Fat 19g (Saturated 3g); Cholesterol 56mg; Sodium 144mg; Carbohydrate 37g (Dietary Fibre 4g); Protein 10g. Approx. Salt (g) 0.4.

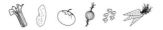

Mmmmmuffins

Home-baked breakfast muffins take a little time to make, but they're worth it to savour over coffee with the Sunday papers, especially when eaten hot straight from the oven! As an added bonus, any extras can be a quick and healthy breakfast the next day or a good snack between meals.

Carrot Breakfast Muffins

These muffins are a good excuse to air your baking skills and the results are not only very tasty and feel indulgent, but are also nutritious to boot! The linseeds and wholemeal flour make these a good source of fibre too.

Preparation time: *15 minutes*

Cooking time: *25 minutes*

Makes: *6 muffins*

125 grams (5 ounces/1 cup) wholemeal self-raising flour

¼ teaspoon bicarbonate of soda (baking soda)

¼ teaspoon baking powder

1½ teaspoons ground cinnamon

1 egg

50 grams (2 ounces/¼ cup) soft light brown or golden granulated sugar

2 tablespoons sunflower oil

3 small carrots, finely grated

1 tablespoon linseeds

Juice and grated zest of 1 orange

100 grams (4 ounces/½ cup) low-fat cream cheese (optional)

4 tablespoons apricot jam (optional)

1 Preheat the oven to 200°C/400°F/Gas Mark 6. Line 6 cups of a deep muffin tin with cupcake paper liners.

2 Mix the flour, bicarbonate of soda, baking powder, and cinnamon together into a large mixing bowl.

3 Break the egg into another mixing bowl and add the sugar and oil; whisk together. Stir the grated carrots and linseeds into this mixture and then fold the dry ingredients into it, a spoonful at a time.

4 Spoon the mixture into the prepared muffin cases and bake in the centre of the oven for 20 to 25 minutes, until golden. Remove from oven and leave the muffins to cool in their cases.

5 Meanwhile, make the optional filling if desired. Mix the cream cheese with the apricot jam and set aside. To serve, break open the muffins while still warm and spread with the cream cheese mixture.

Tip: *Although linseeds add some extra fibre, they also add an extra crunch. If you don't like this texture, just leave them out!*

Per serving: *Calories 177 (From Fat 58); Fat 6g (Saturated 1g); Cholesterol 35mg; Sodium 252mg; Carbohydrate 28g (Dietary Fibre 4g); Protein 4g. Approx. Salt (g) 0.6.*

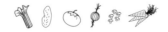

Blueberry Muffins

Blueberry muffins are the classic muffin; I recommend that you eat these melt-in-the-mouth muffins while still warm.

Preparation time: _25 minutes_

Cooking time: _15 minutes_

Makes: _12_

2 cups plain wholemeal (wholewheat) flour	Pinch ground cloves	120 millilitres (4 ounces/½ cup) semi-skimmed milk
¾ cup brown sugar	1½ cups fresh blueberries	2 large eggs
1 tablespoon baking powder	1 tablespoon flour	1 teaspoon vanilla extract
½ teaspoon ground cinnamon	⅓ cup low-fat margarine	A little sunflower oil to grease
Pinch ground nutmeg	200 grams (8 ounces) block low-fat cream cheese	1½ tablespoons sugar

_1_ Preheat oven to 220°C/425°F/Gas Mark 7 and grease 12 cups of a muffin tray.

_2_ Combine the wholemeal flour with the brown sugar, baking powder, cinnamon, nutmeg, and cloves in a large bowl and mix well.

_3_ Make a well in the centre of the mixture.

_4_ Place blueberries in a small bowl. Sprinkle the 1 tablespoon flour over them and toss to coat.

_5_ Place the margarine and cream cheese in a food processor and blend (or mix in a medium bowl).

_6_ Add the milk, eggs, and vanilla to the margarine and cream cheese mixture, mixing (or beating) continuously.

_7_ Add the liquid mixture to the flour mixture; adding a little bit at a time into the well, folding in the dry ingredients.

_8_ Gently fold in the floured blueberries.

_9_ Spoon the final batter mixture into the greased muffin tin.

_10_ Sprinkle 1½ tablespoons sugar evenly over each raw batter mix.

_11_ Bake in the oven for 15 minutes or until muffins spring back when touched lightly in the centre.

_12_ Cool in the tin for 5 minutes then transfer to a wire rack.

Vary It! _Fresh berries are best for these muffins, but you can also use frozen._

Per serving: _Calories 230 (From Fat 74); Fat 8g (Saturated 3g); Cholesterol 46mg; Sodium 232mg; Carbohydrate 35g (Dietary Fibre 3g); Protein 6g. Approx. Salt (g) 0.6._

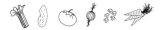

Apple and Prune Muffins

Apples and prunes go well together as the tartness of the apples is offset by the sweetness of the prunes. Prunes are particularly high in fibre and also a good source of several vitamins and minerals.

Preparation time: *20 minutes*

Cooking time: *15 to 20 minutes*

Makes: *12*

100 grams (4 ounces/½ cups) plain wholemeal flour

1 teaspoon baking powder

1 teaspoon bicarbonate of soda

2 tablespoons golden caster sugar

100 grams (4 ounces ¾ cup) ready-to-eat dried prunes, chopped

½ teaspoon ground cinnamon

2 cooking apples, cored, peeled and chopped

1 egg, beaten

50 grams (2 ounces ¼ cup) margarine, melted

200 millilitres (7 ounces/¾ cup) semi-skimmed milk

1 Place 12 large muffin cases in a muffin tin. Preheat oven to 200°C/400°F/Gas Mark 6.

2 Mix flour, baking powder, and bicarbonate of soda together in a large bowl. Stir in sugar, prunes, and apple.

3 In a separate bowl, whisk the remaining ingredients together, and then stir in the flour mixture, making sure you don't beat too much because overbeating spoils the end result.

4 Spoon into muffin cases and bake for 15 to 20 minutes. Cool on a wire rack.

Per serving: *Calories 118 (From Fat 38); Fat 4g (Saturated 1g); Cholesterol 18mg; Sodium 192mg; Carbohydrate 19g (Dietary Fibre 2g); Protein 3g. Approx. Salt (g) 0.5.*

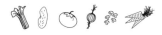

Chapter 7

Let's Do Lunch

In This Chapter

▶ Getting some tips on how to reduce the GI number of your lunch

▶ Being inspired to make your own low-GI lunch

*L*unch needn't just be that slot where you simply grab something to keep you going until your evening meal. Lunch can be an exciting meal in its own right – without having to think too hard about it. You don't have to follow the same formula every day such as having your usual sandwich: break the mould! The right lunch can also help you to avoid, or at least reduce, that afternoon slump (but you can't overcome lack of sleep with food!). And of course a lunch that is nutritious and low GI is going to help put your health back on track.

This chapter gives an overview on how to eat a healthy low-GI lunch. You also find a wide variety of ideas here, from soups to salads and stuffed baked potatoes to pasta dishes. You can be sure that all these recipes are packed full of vitamins and minerals and as low GI as possible!

Note: These recipes are as low GI, and as low in calories, fat, saturated fat, and salt, as possible, and yet retain maximum taste. If you really can't stand wholemeal (wholewheat) flour, use white flour or try half wholemeal and half white instead, so that you don't lose out on the fibre and minerals in wholemeal bread.

Tips for Lunch

It doesn't really matter at what time you have lunch; it depends on what time you got up and had breakfast! Lunch can be as early as midday or else a more relaxed holiday lunch at about 3 p.m. The most important thing is not to skip meals, or leave long gaps between eating. If you do, your body can't perform at its best. You may think that you can save a few calories by skipping a meal, but instead your body tries to make you catch up over the next few meals, and you may actually eat more over time by skipping meals. Skipping meals may also lower your metabolic rate (see Chapter 5 for more about your metabolic rate).

Lunch needs to make up about one third of your total daily calories. If you're on a diet of 1,500 calories, your lunch should provide around 450 calories. Otherwise the average requirement (or Guideline Daily Amount) for calories is 2,000, so your lunch should provide around 600 calories.

Bringing down your lunch's GI

Whatever starchy/carb-containing food you have for lunch, try and make it low GI. If you're having a medium- to high-GI starch food item, try and serve it with another low-GI starchy food, as this helps bring down the overall GI of that meal. The other thing to remember is that having plenty of salad or veggies with your lunch also helps to bring down the GI.

If your favourite lunch turns out to be high GI, don't panic; swapping it for something very similar but lower GI is easy. See Table 7.1 for some 'Swap-it' ideas.

Table 7-1	Swapping High-GI for Lower-GI Lunches
High-GI Lunch	*Lower Alternative*
Baked potato with cheese	Baked potato with beans and some cheese
	Sweet baked potato with a filling of choice
Spaghetti hoops in tomato sauce on toast	Baked beans on toast
White baguette with filling	Granary baguette with filling
Cheese pizza	Thin and crispy pizza with lots of veg topping
White/brown bread sandwich	Granary/multigrain bread sandwich

High-GI Lunch	Lower Alternative
White bread bacon butty	Bacon butty made with white pitta bread
Beefburger in white bun	Beefburger in wholegrain roll/ seeded roll/pitta bread
	Bean/chickpea burger in a white sesame bun
Plain crackers with dip, a little cheese, or pâté	Wholegrain crispbread or oatcakes with dip or little cheese or pâté
Smooth, creamy soup	Chunky vegetable or lentil soup

Out for lunch

Eating out can seem daunting if you don't know some basics:

- ✔ If you're buying a sandwich out, go for a wrap or granary/multigrain bread.

- ✔ Choose chunky vegetable or lentil soups rather than smooth creamy ones.

- ✔ Go for pasta dishes with tomato-based sauce.

- ✔ Any dish with added beans is going to help bring down the GI.

- ✔ Going out for pizza? Then go for a thin and crispy one with lots of veg on top, and don't forget a side salad.

Simple and quick lunch ideas

Lunch is often a meal occasion where you don't have that much time to prepare food but you still want to have something tasty. Here are some ideas for lunches that are a bit different from the usual sandwich or roll, with some tips about how to make them:

- ✔ Pitta bread filled with hummus and salad, fresh fruit, and a small handful of almonds. A recipe for hummus is included in this chapter.

- ✔ Feta cheese (no more than 40 grams or 1½ ounces) and olive salad with two small slices of fruit loaf or tea bread with a thin spreading of low-fat spread. Recipes for tea bread and a fruit loaf are included in Chapter 8.

- ✔ Vegetable soup (if bought check that the fat level isn't too high), two slices of granary bread with low-fat spread, and a piece of fruit. A recipe for a warming curried vegetable soup, which can be made in advance and frozen, is included in this chapter.

✔ A Waldorf salad (you can throw one together with celery, some walnuts, a small piece of Edam cheese chopped up, and a red apple). Bind with some reduced-fat mayonnaise and a skinny muffin. Some muffin recipes are included in Chapter 8.

✔ Pasta with ready-made tomato pasta sauce (low fat of course) and a sprinkle of shaved Parmesan. If time permits, make yourself a side salad too.

✔ Tinned sardines on two pieces of granary toast served with tomato slices and a few black olives dressed with just a little balsamic vinegar and a piece of fruit.

✔ Two-egg omelette served with salad and two slices rye bread, thinly spread with low-fat spread. You can add what you fancy to the omelette such as leftover veg, toms, cooked ham, salmon, or a little grated cheese.

✔ An open sandwich using a low-GI thick slice of bread. Use wafer-thin ham or turkey, salad veg of choice, and top with a little grated cheese and a not-too-ripe banana. The bread can be spread with some mustard first if you like the taste!

✔ For a warming lunch for four, quickly fry an onion in 1 tablespoon of oil and add 4 teaspoons medium curry powder, an apple, some raisins, and a large tin of baked beans. Serve in four baked sweet potatoes. Finish off with yoghurt. An alternative version is to use chilli powder instead of curry powder and to serve in taco shells with a dollop of fromage frais.

Store cupboard essentials for lunch

Below are listed some of the ingredients you need for the recipes in this chapter. You can also keep them as general store cupboard ingredients for making-up your own low-GI lunches. I've included only foods that don't go off very quickly.

✔ Bacon

✔ Variety of canned fish, for example, salmon, sardines, tuna

✔ Cheddar cheese

- ✔ Block Parmesan cheese
- ✔ Walnuts
- ✔ Pine nuts
- ✔ Vegetable and chicken stock cubes
- ✔ Cornflour
- ✔ Tabasco sauce
- ✔ Tomato purée
- ✔ Passata or cans chopped tomatoes
- ✔ Low-fat yoghurt
- ✔ Reduced fat mayonnaise
- ✔ Olive oil
- ✔ Canned chickpeas and mixed beans
- ✔ Dried red lentils
- ✔ Dried split peas
- ✔ Sweet potatoes
- ✔ Onions
- ✔ Garlic
- ✔ Black olives
- ✔ Lemon

Light Lunches: When Just a Bite or Two Will Do

Officially these recipes are starters that work well if you're hosting a dinner party at home. But they also work well as light lunches when you want to stick to something healthy and low GI.

Avocado Dip

Avocados are rich in oil and mono fats (and lots of vitamins and minerals too), so you don't need to add any other oil to this recipe.

Preparation time: *5 minutes*

Serves: *4*

1 large or 2 small very ripe avocados

Juice of ½ lime

1 clove garlic, crushed

Few drops of Tabasco sauce

1 Peel and mash avocado.

2 Add the garlic, lime juice, and Tabasco.

3 Serve with carrot, celery or cucumber sticks, and pitta bread.

Vary It! *Instead of pitta, this recipe makes a great snack with taco chips.*

Tip: *Don't add too much garlic or Tabasco because doing so can kill the taste of the avocado.*

Per serving: *Calories 87 (From Fat 62); Fat 7g (Saturated 1g); Cholesterol 0mg; Sodium 4mg; Carbohydrate 7g (Dietary Fibre 4g); Protein 1g. Salt (g) 0.0*

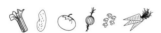

Avocado with Prawns – Slimmer Style

This seafood classic is normally a rich, calorific starter choice. However, this recipe has had the calories trimmed back but still provides the taste. You can get away with using the lowest calorie mayonnaise you can find for this recipe.

Preparation time: *15 minutes*

Serves: *4*

2 medium avocados

100 grams (4 ounces) shelled prawns (medium count shrimp)

4 tablespoons reduced-calorie mayonnaise

1 tablespoon tomato purée

1 to 2 teaspoons lemon juice

Drop or two Tabasco hot pepper sauce

Salt and pepper to taste

1 Mix the mayonnaise with the tomato puree, lemon juice, and Tabasco, and then season with salt and pepper.

2 Mix in the prawns.

3 Shortly before serving, cut the avocados in half lengthwise and remove the stones. Fill with prawn mixture and serve.

Tip: *Serve with some multigrain bread spread with a little reduced-fat spread and cut into quarters.*

Per serving: *Calories 220 (From Fat 162); Fat 18g (Saturated 4g); Cholesterol 48mg; Sodium 323mg; Carbohydrate 9g (Dietary Fibre 8g); Protein 8g. Salt (g) 0.8.*

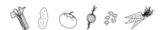

Hummus Dip

This dip is not only a great starter, but also a versatile sandwich filling. Chickpeas are high in fibre and sesame seeds (from which tahina is made) are a good source of calcium.

Preparation time: *20 minutes*

Serves: *8*

1 teaspoon cumin seeds	*2 teaspoons sea salt*
½ teaspoon coriander seeds	*Pinch of cayenne pepper*
1 tablespoon sesame seeds	*125 millilitres (¼ pint/½ cup) water*
2 x 400 grams cans chickpeas drained	*2 teaspoons extra-virgin olive oil*
3 tablespoons tahina	*Chopped coriander leaves and slices of lemon to decorate*
4 tablespoons fresh lemon juice	
4 garlic cloves, minced	

1 Toast the cumin, sesame, and coriander seeds in a small frying-pan until fragrant (about 4 minutes). Crush coarsely in a mortar with a pestle, or use a spice grinder. Set aside.

2 Transfer the chickpeas to a food processor. In a small bowl, whisk together the tahina, garlic, lemon juice, salt, crushed spices, sesame seeds, and the water. Turn the food processor on and add the liquid mixture a tablespoon at the time until a smooth purée is formed.

3 Serve with carrot, cucumber or celery sticks, and pitta bread.

Tip: *If you don't like your hummus too garlicky, reduce the amount of garlic in the recipe*

Per serving: *Calories 118 (From Fat 50); Fat 6g (Saturated 1g); Cholesterol 0mg; Sodium 792mg; Carbohydrate 13g (Dietary Fibre 3g); Protein 5g. Approx. Salt (g) 2.0.*

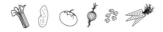

Poached Pears, Cheese, and Walnuts

This recipe is an unusual but impressive starter; the flavours blend very well together. The blue cheese has a strong flavour, so you don't need a lot, which keeps the fat content down.

Preparation time: *15 minutes*

Cooking time: *5 to 10 minutes for the pears and 7 minutes for the bacon*

Serves: *4*

4 pears, peeled, cored, and halved

6 to 8 cubes (3 tablespoons) crystallised ginger

75 grams (3 ounces/¾ cup) blue cheese, crumbled (Danish Blue works well)

75 grams (3 ounces/¾ cup) walnuts

4 slices streaky bacon

Rocket (arugula) salad to serve

1 Poach pears in a little water with ginger for around 5 to 10 minutes or until soft.

2 Drain but reserve 1 tablespoon of the cooking liquor.

3 Mix blue cheese with chopped walnuts.

4 Grill the bacon until crisp but not burnt, chop up and mix with the cheese and walnuts.

5 Serve the pears onto four plates on a bed of rocket, and pour a small amount of the saved liquor on top of each.

Tip: *This recipe can be made in advance and chilled or served with the pears and bacon still warm.*

Vary It! *The pear, cheese, and walnut mixture can be served as a filling for a baked sweet potato.*

Per serving: *Calories 325 (From Fat 178); Fat 20g (Saturated 5g); Cholesterol 19mg; Sodium 377mg; Carbohydrate 29g (Dietary Fibre 4g); Protein 12g. Approx. Salt (g) 0.9.*

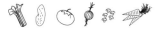

Stuffed Mushrooms

This starter works well as a light lunch or as an accompaniment to grilled meat. This compact dish provides you with something from each of your main food groups – protein, carbs, dairy, and veg.

Preparation time: *20 minutes*

Cooking time: *15 minutes and 5 minutes*

Serves: *4*

8 fairly large mushrooms

4 tablespoons grated cheese, such as a mature cheddar

150 grams (1½ cup) Basmati rice (brown rice is good)

Pinch cumin seeds

Ground black pepper

2 tablespoons toasted pine nuts

1 Clean the mushrooms if necessary and remove and reserve the stalks.

2 Cook the rice according to package instructions, adding the mushroom stalks to the boiling water for the last 5 minutes.

3 Meanwhile, dry bake the mushroom in the oven at 190ºC/375ºF/Gas Mark 5, for 15 minutes.

4 When the rice is cooked, mix the cumin, and pine nuts with the cooked rice and season with black pepper.

5 Put the mushrooms on a large greased oven-proof dish. Top each mushroom with the rice stuffing and cheese.

6 Grill until cheese is browned. Serve hot.

Vary It! *You can substitute peppers for the mushrooms. Serve 1 pepper per person.*

Per serving: *Calories 182 (From Fat 42); Fat 5g (Saturated 2g); Cholesterol 7mg; Sodium 46mg; Carbohydrate 32g (Dietary Fibre 2g); Protein 6g. Salt (g) 0.1*

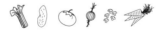

Packed Lunches

Most of the recipes in this chapter can be used as packed lunches, but for ease of eating anywhere, sandwiches, rolls, and wraps are great. Vary the type of bread and filling and always try to include some vegetable sticks or salad.

Even if the weather isn't particularly warm, sandwiches and salads don't stay at their best if kept in a warm room all morning; they may start to grow some unwanted micro-organisms that can lead to food poisoning and really put you off your food for days or even weeks. If you can't refrigerate your lunch as soon as you get to work, you need to use an insulated lunch bag with some ice-packs to help keep everything fresh and prevent nasty bugs from breeding.

Sandwiches

Here are some different types of breads you can use that are low- to medium-GI:

- Coarse barley kernel bread
- Sunflower and barley bread
- Oat bran bread
- Pumpernickel bread
- Wholemeal rye bread
- Cracked wheat kernel bread
- Wholemeal Turkish bread
- Mixed grain/multigrain bread
- Soya and linseed bread
- Oat bran and honey bread with barley
- Pitta bread (wholemeal is lower than white)
- Sourdough wheatbread
- Honey and oat bran bread
- Malted wheat bread
- Tortilla wrap

So what about some suggestions of items to go inside the bread? Here are some fulfilling filling ideas:

- Chicken and avocado
- Lean roast beef and mustard

- ✔ Egg chopped up with reduced-fat mayonnaise and cress
- ✔ Turkey and cranberry jelly/sauce
- ✔ Ham, mustard, and salad
- ✔ Hummus, rocket, and sliced olives
- ✔ Mozzarella cheese and sliced ripe tomatoes with a few sliced olives

You may not always need to use a spread if the filling is moist, for example hummus, peanut butter, or cottage/lower-fat cream cheese. You can try spreading the bread with some mustard or reduced-fat mayonnaise rather than your usual spread. If you are going to use a spread, opt for a reduced-fat spread.

Salad days

For a packed lunch, as a change from sandwiches, you can quickly throw a salad together in a plastic container using whatever you have to hand. Remember to combine lots of green leaves, tomatoes, and other salad items, and add some cheese, hard-boiled egg, meat, tuna, or whatever; but you don't need much of the protein ingredients.

Salad with dressing already added doesn't travel or keep well, and the nuts or seeds added too soon go soggy. So pack some roasted seeds or nuts and some low-fat dressing in separate plastic bags or containers to add to the salad just before you eat it.

Tuna and Mixed Bean Salad

Tuna works very well with cold beans as a salad. This particular salad has a Mediterranean touch and provides all the elements of what makes the Mediterranean diet so healthy – fish, veg, and olive oil. All you need in addition is half a small glass of red wine to drink with it!

Preparation time: *7 to 10 minutes*

Serves: *4*

185 grams (6 ounces) can tuna, drained and flaked

1 small red onion, very finely sliced

2 medium-sized ripe tomatoes or 1 large Spanish tomato, finely sliced

400 grams (16 ounces) can of mixed beans

1 small packet of wild rocket (arugula) leaves

8 black olives cut in half

Dressing

1 crushed clove of garlic

2 tablespoons lemon juice

1 tablespoon extra-virgin olive oil

Freshly ground black pepper

1 Combine the tuna, onion, tomatoes, olives, beans, and rocket in a large bowl.

2 Combine the dressing ingredients together in a screw-top jar. Shake and pour over the salad.

Tip: *Goes well served with some wholemeal pitta bread.*

Per serving: *Calories 209 (From Fat 58); Fat 7g (Saturated 1g); Cholesterol 11mg; Sodium 490mg; Carbohydrate 23g (Dietary Fibre 6g); Protein 15g. Approx. Salt (g) 1.2.*

Sardine and Potato Salad

The sardine is a very neglected fish! Not only is it an oily fish, but also a good source of iron and calcium. Using new potatoes for this tasty recipe keeps the GI value down.

Preparation time: *5 minutes*

Cooking time: *10 to 15 minutes*

Serves: *2*

250 grams (10 ounces) new potatoes in their skin,

125 grams (5 ounces) can sardines, drained

1 tablespoon snipped chives

1 tablespoon chopped coriander or flat leaf parsley

Dressing

1 tablespoon lemon juice

½ tablespoon olive oil

½ teaspoon Dijon mustard

Ground black pepper

1 Boil the potatoes, whole, in their skins until just tender (10 to 15 minutes) and allow to cool a little.

2 Cut each potato in half and, while still warm, combine with the sardines, chives, parsley, or coriander.

3 Combine the dressing ingredients together in a screw-top jar. Shake and pour over the salad.

Vary It! *To allow the flavours to blend more, allow the potatoes to go cold, and combine with the sardines, which you can flake up a little. Add the dressing and allow the mixture to marinade for a couple of hours before eating.*

Per serving: *Calories 294 (From Fat 131); Fat 15g (Saturated 3g); Cholesterol 68mg; Sodium 251mg; Carbohydrate 26g (Dietary Fibre 2g); Protein 15g. Salt (g) 0.6.*

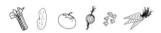

Salmon and Avocado Salad

This salad is a dish rich in healthy mono-unsaturated fats and omega-3s, and so it is great for heart health. Because this recipe makes quite a substantial lunch, it's a good choice if you plan to have a lighter dinner.

Preparation time: *15 minutes*

Cooking time: *10 minutes*

Serves: *4*

440 grams (14 to 15 ounces) can salmon, drained

175 grams (6 ounces/1½ cups) pasta shells, cooked and cooled

1 ripe avocado, peeled, stoned, and diced

125 grams (4 ounces/1 cup) unsalted cashew nuts, toasted

4 tablespoons reduced-fat French dressing

1 tablespoon fresh chopped parsley or basil

Ground black pepper

1 Flake salmon, leave it in fairly large pieces.

2 Mix together the salmon, pasta, avocado, and cashew nuts. Take care not to break up the pieces.

3 Add the dressing, parsley, and seasoning just before serving and mix well.

Tip: *Goes well served with some green young salad leaves.*

Per serving: *Calories 554 (From Fat 262); Fat 29g (Saturated 6g); Cholesterol 37mg; Sodium 592mg; Carbohydrate 47g (Dietary Fibre 6g); Protein 29g. Approx. Salt (g) 1.5.*

New Potato, Watercress, and Bacon Salad

The simple way to make the salad dressing used in this recipe makes a refreshing change to shop-bought versions. Because the dressing is added to the warm potatoes and bacon, it gets absorbed by them and really adds flavour to this salad.

Preparation time: *10 minutes plus 30 minutes standing*

Cooking time: *20 minutes*

Serves: *4*

900 grams (1 pound 13 ounces) baby new potatoes, scrubbed

4 lean back bacon rashers, chopped

1 tablespoon olive oil

1 teaspoon Dijon mustard

Juice of 1 lemon

1 teaspoon clear honey

150 grams (5 ounces/4½ cups) watercress, roughly chopped

Few handfuls rocket (arugula) salad

1 tablespoon pine nuts

Ground pepper

1 Cook potatoes in boiling water for 10 to 15 minutes until tender. Drain and transfer into a serving bowl.

2 Cook the bacon in a dry pan for 3 to 4 minutes, until crisp. Add the oil, mustard, lemon juice, and honey, and stir well.

3 Share the salad leaves between four plates and top with the warm potato and bacon mixture.

4 Sprinkle the pine nuts on top and season well with pepper.

Per serving: *Calories 287 (From Fat 57); Fat 6g (Saturated 1g); Cholesterol 8mg; Sodium 290mg; Carbohydrate 48g (Dietary Fibre 5g); Protein 11g. Approx. Salt (g) 0.7.*

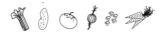

Lunches to Linger Over

Weekends and holidays may give you the time to make a bit more effort over your lunch. These warm, homemade lunches bowl you over with their taste and quality – you can't buy this quality in a can!

The recipes in this section can make quick lunches, too. Just make extra batches for lunches during the week and freeze them for later. If you're freezing soup, freeze it in single serving containers to make lunch preparation that much easier.

Cheddar Onion Soup

This recipe is like French Onion soup. The cheese is the only source of fat in the recipe, but don't be tempted to use too much because it swamps the delicate taste and also bumps up the calories!

Preparation time: *10 minutes*

Cooking time: *35 minutes*

Serves: *4*

1 tablespoon olive oil	*900 millilitres (1½ pints/3¾ cups) chicken stock*	*100 grams (4 ounces/1 cup) strong cheddar cheese, grated*
400 grams (1 pound) peeled onions, cut into rings	*Ground black pepper to taste*	*Chopped parsley for garnish*

1 Cook the onions in the olive oil in a pan slowly for about 20 minutes, until they become caramelised.

2 Add the stock to the pan. Bring to boil, cover, and simmer for 15 minutes.

3 Pour soup into warm dishes and top with cheese. Sprinkle with garnish.

Tip: Serve with some chunky slices of granary French bread.

Per serving: *Calories 207 (From Fat 141); Fat 16g (Saturated 7g); Cholesterol 31mg; Sodium 1108mg; Carbohydrate 9g (Dietary Fibre 2g); Protein 8g. Approx. Salt (g) 2.8.*

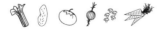

Curried Vegetable Soup

Bursting with oriental spices, this soup is good for a cold winter's day. The vegetables make it a vitamin- and mineral-packed bowlfull.

Preparation time: *10 minutes*

Cooking time: *30 minutes*

Serves: *6*

50 grams (2 ounces/¼ cup) sunflower margarine

1 onion, chopped

2 tablespoons fresh coriander, chopped

1 clove garlic, crushed

1 teaspoon cumin seeds, crushed

¼ teaspoon turmeric powder

¼ teaspoon chilli powder

1 tablespoon plain flour

1¼ litres (2 pints/4 or 5 cups) vegetable stock

800 grams (2 pounds) mixed vegetables such as carrots, parsnips, swede, leeks, broccoli

125 grams (5 ounces/½ cup) low-fat yoghurt

Pepper

1 In a large pan, heat the butter and gently fry the onion and garlic for 2 minutes, until they start to soften. Add the mixed vegetables. Cover and cook for 10 minutes.

2 Stir in the spices and flour and continue cooking for 2 minutes.

3 Stir in the stock and bring to the boil. Cover and simmer until vegetables are tender (15 to 20 minutes).

4 Allow the mixture to cool slightly, and then take half the mixture and purée in a blender. Add the purée back to the unblended mixture.

5 Reheat the soup and stir in fresh coriander. Pour into bowls and add a spoonful of yoghurt.

Per serving: *Calories 141 (From Fat 71); Fat 8g (Saturated 1g); Cholesterol 1mg; Sodium 375mg; Carbohydrate 16g (Dietary Fibre 2g); Protein 3g. Approx. Salt (g) 0.9.*

Lentil Soup

This soup provides you with a good dose of soluble fibre, protein, and about two portions of your fruit and veg for the day: It's both very tasty and filling.

Preparation time: _20 minutes_

Cooking time: _25 minutes_

Serves: _4_

1 tablespoon virgin/cold pressed olive oil

500 grams (1 pound 4 ounces/2½ cups) red lentils

2 medium or one large onion, chopped

1 clove garlic

4 medium carrots, sliced

2 sticks celery, sliced

½ teaspoon ground cumin

½ teaspoon curry powder

1 bay leaf

1½ litres (3 pints/6 cups) of vegetable or chicken stock

1 Rinse the lentils well in cold water.

2 In a large saucepan with the lid on, sweat the onion, garlic, and celery in the oil.

3 Add the stock, carrots, spices, bay leaf, and lentils, and bring to the boil.

4 Simmer gently for about 25 minutes or until the carrot is cooked but still firm.

5 Allow the soup to cool for 10 to 15 minutes, remove the bay leaf, and then liquidise to a smooth consistency.

6 Season with black pepper, and serve with crusty wholegrain bread.

Per serving: _Calories 523 (From Fat 41); Fat 5g (Saturated 1g); Cholesterol 0mg; Sodium 542mg; Carbohydrate 90g (Dietary Fibre 23g); Protein 33g. Salt (g) 1.4_

Minestrone Soup

Although this soup has a lot of ingredients, it's very simple to make and is a very tasty soup packed with antioxidant and vitamin-rich vegetables.

Preparation time: *10 minutes*

Cooking time: *45 minutes*

Serves: *4*

1 onion, roughly chopped

2 cloves garlic

1 tablespoon olive oil

690 grams (1 pound 10 ounces) bottle roughly-chopped passata or two 400 gram (1 pound) cans chopped tomatoes with juice

125 millilitres (5 fluid ounces) water

2 large carrots, peeled and chopped

2 large celery stalks, roughly chopped

Piece (1 cup) of swede (rutabaga), diced

1 courgette (zucchini), chopped

2 tablespoons tomato purée

1½ litre (2½ pints/6 cups) vegetable stock

2 bay leaves

1 teaspoon mixed herbs

Black pepper

50 grams (2 ounces/½ cup) wholemeal small pasta shapes

1 In a large pan, fry the onion and garlic in the olive oil until soft.

2 Add the rest of the ingredients except pasta. Bring to the boil and simmer for 30 minutes, stirring from time to time and adding more water if necessary.

3 Add the pasta and cook until tender (about 15 minutes), again stirring from time to time and adding more liquid if necessary. Serve with warm granary rolls.

Tip: *Sprinkle some Parmesan shavings on top of soup before serving.*

Per serving: *Calories 200 (From Fat 44); Fat 5g (Saturated 1g); Cholesterol 0mg; Sodium 842mg; Carbohydrate 36g (Dietary Fibre 7g); Protein 7g. Approx. Salt (g) 2.1.*

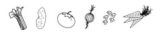

Split Pea and Ham Soup

This recipe is a good way of using up leftover cooked ham from a joint. Don't forget that you need to start this recipe off the night before in order to give the split peas time to soak and soften. Split peas are a good source of soluble fibre.

Preparation time: *20 minutes*

Cooking time: *1 hour 30 minutes*

Serves: *4*

225 grams (9 ounces/1½ cups) cubed cooked ham

450 grams (1 pound/2¼ cups) dried split peas

1½ tablespoons olive oil

1 large onion, chopped

1 clove garlic, crushed

2 carrots, peeled and cubed

2 stalks of celery, thick sliced

2 bay leaves

500 millilitres (1 pint/7 cups) chicken stock

Ground pepper

Some chopped parsley

1 Wash the peas and soak in water over night.

2 Sweat the onion and garlic in the oil in a pan (with the lid on) until they've softened. Add the carrots and celery and continue to sweat in the pan with the lid on until soft.

3 Add the drained peas, bay leaves, and stock. Bring to the boil then leave to simmer for 1 hour.

4 Add the cubes of ham and simmer for a further 10 minutes.

5 Add the ground pepper and garnish with chopped parsley.

Vary It! *You can use leeks instead of celery for a more oniony soup.*

Per serving: *Calories 500 (From Fat 87); Fat 10g (Saturated 2g); Cholesterol 30mg; Sodium 1064mg; Carbohydrate 69g (Dietary Fibre 25g); Protein 37g. Approx. Salt (g) 2.7.*

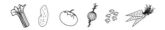

Sweetcorn and Potato Soup

This recipe is a lovely thick and filling soup. The orange colour of the sweet potato and the yellow of the sweetcorn tell you that these ingredients are high in vitamin A and antioxidants.

Preparation time: *5 minutes*

Cooking time: *25 minutes*

Serves: *4*

25 grams (1 ounce/1 tablespoon) sunflower margarine

2 sweet potatoes, diced and par-boiled

1 red pepper, chopped

250 grams (10 ounces/1¾ cups) sweetcorn (can be frozen or canned)

1 onion, chopped

1 tablespoon flour

300 millilitres (½ pint/1¼ cups) vegetable stock

300 millilitres (½ pint/1¼ cups) milk

Ground pepper

Few sprigs of rosemary (optional)

1 Melt sunflower margarine in a large pan. With the lid on, sweat the onion, and pepper for 5 to 10 minutes.

2 Stir in the flour and cook for a further 2 minutes.

3 Gradually blend in the stock and the milk, stirring continuously.

4 Add the par-boiled potato, sweetcorn, and black pepper, cover, and simmer for 15 to 20 minutes.

5 Allow to cool a little. Remove and blend half the mixture. Pour the blended mixture back into the unblended soup and re-heat, adding a few sprigs of rosemary if you like. Serve with crusty granary bread.

Vary It! *You can use ordinary potatoes rather than sweet potatoes for this recipe, but the GI is then medium instead of low.*

Per serving: *Calories 261 (From Fat 78); Fat 9g (Saturated 3g); Cholesterol 11mg; Sodium 197mg; Carbohydrate 42g (Dietary Fibre 4g); Protein 7g. Approx. Salt (g) 0.5.*

Bacon and Walnut Stuffed Sweet Potato

A very simple but tasty baked potato filling, which provides a good source of protein from the bacon and nuts. Sweet potatoes bake very much like ordinary potatoes; just scrub skin and trim off any bruised or woody portions before baking.

Preparation time: 10 minutes

Cooking time: 1 hour for potatoes plus 5 minutes for bacon

Serves: 1

1 large or two small sweet potatoes	25 grams (1 ounce/¼ cup) chopped walnuts
2 slices lean bacon	1 teaspoon walnut oil

1 Bake the potato at 200ºC/400ºF/Gas Mark 6 for 45 minutes to an hour, or until potato skin is crispy and middle is soft (carefully pierce the potato with a knife).

2 Grill bacon until crisp. Chop up, and mix with walnuts and walnut oil.

3 Cut open potatoes, and spoon bacon and walnut mixture inside. Serve with a green salad.

Vary It! The bacon and walnut mixture goes well as a filling for a wrap or sandwich.

Tip: To save time you can microwave the potatoes first for 5 minutes on high or until they start to soften. Remember to score each potato before cooking. However, finishing them off for 20 minutes in the oven is best.

Per serving: *Calories 475(From Fat 225); Fat 25g (Saturated 3g); Cholesterol 27 mg; Sodium 737 mg; Carbohydrate 48g (Dietary Fibre 7g); Protein 18g. Approx. Salt (g) 1.8.*

Creamy Mushrooms

Despite the rich creamy taste, the fat content of this recipe is low if you use low-fat dairy products.

Preparation time: *10 minutes*

Serves: *2*

100 grams (4 ounces) button mushrooms (sliced)

120 millilitres (4 fluid ounces/½ cup) semi-skimmed milk

1 tablespoon low-fat yoghurt

½ teaspoon yeast extract (Marmite)

2 teaspoons cornflour (cornstarch)

Pepper

1 Poach mushrooms in the milk for about 5 minutes until just slightly tender.

2 Blend cornflour with a little water and also blend in the Marmite.

3 Stir the sauce into the mushrooms and heat until the sauce thickens.

4 Add yoghurt and black pepper.

5 Serve on toasted granary or rye bread.

Vary It! *This recipe makes a good breakfast dish too and can be used as a baked potato filling.*

Per serving: *Calories 56 (From Fat 9); Fat 1g (Saturated 1g); Cholesterol 3mg; Sodium 84mg; Carbohydrate 8g (Dietary Fibre 1g); Protein 4g. Approx. Salt (g) 0.2.*

Tomato Tortellini

Having a quick, easy, and tasty pasta dish without resorting to using a jar of sauce makes a change. The fresh ingredients used here work well together and provide a good dose of the antioxidant lycopene.

Preparation time: *5 minutes*

Cooking time: *10 minutes*

Serves: *2*

250 grams (10 ounces) pack fresh spinach and ricotta tortellini

1 tablespoon olive oil

250 grams (10 ounces/2 cups) cherry tomatoes

2 tablespoons parsley leaves, roughly chopped

1 tablespoon finely grated Parmesan

1 Cook pasta for 2 minutes until just cooked.

2 Heat the oil in the frying pan and sizzle the tomatoes until they start to crack and release their juices (this takes about 5 minutes).

3 When pasta is cooked, drain it quickly, reserving some (about ¼ cup) of the cooking water.

4 Put the tomatoes back on a high heat. Add in the pasta, parsley, a splash of cooking water (about 2 tablespoons), and most of the Parmesan into the frying pan. Simmer until it thickens a bit. Add more pasta water, if necessary.

5 Simmer everything together and season with black pepper.

6 Serve with remaining Parmesan.

Tip: *This dish goes well served with rocket salad and some toasted pine nuts.*

Per serving: *Calories 372 (From Fat 142); Fat 16g (Saturated 6g); Cholesterol 31mg; Sodium 372mg; Carbohydrate 45g (Dietary Fibre 4g); Protein 15g. Approx. Salt (g) 0.9.*

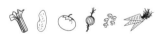

Quick Pizza

This recipe is a quick and simple way to make a healthy version of a family favourite. You can vary the topping, but remember to use only a little of any topping that's fatty or salty.

Preparation time: *5 minutes*

Cooking time: *10 minutes*

Serves: *2*

2 pitta bread

4 teaspoons tomato ketchup

1 small tin (6 ounces) fish in sunflower or olive oil such as salmon or tuna

2 tomatoes, chopped (optional)

1 onion chopped (optional)

About 1 tablespoon of peppers, mushrooms, olives, pineapple, ham (optional)

100 grams (2 ounces/½ cup) grated cheese

Mixed herbs

1 Warm the pittas in an oven for 5 minutes and split in half. Spread tomato ketchup on top.

2 Mash the fish and spread it over the sauce. Cover with tomato and onion and any other ingredients, followed by cheese and mixed herbs.

3 Grill until cheese has turned brown. Serve with a mixed salad.

Per serving: *Calories 647 (From Fat 306); Fat 34g (Saturated 13g); Cholesterol 85mg; Sodium 1752mg; Carbohydrate 38g (Dietary Fibre 2g); Protein 46g. Approx. Salt (g) 4.4.*

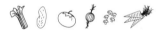

Chapter 8

Snacks: Time for a Little Something

In This Chapter

▶ Understanding why snacking can be good for you

▶ Finding out which snacks are suitable

▶ Tempting you with some delicious, nutritious snack ideas

*1*f you think you're being good by not giving in to those snack attacks, think again! When you get the munchies between meals, you need to allow yourself a wee snack. If you allow yourself to go hungry for too long, or ignore your body telling you that it needs a little something, your resolve weakens, and eventually your body has its way with a vengeance, and you find yourself munching on something unsuitable. Better you control it than allow it to control you!

This chapter helps you out when a snack attack threatens!

To Snack or Not to Snack

In PCOS, you need to avoid feeling extremely hungry because that can drive binge eating, or the eating of the wrong type of snack – both of which can lead to rapid weight gain, which worsens PCOS symptoms. But eating a nutritious, not too calorific, low-GI snack makes good dietary sense.

Being hungry is usually a sign that your blood sugar is falling. Having a low-GI snack gradually raises your blood sugar levels and keeps it on an even keel. Snacks can keep your blood sugars from swinging from high to low, smoothing out the swings. Hunger can also increase during your pre-menstrual period (if you are still having periods) because your metabolic rate actually speeds up at this time.

How much to nibble

If you find yourself in need of a snack between meals (or at bedtime to stop yourself feeling hungry in the middle of the night and raiding the fridge), you don't need a lot to snack on. Don't feel guilty about that bedtime snack: You may feel less groggy in the morning if you have a small snack at bedtime, particularly if you had an early dinner.

The total number of calories you eat over the course of a day matter, not *when* you eat them. So if you feel a little peckish at bedtime, have a snack and don't think it's more fattening than one eaten mid-morning!

Store cupboard essentials for snacks

The list below includes some ingredients that you may find useful to have in store for making some of the recipes in this chapter, or just for putting together your own snack ideas:

- ✔ Dried fruit (raisins, apricots, sultanas, prunes)
- ✔ Mixed nuts (almonds, walnuts)
- ✔ Rolled jumbo oats
- ✔ Wholemeal (wholewheat) flour (plain and self-raising)
- ✔ Apples
- ✔ Nutmeg
- ✔ Cinnamon

Suitable Snacks and a Few Yummy Recipes

A suitable snack for people with PCOS needs to be:

- ✔ Nutritious
- ✔ Low GI
- ✔ Not too high in calories (100–200 calories, depending on how hungry you are and if you're trying to lose weight)
- ✔ Low in fat, particularly saturated fat

The section below has some everyday examples of suitable low-GI snacks and their GI value, where known (remembering that the GI of every food hasn't been measured yet), which are also not too high in fat or calories.

Easy-as-pie snacks that are better for you than, well, pie

This section gives you a feel for suitable snacks. As a general rule, try not to have more than two snacks a day. Save them for the times when you know you get hungry. However, you can squeeze in an extra snack if you're having a particularly ravenous day, or you've been exercising quite hard.

Crispbreads, rich tea biscuits, and crackers

Crispbreads, rich tea biscuits, and crackers make good snacks because they tend to be high in fibre, and they're rich in low-GI carbs that help keep your blood sugars on an even keel:

- Oatcakes (GI: 55)
- Crispbread with mixed grains/seeds
- Rich tea (semi-sweet biscuits) (GI: 55)

Bread/toast

You can serve these with a little low-fat margarine and some jam, or a thin spread of peanut butter or hummus:

- Mixed grain type bread, including barley kernel, pumpernickel, kibbled wheat, oatbran (GI: 34–47)
- Pitta bread (white) (GI: 57)
- Fruit bread (GI: 45)
- Mexican corn tortillas (GI: 52)

Breakfast cereal

You probably only need half your normal breakfast portion of these if you're eating them as a snack:

- Bran type (GI: 42)
- Porridge, jumbo oats (GI: 42)
- Toasted muesli (GI: 43)

Dairy foods

The dairy group of foods helps to keep your calcium reserves topped up, which prevents brittle bones. Low-fat dairy products are associated with lower blood pressure. The GI values are:

- Low-fat custard (GI: 45)
- Yoghurts, low-fat and sugar-free (GI: 25)
- Reduced fat dairy ice-cream (GI: 50)
- Milk, semi-skimmed (GI: 30)
- Low-fat milk shakes/smoothies (GI: 30)
- Probiotic milk-based yoghurt shot (GI: 45)

Fruit and fruit juice

Aim to eat at least five helpings of fruit and veg every day. Eating fruit as a snack helps you to achieve this amount.

- All fruit except pineapple, over-ripe bananas, and watermelon are medium to low GI
- Dried fruit
- For juices, apple (GI: 40), orange (GI: 50), and pineapple (GI: 46) are low, while tomato juice is exceptionally low (GI: 38)

Other snacks

- Plain popcorn (GI: 55)
- Reduced fat mousse (GI: 34)
- Soup, low-fat (varies but around GI: 50). Home-made can be lower because it is typically less processed
- Instant noodles (GI: 47)
- Low-fat dips served with crudités/oat-cakes
- Small handful mixed nuts and seeds
- Small handful nuts and dried fruit mix

Recipes

The snack recipes in this section have been developed to be low to medium GI. To make them as healthy as possible they have been kept as low in fat, sugar, and salt and as high in fibre as possible, while still retaining full flavour (otherwise you wouldn't eat them, would you?). The recipes use wholemeal/wholewheat flour because this provides more fibre and minerals.

However, you can use white flour if you must, or why not try half and half? If you need to lose weight, don't have more than one helping of these baked goodies each day.

These snacks all freeze well, so you can bake ahead for the week. You can take a nutritious treat with you to work and save yourself from grabbing a sweet pastry or a chocolate bar in the middle of the morning or afternoon.

Chocolate and Cherry Muffins

Chocolate isn't banned if you're on a healthy diet, depending on the amount and frequency! Try this low-fat but still decadent chocolaty muffin – but not too many and not too often!

Preparation time: *20 minutes*

Cooking time: *20 minutes*

Makes: *12 muffins*

210 grams (8 ounces/1 cup) self-raising flour (wholemeal (wholewheat) if possible)

40 grams (2 ounces/¼ cup) cocoa powder

150 grams (5 ounces/¾ cup) sugar

250 millilitres (8 fluid ounces/1 cup) semi-skimmed milk

60 grams (2 ounces) low-fat margarine

1 teaspoon vanilla essence

100 grams (4 ounces/½ cup) chocolate chips

100 grams (4 ounces/½ cup) glace cherries, chopped

1 Preheat the oven to 180°C/350°F/Gas Mark 4. Grease a 12-cup cake tin and set out cake cases (baking cups) or greaseproof paper.

2 Mix the flour, cocoa, and sugar together in a bowl.

3 In a separate small bowl, mix the milk, melted margarine, and vanilla together.

4 Make a well in the dry mixture and pour in the milk mixture. Mix well.

5 Add chocolate chips and cherries and fill each muffin tin or cake case three-quarters full.

6 Cook for 20 minutes in the oven.

7 Eat straight from the tin while warm (allow to cool a little first!), or remove from tin and allow to cool completely. You can also freeze the muffins and heat up in the microwave for about 20 seconds on high when you're ready to eat them.

Vary It! *You can use sultanas and a few chopped hazelnuts instead of the glace cherries.*

Per serving: *Calories 185 (From Fat 57); Fat 6g (Saturated 2g); Cholesterol 1mg; Sodium 303mg; Carbohydrate 34g (Dietary Fibre 2g); Protein 3g. Approx. Salt (g) 0.8.*

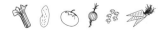

Tea Bread

In Wales, this dish is known as *Bara Brith* and is still served up at tea-time on the farms to sustain the farm folk during milking, because supper can't be had until the evening when all the milking is done. Traditionally it was served sliced and buttered but you may find it so moist that you can get away with eating it plain – or maybe just a thin spread of reduced fat margarine.

Preparation time: *15 minutes*

Cooking time: *1 hour*

Makes: *1 loaf*

300 millilitres (½ pint/1¼ cups) cooled tea

100 grams (4 ounces/½ cup) sunflower margarine

125 grams (5 ounces/1 cup) brown sugar

175 grams (7 ounces/1¼ cups) self-raising wholemeal (wholewheat) flour

75 grams (3 ounces/½ cup) rolled oats

½ teaspoon baking powder

Pinch nutmeg

125 grams (5 ounces/1 cup) mixed dried fruit

½ teaspoon ground cinnamon

½ teaspoon bicarbonate of soda (baking soda)

1 Preheat the oven to 190°C/375°F/Gas Mark 5. Grease a 20-centimetre (8-inch) cake tin.

2 Place tea in a large saucepan and add sugar, margarine, and fruit. Heat gently until margarine has melted.

3 Cool, and then add other ingredients. Stir until well mixed and pour into the cake tin.

4 Cook for 60 minutes, or until firm.

5 Turn out and cool on a wire rack. Store in an airtight container.

Per serving: Calories 198 (From Fat 67); Fat 7g (Saturated 1g); Cholesterol 0mg; Sodium 315mg; Carbohydrate 32g (Dietary Fibre 3g); Protein 3g. Based on 12 servings. Approx. Salt (g) 0.8.

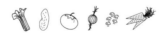

Low-Fat Fruit Cake

This cake can substitute for a Christmas cake, because the mincemeat and condensed milk make it rich and it's spicy. This cake is also gluten and wheat free! Because of the richness you only need a thin slice of this at a time. It also keeps for a month.

Preparation time: *20 minutes*

Cooking time: *2 to 2½ hours*

400 grams (1 pound/1¾ cups) fruit mincemeat

350 grams (12 ounces/2¼ cups) mixed dried fruit

50 grams (2 ounces/½ cup) mixed chopped peel

100 grams (4 ounces/1 cup) halved glace cherries, washed and dried

100 grams (4 ounces/1 cup) walnut halves, chopped

200 grams (8 ounces/5¾ cups) corn-flakes, crushed into fine crumbs

3 standard eggs, beaten

1 large can sweetened skimmed condensed milk

1 level teaspoon each mixed spice and baking powder

1 Grease a 20-centimetre (8-inch) round cake tin and line with greaseproof paper. Pre-heat the oven to 150°C/300°F/Gas Mark 2.

2 Place all the ingredients into a large bowl. Mix slowly but thoroughly. Transfer to the prepared tin and flatten the top evenly with a knife.

3 Bake in oven for 2 to 2½ hours.

4 Leave in the tin 10 minutes. Turn out and cool on a wire rack. Wrap and store in an air-tight tin.

Tip: *This cake keeps fresh and moist for several weeks.*

Per serving: Calories 283 (From Fat 47); Fat 5g (Saturated 1g); Cholesterol 42mg; Sodium 169mg; Carbohydrate 55g (Dietary Fibre 3g); Protein 6g. Based on 16 servings. Approx. Salt (g) 0.4.

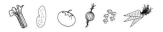

Fruit and Seed Loaf

This loaf is packed with nuts, seeds, and dried fruits, and so a little goes a long way. Each mouthful provides loads of vitamins, minerals, antioxidants, and fibre.

Preparation time: *15 minutes, plus 50 minutes standing time*

Cooking time: *50 minutes*

25 grams (1 ounce) dark chocolate, grated

200 grams (8 ounces/2 cups) wholewheat/wholemeal flour

100 grams (4 ounces/¾ cup) jumbo oats

100 grams (4 ounces/¾ cup) linseeds

50 grams (2 ounces/½ cup) sunflower seeds

50 grams (2 ounces/½ cup) pumpkin seeds

50 grams (2 ounces/½ cup) sesame seeds

50 grams (2 ounces/½ cup) walnuts, chopped

2 pieces stem ginger, finely chopped

75 grams (3 ounces/½ cup) dried cranberries

100 grams (4 ounces/¾ cup) dried fruit such as raisins, finely chopped apricots or chopped figs

½ teaspoon nutmeg

½ teaspoon cinnamon

½ teaspoon ground ginger

2 eggs

250 millilitres (8 fluid ounces/1 cup) semi-skimmed milk

2 tablespoons cranberry, grape, or apple juice

2 tablespoons walnut oil

1 tablespoon black treacle

1 Heat oven to 190°C/375°F/Gas Mark 5.

2 Line an 18-centimetre (7½-inch) round cake tin.

3 Put all dry ingredients in a mixing bowl.

4 Beat together the egg and oil, and then add the fruit juice, treacle, and milk.

5 Beat in the liquid ingredients to the dry mixture.

6 Leave to stand for 50 minutes.

7 If mixture is stiff, add more milk.

8 Spoon the mixture into the tin. Bake for 50 minutes or until a skewer comes out dry.

9 Allow to cool for 30 minutes in the tin, and then turn out.

Tip: *You can eat a slice of this for a quick but filling breakfast.*

Per serving: *Calories 252 (From Fat 113); Fat 13g (Saturated 2g); Cholesterol 27mg; Sodium 23mg; Carbohydrate 30g (Dietary Fibre 5g); Protein 8g. Based on 16 servings. Approx. Salt (g) 0.1.*

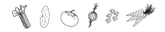

Fruit Bars

Although containing some butter (to make the bars set), this recipe is still healthy and low GI with a lovely orangey tang.

Preparation time: *15 minutes, plus 15 minutes standing time*

Cooking time: *40 minutes*

Serves: *8*

150 millilitres (¼ pint/¾ cup) semi-skimmed milk

1 orange, zested, peeled, segmented, and chopped

150 grams (6 ounces/1½ cups) wholemeal/wholewheat self-raising flour

100 grams (4 ounces/1 cup) dried dates or dried apricots (stoned and chopped)

½ teaspoon ground cinnamon

1 egg

50 grams (2 ounces/¼ cup) butter, melted

½ teaspoon baking powder

1 Preheat oven to 180°C/350°F/Gas Mark 4. Mix together the flour, baking powder, and cinnamon in a bowl. Put to one side.

2 Warm milk, add dates or apricots, and leave to stand for 15 minutes.

3 Add egg, melted butter, and 1 teaspoon of the grated orange rind to milk and beat. Stir into the dry ingredients with chopped orange flesh and mix well.

4 Spoon into a greased, lined 18-centimetre (7½ inch) square tin. Bake for 40 minutes (test at 30 minutes) until risen and golden brown.

5 Cool on a wire rack and cut into bars.

Per serving: Calories 207 (From Fat 59); Fat 7g (Saturated 4g); Cholesterol 41mg; Sodium 380mg; Carbohydrate 34g (Dietary Fibre 5g); Protein 6g. Approx. Salt (g) 1.0

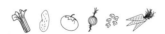

Fruit Scones

Adding fruit to any recipe reduces the GI. These scones make a lovely tea-time treat, but don't add the clotted cream!

Preparation time: *15 minutes*

Cooking time: *15 minutes*

Makes: *10 to 12 scones*

450 grams (1 pound) wholemeal (wholewheat) self-raising flour

100 grams (4 ounces/½ cup) fat-reduced sunflower margarine

Dash of semi-skimmed milk

100 grams (4 ounces/¾ cup) sultanas

50 grams (2 ounces/½ cup) brown sugar

½ teaspoon bicarbonate of soda

1 Preheat oven to 190°C/375°F/Gas Mark 5.

2 Rub the butter lightly into flour, lifting the mixture to add air, until the mixture resembles breadcrumbs.

3 Add the sugar and sultanas, and then add the bicarbonate of soda, mixing in enough milk to make a soft dough.

4 Pat or roll out the dough on a lightly floured surface until about 1.5 centimetres (½ inch) thick. Cut into 4-centimetre (1½ inch) rounds.

5 Bake for 12 to 15 minutes.

Vary It! *You can use cherries or walnuts instead of sultanas.*

Per serving: Calories 246 (From Fat 63); Fat 7g (Saturated 1g); Cholesterol 0mg; Sodium 296mg; Carbohydrate 45g (Dietary Fibre 6g); Protein 7g. Based on 10 servings. Approx. Salt (g) 0.7.

Chapter 9

Dining In and Eating Out: Main Meals and a Few Yummy Desserts

. . . .

In This Chapter

▶ Discovering lots and lots of lovely low-GI recipes

▶ Avoiding falling into diet traps when eating out

. . . .

Dinner is a social meal you can relax over, so you can spend a bit of time preparing for it. The recipes in this chapter aren't hard, and don't take hours of fiddling around. So spend the little effort it takes to make these recipes, and then reap the rewards in the pleasure of the meal and the difference it makes to your health.

This chapter also includes a few low-GI and lower-calorie versions of some of your favourite desserts such as cheesecake, trifle, and even Christmas pudding.

Sorting Out Your Main Meal of the Day

When you eat your evening meal doesn't matter too much, but try to leave a couple of hours after eating before going to bed so that you don't get indigestion. This section gives you a wide variety of ideas for your main meal of the day; some are based on veggie ingredients such as beans and pulses whereas others contain a little meat or fish. Some use meat or fish as the main ingredient. The recipes also indicate where you can substitute the meat for a veggie equivalent. And, as always, all these recipes are packed full of vitamins and minerals and are as low GI as possible!

Vegetarian main dishes

A vegetarian diet is usually a healthy diet, provided that you take a little bit more care ensuring that you eat a variety of foods from all the main food groups (see Chapter 3). A vegetarian diet tends to be higher in fibre and lower in fat than a carnivorous diet. So even if you're not veggie, trying some of these yummy veggie dishes isn't going to hurt you!

Bean and Vegetable Bake

The different colour vegetables in this dish make it an excellent source of several antioxidants. (Highly coloured vegetables contain antioxidants, and each different colour veg provides a different type of antioxidant.) The cheese, sesame seeds, and beans ensure that the bake is also a good source of calcium.

Preparation time: *20 minutes*

Cooking time: *40 minutes*

Serves: *6*

1 onion, chopped

1 carrot, grated

1 tablespoon olive oil

400 grams (14 ounces/2¼ cups) can diced tomatoes

Ground black pepper

2 teaspoons cornflour (masa harina), blended with a little cold water

400 grams (14 ounces/2¼ cups) can red kidney beans, drained

150 grams (6 ounces/1½ cups) granary breadcrumbs

100 grams (4 ounces/1 cup) cheddar cheese, grated

2 tablespoons sesame seeds

2 tablespoons freshly chopped parsley

200 grams (8 ounces) aubergines (eggplant), sliced and blanched

200 grams (8 ounces) courgettes (zucchini), sliced and blanched

1 Preheat oven to 200ºC/400ºF/Gas Mark 6. Fry the onion and carrot in a little oil for 2 to 3 minutes. Stir in canned tomatoes and season well with black pepper. Simmer, uncovered for 10 minutes. Add cornflour and bring to the boil to thicken.

2 Add the kidney beans to the vegetable mixture.

3 In a small bowl, mix together the breadcrumbs, cheese, sesame seeds, and parsley.

4 Place half the aubergines and courgettes in the base of a greased 1½ litre (3 pint) oven-proof dish. Cover with a layer of tomato sauce and then a layer of breadcrumb mixture. Repeat with remaining ingredients.

5 Cover and cook for 40 minutes, removing cover for final 10 minutes.

Per serving: Calories 258 (From Fat 95); Fat 11g (Saturated 4g); Cholesterol 18mg; Sodium 412mg; Carbohydrate 32g (Dietary Fibre 7g); Protein 12g. Approx. Salt (g) 1.0.

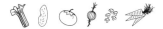

Baked Bean Lasagne

A quick variation on the traditional lasagne, which is a good source of fibre but still packed with flavour.

Preparation time: *15 minutes*

Cooking time: *30 minutes*

Serves: *4*

1 onion	*100 grams (4 ounces) mushrooms, sliced*
1 tablespoon olive oil	*100 grams (4 ounces) lasagne (wholewheat if possible)*
400 grams (14 ounces) can baked beans (buy the reduced salt version if available)	*150 grams (6 ounces/1½ cups) cottage cheese*
400 grams (1 pound) can chopped tomatoes	*2 tablespoons natural yoghurt*
2 teaspoons dried mixed herbs	*100 grams (4 ounces/1 cup) grated cheese*

1 Preheat oven to 200ºC/400ºF/Gas Mark 6. Fry onion in oil until tender. Add baked beans, tomatoes, herbs, and mushrooms.

2 Cover bottom of an ovenproof dish with this mixture. Layer on lasagne, another layer of the baked bean mixture, another layer of lasagne, and so on until everything is used up, ensuring that the top layer is lasagne.

3 Mix cottage cheese and yoghurt in a separate bowl, and smooth over the top of the lasagne. Sprinkle grated cheese over the top. Cook for 20 to 30 minutes or until pasta is soft.

Per serving: Calories 410 (From Fat 119); Fat 13g (Saturated 6g); Cholesterol 24mg; Sodium 754mg; Carbohydrate 50g (Dietary Fibre 12g); Protein 27g. Approx Salt (g) 1.9.

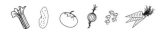

Chunky Vegetable Cassoulet

This recipe is a one pot, all-in-one meal – and so saves on washing up lots of pots and pans – and it's also jam-packed with an assortment of different antioxidant rich veggies.

Preparation time: *15 minutes*

Cooking time: *50 minutes plus 10 minutes*

Serves: *4*

1 onion, chopped

1 clove garlic

1 tablespoon cold pressed/virgin olive oil

200 grams (8 ounces) sweet potatoes, diced

200 grams (8 ounces) swede (rutabega), diced

1 leek, chopped into rounds

200 grams (8 ounces) carrots diced

2 tablespoons chopped coriander (cilantro)

2 tablespoons tomato purée

425 millilitres (¾ pint/1¾ cups) hot vegetable stock

2 medium ripe tomatoes, chopped

400 grams (14 ounces) can borlotti beans (cranberry or pinto beans), drained

100 grams (4 ounces/1 cup) granary breadcrumbs

75 grams (3 ounces/¾ cup) strong cheddar cheese, grated

1 Cook the onions and garlic in oil until just softened in a large ovenproof casserole dish.

2 Throw in the potatoes, onions, swede, leek, carrots, and coriander, and toss well with the onions.

3 Stir in the purée and stock, cover with a lid, and cook over a low heat for 45 minutes.

4 Turn off the heat and turn on oven to 220ºC/425ºF/Gas Mark 7.

5 Stir in the tomatoes and borlotti beans.

6 Mix the breadcrumbs with the cheese and scatter over the top of the vegetables. Bake in the hot oven for 15 minutes so that the topping is browned.

Per serving: *Calories 372 (From Fat 107); Fat 12g (Saturated 5g); Cholesterol 20mg; Sodium 653mg; Carbohydrate 55g (Dietary Fibre 11g); Protein 14g. Approx Salt (g) 1.6.*

Mixed Bean Hotpot

This recipe is quick to make but you do need to allow an hour to cook. The cooking time allows the flavours to blend well together to make a lovely warming and filling autumn or winter dish.

Preparation time: *10 minutes*

Cooking time: *1 hour*

Serves: *4*

400 grams (14 ounces/2 cups) can mixed beans, drained and rinsed

100 grams (4 ounces/1 cup) green beans, sliced

400 grams (14 ounces) can diced tomatoes

1 tablespoon tomato purée

1 garlic clove, crushed

1 teaspoon mixed herbs

Ground black pepper

450 grams (1 pound) sweet potatoes, peeled, parboiled, and cooled

100 grams (4 ounces/1 cup) cheddar cheese, grated

1 Preheat oven to 170ºC/325ºF/Gas Mark 3. Put the beans in an ovenproof casserole dish.

2 Mix together remaining ingredients except potatoes and cheese.

3 Pour over beans, mix well.

4 Thinly slice the potatoes, and lay the sliced potatoes on top of the bean mixture.

5 Sprinkle with the cheese.

6 Cook for 1 hour, with no lid, until the potatoes are cooked

Per serving: *Calories 264 (From Fat 76); Fat 8g (Saturated 5g); Cholesterol 26mg; Sodium 414mg; Carbohydrate 36g (Dietary Fibre 8g); Protein 13g. Approx Salt (g) 1.0.*

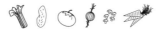

Vegetable Crumble

This recipe can be a meat-free or a bacon-containing dish; either way the bread and beans make it rich in fibre and the peppers and tomatoes make it rich in vitamin C and antioxidants.

Preparation time: *15 minutes*

Cooking time: *30 minutes*

Serves: *4*

1 tablespoon cold pressed/virgin olive oil

1 large onion, chopped

2 peppers (any colours)

150 grams (5 ounces) mushrooms, sliced (or if you eat meat, 4 rashers (slices) back bacon)

400 grams (16 ounces) can tomatoes

400 grams (16 ounces) can baked beans

8 slices granary (or low-carb) bread

100 grams (4 ounces) strong cheddar cheese

1 Preheat oven to 200ºC/400ºF/Gas Mark 6.

2 Fry onions in oil for 3 to 4 minutes, until soft.

3 Add peppers and bacon (or mushrooms if using). After pepper is tender (around 5 minutes) mix in tomatoes and beans. Spoon into an ovenproof dish.

4 In a food processor, combine the bread and the cheese to make a cheesy breadcrumb crumble topping and spread over the top of the tomato mixture.

5 Cover, and place in the oven for 30 minutes, removing the lid for the last 10 minutes so that the breadcrumbs go golden brown.

Per serving: *Calories 478 (From Fat 140); Fat 16g (Saturated 7g); Cholesterol 30mg; Sodium 957mg; Carbohydrate 59g (Dietary Fibre 12g); Protein 20g. Approx Salt (g) 2.4.*

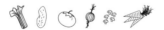

Mushroom Risotto

This dish is a traditional Italian recipe that has been adapted to be lower in fat. Try to get the dried porcini mushrooms if you can, because they impart the lovely and distinctive flavour.

Preparation time: *10 minutes*

Cooking time: *15 minutes*

Serves: *4*

1 tablespoon dried porcini mushrooms (if not available, add an extra 50 grams/2 ounces fresh mushrooms)

2 tablespoons cold pressed/virgin olive oil

1 onion, chopped

2 garlic cloves, finely chopped

225 grams (8 ounces) mushrooms (chestnut are good here), sliced

350 grams (12 ounces/1¾ cups) risotto rice

150 millilitres (¼ pint/½ cup) dry white wine

1.2 litres (2 pints/4 cups) hot vegetable stock

2 tablespoons chopped fresh parsley

Freshly ground black pepper

Freshly grated Parmesan cheese to serve

1 If using dried mushrooms, soak the mushrooms in hot water for 10 minutes, and then drain well.

2 Heat the oil in a large saucepan and add the onion and garlic. Fry over a gentle heat for 2 to 3 minutes, until softened. Add the mushrooms and fry for a further 2 to 3 minutes, until browned.

3 Stir in the rice and coat in the oil. Pour in the wine and simmer, stirring, until the liquid has been absorbed. Add some of the stock and simmer, stirring again, until the liquid has been absorbed. Continue adding the stock in this way, until all the liquid has been absorbed and the rice is plump and tender.

4 If used, roughly chop the soaked mushrooms and stir into the risotto, along with the parsley, and ground black pepper. Serve with freshly grated Parmesan cheese.

Per serving: *Calories 434 (From Fat 87); Fat 10g (Saturated 2g); Cholesterol 0mg; Sodium 357mg; Carbohydrate 77g (Dietary Fibre 3g); Protein 12g. Parmesan not included in analysis. Approx Salt (g) 0.9.*

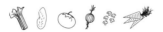

Brazil Nut Burgers

Brazil nuts are an excellent source of the antioxidant mineral, selenium, which is sometimes in short supply in the diet. These burgers make a tasty alternative to the ground beef version and are lower in saturated fat.

Preparation time: *15 minutes, chill for 20 minutes*

Cooking time: *7 minutes each side*

Serves: *4*

75 grams (3 ounces/½ cup) shelled Brazil nuts

100 grams (4 ounces/1 cup) granary bread crumbs

1 tablespoon cold pressed/virgin olive oil

1 small onion, peeled and chopped

½ stick of celery, finely chopped

75 grams (3 ounces/¾ cup) carrots, grated

2 tablespoons tomato purée

Pinch dried thyme

1 egg, beaten

Black pepper

To serve:

Granary baps (low-carb buns)

Thinly sliced Emmental cheese

Tomato and cucumber, sliced

Rocket (arugula) salad

1 Grind the nuts in a food processor (or, if you don't have a food processor, place in a strong plastic bag and crush with a rolling pin). Mix nuts with the breadcrumbs.

2 Heat the oil, fry the onion and celery, and cook gently until onion is soft. Add the nut mixture with the carrots, tomato purée, and thyme.

3 Add the beaten egg, and season with pepper and mix.

4 Divide the mixture into four portions (not too thick), shape into rounds, and chill for 20 minutes.

5 Lay some greased aluminium foil on the bottom of a grill pan and grill or barbecue the burgers on a medium heat for 7 minutes on each side.

6 Serve in a granary bap with salad and cheese.

Per serving: *Calories 433 (From Fat 220); Fat 24g (Saturated 9g); Cholesterol 66mg; Sodium 432mg; Carbohydrate 42g (Dietary Fibre 8g); Protein 16g. Approx Salt (g) 1.1.*

Curried Chickpeas

This recipe is a mild and creamy curry with a taste that's quite delicate and not overly spicy. Chickpeas are a good source of fibre and calcium.

Preparation time: *15 minutes*

Cooking time: *25 minutes*

Serves: *4*

1 tablespoon cold pressed/virgin olive oil

1 onion, sliced

2 cloves of garlic, crushed

1 tablespoon mild curry powder

1 tablespoon wholemeal (wholewheat) flour

400 grams (15 ounces/2 cups) can chickpeas, drained

200 grams (10 ounces/1¼ cups) can pineapple pieces in natural juice (keep juice)

75 grams (3 ounces/½ cup) raisins

50 grams (2 ounces/½ cup) ground almonds (optional)

300 millilitres (½ pint/1¼ cups) semi-skimmed (2 per cent) milk

1 eating apple, peeled, cored, and cut into small pieces

1 tablespoon lemon juice

300 grams (12 ounces/1¾ cups) basmati rice

1 Heat the oil in a saucepan, and fry the onion and garlic until softened. Stir in the curry powder and flour, and cook on a gentle heat for 2 minutes.

2 Add the chickpeas and mix in with the curry mixture. Stir in the pineapple with its juice, raisins, ground almonds (if using), and milk. Season, and bring to the boil. Cover and simmer for 20 minutes, stirring occasionally to prevent sticking. If the mixture gets too thick, add more milk. Add the apple to the curry with the lemon juice and cook for 5 minutes.

3 Cook rice according to packet instructions and serve with the curry.

Per serving: Calories 512 (From Fat 63); Fat 7g (Saturated 2g); Cholesterol 6mg; Sodium 266mg; Carbohydrate 104g (Dietary Fibre 8g); Protein 12g. Approx Salt (g) 0.7.

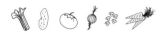

Homemade Pizza

Making your own dough for this pizza is really worth the effort. The resultant base really does melt in the mouth and is much nicer than the often hard dough base you get with bought pizzas. You can vary your topping to suit your taste.

Preparation time: *20 minutes plus 1 hour 10 minutes rising time*

Cooking time: *30 minutes*

Serves: *4*

Base:

1 heaped teaspoon (7 grams) dried yeast or 1 sachet dried yeast for breadmaking	250 millilitres (½ pint/1 cup) lukewarm water	75 grams (3 ounces/⅓ cup) rolled oats
Pinch sugar	425 grams (15 ounces/4 ½ cups) wholemeal (wholewheat) flour	4 tablespoons cold pressed/virgin olive oil
		Pinch salt

Sauce:

400 grams (14 ounces) can chopped tomatoes	¼ teaspoon oregano	1 small onion, finely chopped
¼ teaspoon mixed herbs	1 clove garlic, chopped	**Topping – ideas to choose from:**
	Pepper to taste	

100 grams (4 ounces/1 cup) cheddar cheese, grated

2 slices of ham and 2 rings of pineapple, chopped	50 grams (2 ounces) mushrooms and ½ green pepper, sliced thinly	Small tin (120 grams/5 ounces) tuna, flaked, or small tin sardines
	4 to 5 sliced black olives	

1 Mix yeast with sugar and a little of the lukewarm water and let it sit for 10 minutes, until it gets a little foamy.

2 Mix together oil, flour, oats, and salt.

3 Add yeast to flour, and rest of water. Knead until smooth, adding more water if it doesn't bind.

4 Place in a bowl, cover, and let rise in a warm place for an hour until doubled in size.

5 On a pizza stone or inverted baking tray, roll out the dough to form pizza base, about 2 centimetres thick with slightly thicker edges.

6 Preheat oven to 180°C/350°F/Gas Mark 4. Put tomatoes, herbs, pepper, garlic, and onion in a saucepan, and boil gently until juice has evaporated.

7 Spread sauce over pizza base, leaving a small gap around the edge.

8 Sprinkle on your topping of choice. Sprinkle cheese over the top.

9 Cook in the oven for 20 to 30 minutes, until cheese is brown and crust is browned.

Vary It! *You can use mozzarella cheese instead of cheddar. You cut the fat level a little, but the flavour is milder.*

Per serving: Calories 695 (From Fat 235); Fat 26g (Saturated 8g); Cholesterol 30mg; Sodium 455mg; Carbohydrate 97g (Dietary Fibre 17g); Protein 26g. This analysis is based on crust, sauce, and cheese. Approx. Salt (g) 1.1.

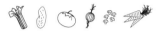

Mediterranean Pasta

Lots of colours and flavours are present in this typical Mediterranean pasta dish. You get tons of antioxidants, vitamins, and minerals in this dish so that, with luck, like many Mediterraneans you can live until you're 100!

Preparation time: *10 minutes*

Cooking time: *10 minutes*

Serves: *4*

2 tablespoons cold pressed/virgin olive oil

1 medium onion

1 clove garlic, minced

1 red pepper, de-seeded and chopped

1 green pepper, de-seeded and chopped

2 courgettes (zucchini), diced

8 mushrooms, chopped

6 cooked veggie sausages (or 6 rashers cooked streaky bacon)

400 grams (14 ounces) can chopped tomatoes

1 tablespoon tomato purée

Pinch dried tarragon

125 millilitres (¼ pint) stock

300 grams (12 ounces/5 cups) pasta shapes

25 grams (1 ounces/1 heaped tablespoon) grated Parmesan cheese

1 Heat the oil in a large saucepan; add the onion, garlic, both peppers, and courgettes.

2 Cook for 4 to 5 minutes until soft. Add the sausages and mushrooms and cook for a further 3 to 4 minutes. Add the tomatoes, tomato purée, stock, and tarragon, and simmer for 10 minutes, stirring occasionally.

3 Meanwhile, cook pasta in a large pan of boiling water according to instructions. Mix with sauce and place in dishes. Top with cheese and serve with a green salad.

Per serving: Calories 483 (From Fat 140); Fat 16g (Saturated 3g); Cholesterol 1mg; Sodium 542mg; Carbohydrate 70g (Dietary Fibre 8g); Protein 19g. Approx Salt (g) 1.4.

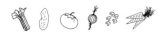

Seafood dishes

Seafood is an ideal protein source if you have PCOS because it's low in fat and the oil it contains is the sort that helps to protect you from heart disease. If you're not used to eating fish or other seafood, start with the less obviously fishy dishes like the fish cakes and work up to the smoked fish. Once you've tasted a really good seafood dish, you're going to want to keep it in your recipe favourites file!

Herby Fish Cakes

Sweet potato works well in this recipe. Using canned fish saves time on cooking the fish to make this a relatively low fuss meal, which goes equally well with a salad or cooked veg.

Preparation time: *10 minutes plus 30 minutes chill time*

Cooking time: *20 minutes*

Serves: *4*

200 grams (8 ounces) sweet potato, cooked and mashed

150 grams (6 ounces/1 cup) sweetcorn

2 tablespoons fresh parsley, chopped

1 teaspoon fresh thyme

400 grams (14 ounces) can of fish (tuna or salmon, for example)

Ground black pepper

½ tablespoon sunflower oil

1 egg (beaten)

100 grams (4 ounces/1 cup) granary breadcrumbs

1 Mix sweet potato, sweetcorn, parsley, thyme, and tuna in a bowl and season with pepper.

2 Divide into 8 portions and shape into cakes.

3 Place on a baking tray and chill for 30 minutes.

4 Put oven to warm at 200ºC/400ºF/Gas Mark 6.

5 Put ½ tablespoon sunflower oil on a baking tray and put in oven for 5 minutes to heat-up.

6 Dip the cakes in the beaten egg and coat both sides of the cake with breadcrumbs.

7 Take warm tray out of oven and place cakes immediately on tray.

8 Cook for 20 minutes until golden brown.

Per serving: Calories 305 (From Fat 48); Fat 5g (Saturated 1g); Cholesterol 83mg; Sodium 488mg; Carbohydrate 34g (Dietary Fibre 4g); Protein 32g. Approx Salt (g) 1.2

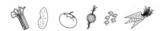

Smoked Fish Pie

The sweet potato goes particularly well with the stronger taste of smoked fish. You can use just one type of fish but a mixture of fish does add more flavour and variety. Try to include one that is oily so that you get your omega-3s!

Preparation time: *20 minutes*

Cooking time: *20 minutes*

Serves: *4*

500 grams (1 pound 2 ounces) sweet potatoes, peeled and diced

500 grams (1 pound 2 ounces) ordinary potatoes, peeled and diced

Total of 680 grams (1½ pounds) mixture of smoked fish such as smoked cod, smoked haddock, and smoked mackerel

300 millilitres (½ pint/1¼ cups) milk

1 tablespoon (20 grams/1 ounce) cornflour/maize flour (masa harina)

2 hard boiled eggs, cut into small pieces

1 tablespoon parsley, chopped

20 grams (1 ounce) low-fat spread

1 Preheat oven to 200ºC/400ºF/Gas Mark 6. Boil all potatoes for 15 to 20 minutes, until soft.

2 Poach or microwave fish in milk until tender and flaky. Break into flakes with a fork.

3 Thicken the fish and milk mixture with cornflour, by blending the cornflour with a little cold milk and then adding to the rest. Stir well and bring to the boil to thicken. Mix with the fish and hard-boiled egg in an ovenproof dish.

4 Mash up potato and add the low-fat spread and the parsley. If the mixture seems dry, add a little milk. Spoon over fish and cook for 20 minutes. Serve with peas and carrots.

Tip: When poaching the fish in milk you can add some slices of onion, a clove of garlic, and sage and coriander leaves to the milk to add a subtle flavour. Remove after poaching.

Per serving: Calories 452 (From Fat 77); Fat 9g (Saturated 4 g); Cholesterol 173mg; Sodium 1836mg; Carbohydrate 44g (Dietary Fibre 5g); Protein 48g. Approx Salt (g) 4.6.

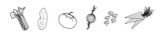

Kedgeree

This dish is rich in omega-3s due to the mackerel, and is quick and easy to make too.

Preparation time: *15 minutes*

Cooking time: *20 minutes*

Serves: *4*

300 grams (12 ounces/1¾ cups) basmati rice (brown if possible)

2 small onions, chopped

2 tablespoons cold pressed/virgin olive oil

2 cloves garlic, crushed

1 tablespoon mild curry powder

4 eggs (omega-3 enriched if possible), boiled and cut into quarters

300 grams (12 ounces) smoked mackerel fillets, flaked, with skin removed

1 fish stock cube, dissolved in 300 millilitres (½ pint) boiling water

1 Boil the rice according to instructions on packet.

2 Meanwhile, fry onion in oil, for 3 to 4 minutes, adding garlic after about one minute.

3 Add curry powder, and then add eggs and mackerel.

4 Add enough stock to make the mixture moister, and stir in rice, allowing the mixture to simmer for about five minutes to allow the rice to soak up the flavours.

Vary It! *If you're cooking this up for breakfast, try it instead with some kippers.*

Per serving: *Calories 538 (From Fat 206); Fat 23g (Saturated 5g); Cholesterol 261mg; Sodium 626mg; Carbohydrate 59g (Dietary Fibre 4g); Protein 26g. Approx Salt (g) Salt (g) 1.6.*

Fragrant Prawn Curry

The combination of spices in this dish make it a bit involved to put together, but the result has a beautiful flavour that doesn't drown out the prawns, so the effort is well worthwhile.

Preparation time: *15 minutes*

Cooking time: *10 minutes*

Serves: *4*

6 spring onions (scallions), chopped

1 to 2 fresh green chillies, halved

2 garlic cloves, crushed

2 teaspoons cold pressed/virgin olive oil

1 teaspoon turmeric

1 teaspoon cumin seeds

1 teaspoon ground cumin

1 teaspoon mustard seeds

1 teaspoon ground coriander

5 medium tomatoes, chopped

2 tablespoons water

4 tablespoons reduced-fat double cream

50 grams (2 ounces) creamed coconut ('lite' coconut milk), dissolved in 100 millilitres (½ cup) boiling water

400 grams (1 pound) cooked, peeled prawns

2 tablespoons chopped fresh coriander (cilantro)

Basmati rice, cooked, to serve

1 Put the spring onions, chillies, and garlic in a mortar, and grind with a pestle to make a paste, or purée in a food processor or blender.

2 Heat the oil in a saucepan, add the turmeric, cumin seeds, ground cumin, mustard seeds, and ground coriander, and fry gently for 30 seconds to 1 minute until spices are fragrant (don't burn). Add the spring onion paste to the pan and fry for a further 2 to 3 minutes.

3 Add the tomatoes and water to the pan and simmer for 5 minutes until soft and well-blended. Add the double cream and creamed coconut and simmer for a further 2 minutes. Stir in the prawns and fresh coriander, heat through, and serve with boiled rice.

Tip: *This recipe freezes well.*

Per serving: *Calories 228 (From Fat 64); Fat 7g (Saturated 2g); Cholesterol 227mg; Sodium 276mg; Carbohydrate 14g (Dietary Fibre 3g); Protein 27g. Approx. Salt (g) 0.7.*

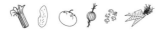

Tuna Lasagne

This recipe makes a lovely 'meaty' tasting lasagne, which is less dense and heavy than the minced beef version.

Preparation time: *30 minutes*

Cooking time: *45 minutes*

Serves: *4*

200 grams (6 ounces) can tuna (in spring water if possible), drained

1 clove garlic, crushed

1 green pepper, sliced

100 grams (4 ounces) mushrooms, sliced

1 teaspoon dried marjoram

400 grams (14 ounces) can diced tomatoes

1 tablespoon tomato purée

Ground black pepper

100 grams (4 ounces) lasagne pasta

300 millilitres (½ pint/1¼ cups) semi-skimmed or skimmed milk

1 tablespoon cornflour (masa harina)

100 grams (4 ounces/1 cup) half-fat cheddar type cheese, grated

1 Preheat oven to 180ºC/350°F/Gas Mark 4.

2 Drain the tuna and break up using a fork. Mix the tuna with the garlic, green pepper, mushrooms, marjoram, tomatoes, and tomato purée. Season with ground black pepper.

3 Spoon half of the tuna mixture in the bottom of an ovenproof dish. Cover with lasagne (break to fit). Spread the remaining tuna over. Blend the cornflour with a little of the milk, and then add the remaining milk. Bring to the boil, stirring continuously.

4 Stir in 75 grams (3 ounces) of the cheese. Pour on top of the tuna. Sprinkle with the remaining cheese. Bake for 45 minutes.

Per serving: Calories 277 (From Fat 41); Fat 5g (Saturated 2g); Cholesterol 22mg; Sodium 460mg; Carbohydrate 36g (Dietary Fibre 4g); Protein 25g. Approx. Salt (g) 1.2.

Tuna Pasta

This dish is a favourite in my household due to its lovely taste and ease of making; it's also quite filling. Serve with a green salad.

Preparation time: *10 minutes*

Cooking time: *10 minutes*

Serves: *4*

225 grams (9 ounces/2½ cups) pasta

1 large onion

1 tablespoon olive oil

1 clove garlic, crushed

200 grams (8 ounces) mushrooms, sliced

400 grams (14 ounces) can tuna in spring water if available, drained

150 millilitres (¼ pint/½ cup) low-fat crème fraîche (or low-fat sour cream)

Handful of grated cheese

1 Boil pasta according to instructions on packet.

2 Fry onion in oil. Add garlic after onion has begun to go tender.

3 Add mushrooms. Once mushrooms have cooked, add tuna and crème fraîche. Drain pasta and stir in. Serve sprinkled with grated cheese.

Tip: *Instead of crème fraîche and mushrooms, you can use a tin of condensed mushroom soup.*

Per serving: *Calories 448 (From Fat 118); Fat 13g (Saturated 6g); Cholesterol 46mg; Sodium 472mg; Carbohydrate 49g (Dietary Fibre 3g); Protein 35g. Approx. Salt (g) 1.2.*

Tuna Niçoise

This dish is a posher version of the recipe using canned tuna, and is upper class enough to serve at a dinner party without having to ply your guests with too many calories!

Preparation time: *5 minutes*

Cooking time: *5 to 10 minutes for beans plus 4 minutes for eggs and 5 to 10 minutes for tuna*

Serves: *1*

50 grams (2 ounces/½ cup) fine green beans, chopped

1 large tomato, sliced

6 black olives

2 tablespoons low-fat vinaigrette style dressing

1 tablespoon snipped fresh chives or spring onions

Ground black pepper

1 large egg

100 grams (4 ounces) tuna steak (approximate weight)

½ teaspoon olive oil

Slice of lemon

1 Cook the beans in a small pan of boiling water until just tender (about 2 minutes). Drain and rinse in cold water. Mix the beans with the tomato, olives, dressing, and chives. Season with ground black pepper.

2 Place the egg in a small pan of cold water. Bring slowly to the boil, and then cook for 5 minutes. Drain, rinse in cold water, and then tap the shell all over and remove.

3 Brush the tuna steak on both sides with the oil. Heat a griddle or frying pan until hot, and then cook the tuna steak for 1 to 2 minutes on both sides or until cooked right through. Place the tuna, while still hot, on top of the tomato, olive, and bean mixture, and top with a squeeze of lemon juice and the soft-boiled egg and serve immediately. Grind some more black pepper over the egg and tuna.

Per serving: Calories 417 (From Fat 174); Fat 19g (Saturated 3g); Cholesterol 278mg; Sodium 821mg; Carbohydrate 18g (Dietary Fibre 4g); Protein 43g. Approx. Salt (g) 2.1.

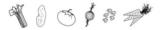

Poultry dishes

Poultry is a low-fat and low-calorie protein source, and very versatile. Chicken and particularly turkey can sometimes be a bit dry, but these recipes all involve cooking the meat with some really tasty low-fat sources, which overcomes the dryness.

Spicy Turkey Tacos

This dish is fun, quick to assemble, and really tasty. You're going to want to eat more than your allotted two tacos, but try to resist!

Preparation time: *10 minutes*

Cooking time: *15 to 20 minutes*

Serves: *6*

1 small onion

1 tablespoon oil

1 clove garlic

450 grams (1 pound) fresh turkey mince or Quorn mince (soy crumbles)

1 teaspoon chilli powder

1 green pepper, de-seeded and cut into small strips

400 grams (14 ounces) can chopped tomatoes

1 tablespoon freshly chopped oregano or 1 teaspoon dried oregano

220 grams (8 ounces/1¼ cups) can red kidney beans, rinsed and drained

125 millilitres (¼ pint/½ cup) vegetable or chicken stock

6 spring onions, trimmed and chopped

To serve:

12 taco shells

¼ iceberg lettuce, shredded

8 tablespoons fromage frais (or low-fat sour cream)

50 grams (2 ounces/½ cup) half-fat Cheddar cheese, grated

1 Fry the onion in the oil in a non-stick frying pan. When the onion begins to go soft, add the garlic clove.

2 Add the mince with the chilli powder and fry for a further 3 minutes, stirring frequently, until sealed.

3 Add the green pepper, chopped tomatoes (with their juice), herbs, and red kidney beans.

4 Pour in the ¼ pint stock.

5 Bring to the boil, and then simmer for 5 to 8 minutes or until the turkey is thoroughly cooked and most of the juice is absorbed. Stir in the spring onions.

6 Meanwhile heat the taco shells as directed on the packet. Place a spoonful of shredded lettuce in the taco shells, top with the mince and a spoonful of fromage frais, and sprinkle with the grated cheese.

Per serving: Calories 326 (From Fat 139); Fat 15g (Saturated 4g); Cholesterol 53mg; Sodium 441mg; Carbohydrate 32g (Dietary Fibre 6g); Protein 18g. Approx. Salt (g) 1.1

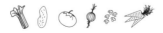

Chicken Curry with Dhal

This traditional curry is based on an Indian recipe, and is a great one to serve up to curry loving guests: They won't believe it's light on the fat too!

Preparation time: *30 minutes*

Cooking time: *20 minutes*

Serves: *4*

For the curry:

1 tablespoon sunflower oil

3 cloves garlic, crushed

1 medium onion, finely chopped

2 teaspoons medium curry powder

2 tablespoons garam masala

1 teaspoon ground coriander

½ teaspoon dried mint (optional)

570 grams (1 pound 7 ounces) boneless, skinless chicken breast, diced

200 millilitres (¼ pint/¾ cup) water in which half a chicken stock cube has been dissolved

For the Dhal:

400 grams (14 ounces/2 cups) canned puy lentils (green French lentils), drained

½ teaspoon turmeric

½ teaspoon mixed spice

½ teaspoon cumin seeds

½ teaspoon coriander seeds

½ teaspoon curry powder

30 grams (1 ounce/½ cup) fresh mint, chopped (optional)

30 grams (1 ounce/½ cup) fresh coriander, chopped

Freshly ground black pepper

Juice of one lemon

125 millilitres (¼ pint) water in which half a chicken stock cube has been dissolved

140 grams (5 ounces/½ cup) low-fat natural yoghurt

1 Heat the oil in a wok or large, heavy frying pan. Add the garlic and onion and stir-fry for about 5 minutes until onion is golden.

2 Stir in the curry powder, garam masala, coriander, and mint, if using. Add the chicken and cook over a moderate heat for 5 minutes, stirring occasionally.

3 Add the stock, stir, and simmer with the lid on for 10 minutes, and then with the lid off for another 5 minutes until the chicken is cooked and the sauce has thickened.

4 Place the lentils, spices and, stock in a pan, and gently heat.

5 When the lentils are very soft (after about 20 minutes), add the fresh coriander, lemon juice, and black pepper. Cook for a further 2 minutes.

6 Serve with the curry. Put the yoghurt in a serving dish. Serve with naan bread or rice.

Per serving: Calories 295 (From Fat 74); Fat 8g (Saturated 2g); Cholesterol 81mg; Sodium 467mg; Carbohydrate 19g (Dietary Fibre 7g); Protein 36g. Approx. 1.2.

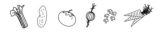

Stir-fry Chicken and Noodles

A really quick Chinese dish for you to make, which is low in saturated fats yet packed with protein and antioxidants.

Preparation time: *10 minutes*

Cooking time: *10 minutes*

Serves: *4*

4 portions (240 grams/8½ ounces) noodles

1½ tablespoons sunflower oil

2 teaspoons (10 millilitres) nut or seed oil such as sesame or walnut

4 (400 to 500 grams/16 to 20 ounces) chicken breasts, sliced

1 red pepper, thinly sliced

100 grams (4 ounces) mushrooms, sliced

100 grams (4 ounces) ladies fingers (ochra), sliced

100 grams (4 ounces) mange tout (sugar snap peas)

60 grams (2½ ounces/½ cup) unsalted cashew nuts, toasted (optional)

1 packet (1 cup) Chinese stir-fry sauce of choice

1 Boil the noodles according to packet instructions, drain, stir in nut or seed oil, cover, and set aside.

2 Fry the chicken in the sunflower oil, until starting to go golden.

3 Add the pepper, and then after about a minute, add the mushrooms, ladies fingers, and mange tout, stirring as needed.

4 Once the vegetables are all tender, stir in the cashew nuts (if using) and noodles.

5 Mix in preferred stir-fry sauce. Serve immediately.

Vary It! *Instead of the peppers, mushrooms, ladies fingers, and mange tout you can use similar quantities of your favourite stir-fry vegetables including bean sprouts and water chestnuts.*

Per serving: *Calories 472 (From Fat 92); Fat 10g (Saturated 2g); Cholesterol 55mg; Sodium 2277mg; Carbohydrate 66g (Dietary Fibre 3g); Protein 28g. Approx. Salt (g) 5.7.*

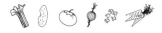

Yellow Bean Stir-fry

The three different colour peppers in this recipe add loads of vitamin C and cancer-fighting carotenes. The chilli adds a bite and is supposed to help protect against heart disease and certain cancers.

Preparation time: *15 minutes*

Cooking time: *15 minutes*

Serves: *4*

300 grams (12 ounces/1¼ cups) basmati rice (brown is good)

1 red pepper, sliced

1 yellow pepper, sliced

1 green pepper, sliced

3 tablespoons cold pressed/virgin olive oil

1 garlic clove, crushed

4 spring onions, chopped

1 red chilli, de-seeded and chopped

450 grams (1 pound) turkey mince or Quorn

125 millilitres (¼ pint/½ cup) vegetable stock added with the yellow bean sauce if using Quorn

150 millilitres (¼ pint/¾ cup) bottle yellow bean (or sweet and sour) stir-fry sauce

1 Boil rice according to instructions on packet.

2 Cook peppers in oil for 3 minutes. Add garlic, spring onions, chilli, and turkey mince or Quorn.

3 Stir-fry for 5 minutes until mince is cooked through.

4 Add yellow bean sauce (plus some vegetable stock if using Quorn) and stir-fry for 3 minutes.

5 Serve with rice.

Per serving: *Calories 467 (From Fat 181); Fat 20g (Saturated 3g); Cholesterol 67mg; Sodium 2585mg; Carbohydrate 53g (Dietary Fibre 8g); Protein 24g. Approx. Salt (g) 6.5.*

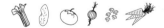

Meat dishes

You can include red meat in your diet two to three times a week, but stick to a 120-gram (5-ounce) portion at a time. Choose the leaner cuts and the least fatty mince. Red meat provides a good source of iron and zinc.

Sausage and Chunky Vegetable Casserole

Sausages are a great tasting invention but are often given the thumbs down health-wise due to their high fat and salt content. Go for good quality sausages, which are lower in fat. Or try some veggie sausages, which are really quite good these days – and lots of varieties are available to choose from. When you add plenty of veg to a sausage dish, nothing is wrong with having a few sausages now and then.

Preparation time: *15 minutes*

Cooking time: *35 minutes*

Serves: *4*

2 tablespoons cold pressed/virgin olive oil

8 sausages (or use veggie sausages if preferred) cut into pieces

1 red onion, peeled and cut into wedges

2 garlic cloves, peeled and crushed

2 carrots, peeled, cut into chunks

150 grams (5 ounces) mushrooms, halved

4 small parsnips, peeled and chopped

8 baby turnips, stalks trimmed, or swede (rutabaga), chopped

900 millilitres (½ pint/3 cups) hot vegetable stock

1 teaspoon mixed herbs

Ground black pepper

150 grams (6 ounces/1 cup) broad beans (fava beans), popped from their outer skins (or 300-gram can)

1 tablespoon cornflour

115 millilitres (¼ pint/½ cup) low-fat crème fraîche (or sour cream)

2 tablespoons chopped parsley

Crusty granary bread (or low-carb bread) to serve

1 Heat oil in a large saucepan, add the raw sausages, and cook for 15 minutes over a medium heat, stirring frequently, until softened. Remove from heat.

2 Add the onion and garlic to the pan and fry over a medium heat for 5 minutes until softened. Add the carrots, mushrooms, parsnips, and turnips or swede and cook, stirring for 5 minutes until beginning to brown.

3 Add the stock, mixed herbs, and pepper and bring to the boil, cover, and simmer for 30 minutes, until all the vegetables are tender, adding more stock if the mixture gets too dry and starts to stick. Add the broad beans.

4 Mix 2 tablespoons water with the cornflour, add to the pan and cook until thickened. Return the sausages to the pan and stir in the crème fraîche. Heat for a further 2 minutes until everything is piping hot. Serve sprinkled with the parsley, and crusty bread.

Per serving: Calories 451 (From Fat 166); Fat 19g (Saturated 5g); Cholesterol 31mg; Sodium 762mg; Carbohydrate 63g (Dietary Fibre 11g); Protein 15g. Approx. Salt (g) 1.9.

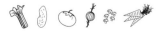

Bacon Risotto

Not a recipe to follow if you're on a strict low-salt diet, but a flavour-packed risotto to try now and then, which is quick to knock-up.

Preparation time: *10 minutes*

Cooking time: *25 minutes*

Serves: *4*

900 millilitres (1½ pints/4 cups) chicken stock

1 tablespoon Worcestershire sauce

350 grams (13 ounces/2¼ cups) basmati rice

1 tablespoon sunflower oil

1 large onion, chopped

225 grams (8 ounces) rindless back bacon, chopped

175 grams (6 ounces) sausages, chopped

125 grams (4 ounces) button mushrooms, halved

1 red pepper, sliced

1 green pepper, sliced

Green salad, to serve

1 Bring the stock and Worcestershire sauce to the boil, and add the rice. Bring both to the boil, and simmer for 15 minutes or until the water has been absorbed.

2 Meanwhile, heat the oil in a frying pan, add the onion, fry for 3 minutes, and then add the bacon and sausage. Fry until brown over a moderate heat.

3 Add the mushrooms and peppers. Cook for a further 5 minutes, until all ingredients are tender.

4 Remove rice (don't strain) and place in a large serving dish. Add the bacon mixture and toss to gently combine all ingredients.

Tip: *For a vegetarian version, omit bacon and double up on veggie sausages; use vegetable instead of chicken stock.*

Per serving: *Calories 626 (From Fat 226); Fat 25g (Saturated 7g); Cholesterol 62mg; Sodium 2109mg; Carbohydrate 76g (Dietary Fibre 4g); Protein 26g. Approx. Salt (g) 5.3.*

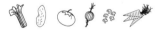

Spaghetti Carbonara

Normally this recipe is packed with fat, and the saturated type too. This recipe provides a much lower-fat version, but still retains the creamy taste of the original version.

Preparation time: *10 minutes*

Cooking time: *30 minutes*

Serves: *4*

225 grams (8 ounces) spaghetti

1 vegetable stock cube

1 tablespoon olive oil

6 spring (green) onions, finely chopped

1 garlic clove, crushed

1 tablespoon plain flour

300 millilitres (½ pint/1¼ cups) semi-skimmed milk

115 grams (4 ounces) smoked ham, cut into strips

1 teaspoon Dijon mustard

Freshly ground black pepper

50 grams (2 ounces) Parmesan, grated

Chopped parsley to garnish

1 Cook the spaghetti with the stock cube in a large pan of boiling water according to packet instructions, and drain.

2 Meanwhile, in a non-stick pan, fry the onions and garlic in the olive oil until soft.

3 Stir in the flour to make a roux and cook for 1 minute.

4 Gradually stir in the milk until it thickens. Add some of the spaghetti water if too thick.

5 Add the ham to the sauce along with the mustard and black pepper.

6 Toss the sauce with the spaghetti and add the Parmesan, mix well, and heat through.

7 Garnish with chopped parsley and serve with salad.

Vary It! *This recipe works well with wholemeal spaghetti too.*

Per serving: *Calories 365 (From Fat 98); Fat 11g (Saturated 4g); Cholesterol 30mg; Sodium 825mg; Carbohydrate 47g (Dietary Fibre 3g); Protein 20g. Approx. Salt (g) 2.1.*

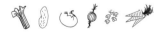

Chilli Con Carne

This chilli uses the real thing – two whole green chillies; chillies are supposed to have several medical properties, but besides the health benefit, this dish is very tasty dish and low in fat too.

Preparation time: *15 minutes*

Cooking time: *15 minutes*

Serves: *4*

300 grams (12 ounces/2 cups) basmati rice/tortilla chips

1 tablespoon cold pressed/virgin olive oil

2 small onions, finely chopped

1 teaspoon cumin seeds

2 cloves garlic, crushed

2 green chillies, de-seeded and chopped

2 x 400 grams (1 pound) can chopped tomatoes

400 grams (1 pound) lean minced beef (or Quorn (soy crumbles) if preferred)

Red wine or stock if needed

2 x 400 grams (1 pound) can kidney beans, drained

2 tablespoons coriander, roughly chopped (optional)

Ground black pepper to taste

125 grams (5 ounces) fromage frais (or sour cream)

1 If using rice, cook according to packet instructions.

2 Heat a non-stick pan and add oil. Gently sauté the chopped onion in the oil for 3 to 4 minutes.

3 Add the cumin seeds, garlic, chilli, and chopped tomato with juices. Stir and allow to cook for a few minutes.

4 Add the beef or Quorn, with some stock or red wine if needed. Stir well, cover, and cook for about 10 to 15 minutes.

5 Stir in the kidney beans and continue cooking for a few minutes until the beef is fully cooked.

6 Add the coriander, if using, season to taste with black pepper and serve with tortilla chips or rice and a dollop of fromage frais on top.

Per serving: Calories 669 (From Fat 173); Fat 19g (Saturated 8g); Cholesterol 45mg; Sodium 641mg; Carbohydrate 94g (Dietary Fibre 14g); Protein 34g. Approx. Salt (g) 1.6.

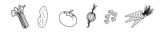

Spiced Bean Bake

This recipe is a really tasty minced beef dish, which warms you up and fills you up on colder evenings: It can be adapted to be veggie too!

Preparation time: *20 minutes*

Cooking time: *25 minutes*

Serves: *4*

400 grams (1 pound) minced (ground) beef or minced Quorn (soy crumbles)

1 tablespoon olive oil if using Quorn

1 onion, chopped

1 clove garlic, crushed

1 teaspoons curry powder

¼ pint vegetable stock

2 apples, cored and thinly sliced

1 tablespoon Worcestershire sauce

400 grams (1 pound) can baked beans

1 Preheat oven to 190ºC/375ºF/Gas Mark 5.

2 Fry mince, onion, and garlic in a large pan until meat is brown. If using Quorn, pre-fry onion and garlic in 1 tablespoon oil before adding mince.

3 Stir in curry powder and add stock.

4 Add slices from one apple and stir in, along with the Worcestershire sauce, and bring to the boil.

5 Add baked beans and heat through.

6 Pour into an ovenproof dish and arrange second apple slices on top of bean mixture.

7 Cover and cook for 25 minutes.

Tip: *Boiled basmati rice goes well with this recipe.*

Per serving: *Calories 330 (From Fat 108); Fat 12g (Saturated 4g); Cholesterol 31mg; Sodium 535mg; Carbohydrate 36g (Dietary Fibre 8g); Protein 23g. Approx. Salt (g) 1.3.*

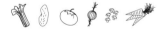

Cheesy Beef and Sweet Potato Bake

This recipe makes a lovely hotpot for a winter evening. The tastes blend well together so don't be afraid to serve this up at a dinner party.

Preparation time: *10 minutes*

Cooking time: *25 minutes and 20 minutes*

Serves: *4*

1 tablespoon cold pressed/virgin olive oil

1 onion, chopped

1 clove garlic, crushed

400 grams (1 pound) lean minced (ground) beef (or veggie mince if preferred)

200 grams (8 ounces) carrots, grated

1 apple, cored and grated

2 tablespoons brown sauce

1 tablespoon Worcestershire sauce

Ground black pepper to taste

400 grams (1 pound) can chopped tomatoes

1 beef stock cube dissolved in 4 tablespoons hot water

600 grams (1½ pound) sweet potatoes, cooked and mashed

100 grams (4 ounces) mature cheddar, grated

1 Preheat oven to 190ºC/375°F/Gas Mark 5.

2 Heat oil in a large pan. Add onion and garlic and fry until soft (3 to 4 minutes).

3 Add minced beef and fry until cooked (10 minutes).

4 Add all remaining ingredients except potatoes and cheese.

5 Bring to the boil and simmer for 10 minutes. Add stock as necessary to prevent mixture getting too dry.

6 Spoon the meat mixture into an ovenproof dish.

7 Combine mashed potato and cheese and spread over the meat.

8 Cook for 20 minutes with lid off, until golden brown on top.

Tip: *Goes nicely with fresh green vegetables.*

Per serving: *Calories 474 (From Fat 184); Fat 20g (Saturated 9g); Cholesterol 58mg; Sodium 1057mg; Carbohydrate 45g (Dietary Fibre 7g); Protein 28g. Approx. Salt (g) 2.6.*

Beef Stroganoff

The original Beef Stroganoff is quite a creamy and rich dish. This recipe retains all the flavour and is slightly tangier than its more calorie laden parent dish!

Preparation time: *30 minutes*

Cooking time: *12 minutes*

Serves: *4*

400 grams (1 pound) lean beef grilling steak

1 tablespoon sunflower oil

1 onion, finely chopped

200 grams (8 ounces) button mushrooms sliced and lightly poached in a little chicken stock

125 grams (5 ounces/½ cup) low-fat natural yoghurt

65 grams (2½ ounces/¼ cup) reduced-fat crème fraîche or fromage frais (or low-fat sour cream)

2 teaspoons lemon juice

Ground black pepper

1 Trim away any fat from the steak. Cut the meat into matchstick strips.

2 Heat the oil in a large frying pan and brown the meat in it. Add the onion and cook gently for another 2 to 3 minutes.

3 Add the mushrooms and cook until they are tender and the meat is cooked through (about 8 minutes).

4 Mix the yoghurt, crème fraîche/fromage frais, and lemon juice, and stir into the pan.

5 Simmer for 2 to 3 minutes, and then add some ground black pepper.

Tip: Serve with some basmati rice and lightly cooked carrots and peas.

Per serving: *Calories 253 (From Fat 111); Fat 12g (Saturated 4g); Cholesterol 64mg; Sodium 69mg; Carbohydrate 10g (Dietary Fibre 1g); Protein 25g. Approx. Salt (g) 0.2.*

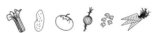

Pork Goulash

Lean pork is a low-fat meat, but it can tend to get a little dry so is best cooked in a sauce as in this recipe. The goulash spices complement the pork well.

Preparation time: *15 minutes*

Cooking time: *30 minutes*

Serves: *3*

1 medium onion, chopped	*1 tablespoon paprika*
2 cloves garlic, chopped	*½ teaspoon caraway seeds*
400 grams (1 pound) lean pork cubed	*1 tablespoon lemon juice*
3 medium tomatoes, cut into wedges	*Ground black pepper*
100 grams (4 ounces) button mushrooms	*125 grams (5 ounces/½ cup) natural yoghurt*
1 tablespoon tomato purée	

1 Fry the onion and garlic in oil until translucent, add the pork, and brown gently. Stir in remaining ingredients (except yoghurt), including the spices, lemon juice, and tomato purée.

2 Simmer for 20 minutes, stirring occasionally. If the mixture gets too dry, add a little water or chicken stock.

3 When cooked, remove from heat and stir in the yoghurt.

Tip: Goes well with new potatoes, green beans, and carrots.

Per serving: Calories 259 (From Fat 74); Fat 8g (Saturated 3g); Cholesterol 81mg; Sodium 101mg; Carbohydrate 16g (Dietary Fibre 3g); Protein 31g. Approx. Salt (g) 0.3.

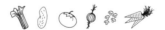

Desserts

Proper desserts aren't strictly necessary at mealtimes, especially if you're trying to lose weight, in which case some fruit or a yoghurt after dinner is probably enough. But at the weekend, special occasions, or when entertaining, try out some of these indulgences. These desserts all have less fat and calories than their fully loaded sisters, but you and your guests would never know!

Apple and Hazelnut Crunch

This recipe is an instant but tasty pudding, which is nutritious and not too hefty on the calories to boot!

Preparation time: *10 minutes*

Cooking time: *10 minutes*

Serves: *4*

400 grams (1 pound) apples, peeled, cored and chopped

1 tablespoon brown sugar

125 grams (5 ounces/½ cup) hazelnut or toffee yoghurt

2 fruit and nut crunchy bars

1 Place apples in a saucepan with 3 tablespoons water and the brown sugar.

2 Cover and simmer on low heat until tender (about 10 minutes). Leave to cool.

3 Stir yoghurt and apple together and spoon into 4 bowls. Crush fruit and nut bar and sprinkle over top.

4 Chill and serve.

Per serving: Calories 159 (From Fat 32); Fat 4g (Saturated 2g); Cholesterol 2mg; Sodium 58mg; Carbohydrate 31g (Dietary Fibre 3g); Protein 3g. Approx. Salt (g) 0.1.

Pears in Chocolate Sauce

Pears go surprisingly well with chocolate sauce; the bitter dark chocolate works well with the sweeter pears.

Preparation time: *10 minutes*

Cooking time: *20 minutes*

Serves: *6*

750 millilitres (1¼ pints/3 cups) water

100 grams (4 ounces/¾ cup) sugar

1 cinnamon stick

Juice and zest of ½ lemon

6 medium size pears, peeled, cored and quartered

For the sauce:

130 grams (5 ounces/¾ cup) dark chocolate, chopped into small pieces

1 tablespoon sunflower oil

25 millilitres (2 tablespoons) cold water

1 Heat the water, sugar, cinnamon stick, lemon juice, and zest in a large saucepan with high sides, and simmer for 5 minutes. Add the pears and simmer for 20 minutes, uncovered (keep an eye on the level of the sauce).

2 Spoon out the pears with just a little of the remaining liquor.

3 Make the sauce by placing all the ingredients in a small saucepan. Heat gently, stirring occasionally. When combined, pour over the pears. Serve immediately.

Vary It! *You can serve the chocolate sauce with bananas and a dollop of low-fat crème fraîche, but no need to cook the bananas first.*

Per serving: *Calories 280 (From Fat 85); Fat 10g (Saturated 5g); Cholesterol 2mg; Sodium 3mg; Carbohydrate 50g (Dietary Fibre 5g); Protein 1g. Approx. Salt (g) 0.0.*

Apple and Rhubarb Crumble

Use whatever fruit can be stewed and that is in season for this recipe, which combines several highly nutritious foods in one dish; fruit, nuts, and a wholegrain cereal.

Preparation time: *20 minutes*

Cooking time: *40 minutes*

Serves: *8*

600 grams (1 pound 5 ounces; about 1½) apples peeled, cored, and cut into eighths

670 grams (1½ pounds; about 4 stalks) rhubarb, ends trimmed, washed and cut into 4-centimetre lengths

Other fruit can be used instead of apple and rhubarb such as gooseberries or plums

2 tablespoons caster sugar (superfine sugar)

Topping:

75 grams (3 ounces/¾ cup) plain wholemeal (wholewheat) flour

100 grams (4 ounces/1 cup) ground almonds

100 grams (4 ounces/1 cup) reduced-fat margarine

100 grams (4 ounces/1 cup) muesli

95 grams (4½ ounces/¾ cup) brown sugar

1 Preheat oven to 200ºC/400°F/Gas Mark 6 and lightly grease a 2-litre ovenproof dish.

2 Layer the apples and rhubarb in the dish, sprinkling a little caster sugar between layers.

3 Combine flour and almonds in a bowl. Use your hands to rub in the margarine until well-mixed and large crumbs start to form. Mix in the muesli and brown sugar.

4 Sprinkle the topping evenly over the fruit. Cover the crumble with aluminium foil and bake for 20 minutes. Remove the foil and continue to cook for a further 10 to 20 minutes or until the fruit is tender and the crumble is golden brown. Set aside for 5 minutes before serving.

Per serving: *Calories 308 (From Fat 135); Fat 15g (Saturated 2g); Cholesterol 0mg; Sodium 127mg; Carbohydrate 46g (Dietary Fibre 6g); Protein 6g. Approx. Salt (g) 0.3.*

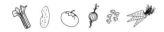

Sherry Trifle

Just because you're trying to eat healthily doesn't mean you can't have trifle! This version has all the taste but is surprisingly low in fat and sugar.

Preparation time: *20 minutes plus setting time for jelly*

Serves: *6*

3 trifle sponges

Sugar-free strawberry or raspberry jam

2 tablespoons sherry

200 grams (8 ounces) strawberries, raspberries, or peaches (tinned, frozen, or fresh)

1 packet strawberry or raspberry sugar free jelly (jello)

600 millilitres (1 pint/2½ cups) low-fat custard

Low fat squirty (whipped) cream

Handful toasted flaked almonds

1 Slice the sponge and spread with the jam.

2 Arrange in the bottom of a glass serving bowl. Pour the sherry over the sponges.

3 Add the fruit.

4 Prepare the jelly as per the instructions (if using tinned fruit, use the juices instead of water when preparing). Pour the jelly over the fruit and sponge.

5 Place in the refrigerator and allow to set.

6 Make the custard and allow to cool down to room temperature.

7 Pour the custard over the set jelly. Squirt over some cream swirls to decorate and finish off with flaked almonds.

Tip: *You can use tinned low-fat custard to save some time, but this doesn't set like home-made custard and makes a more sloppy trifle, which some people prefer!*

Per serving: *Calories 491 (From Fat 49); Fat 5g (Saturated 2g); Cholesterol 111mg; Sodium 513mg; Carbohydrate 96g (Dietary Fibre 1g); Protein 12g. Approx. Salt (g) 1.3.*

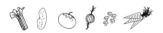

Cheesecake

For a tangy and light version of cheesecake, try out this recipe, which is also remarkably quick to make but looks like you spent ages on it. You can serve this dessert up to dinner guests.

Preparation time: *15 minutes plus chilling time*

Serves: *6*

150 grams (6 ounces/¾ cup) low-fat soft cheese (cream cheese or neufchatel)

100 grams (4 ounces/½ cup) low-fat fruit yoghurt (lemon yoghurt works well)

Juice and grated rind of 1 lemon

2 tablespoons sugar

1 envelope unflavoured gelatine

3 tablespoons boiling water

White of 1 egg, stiffly whisked

Pastry/biscuit base

1 Beat soft cheese with yoghurt, the juice, rind of 1 lemon, and sugar until smooth and creamy (you can do this in a food processor).

2 Dissolve gelatine in boiling water, cool slightly, and add to the mixture. Gently fold in the egg white.

3 Pour into your favourite pastry or biscuit base and chill until set.

Per serving: Calories 231 (From Fat 106); Fat 12g (Saturated 4g); Cholesterol 15mg; Sodium 199mg; Carbohydrate 25g (Dietary Fibre 0g); Protein 6g. Approx. Salt (g) 0.5.

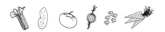

Bread and Butter Pudding

This recipe is a really comforting pudding for a cold evening. The dried fruit and milk helps to lower the GI. This dessert is one to have if you've had a fairly light main course!

Preparation time: *15 minutes*

Cooking time: *45 minutes*

Serves: *4*

1 malt loaf (225 grams/9 ounces)

100 grams (4 ounces/¾ cup) raisins, or other dried fruit

3 eggs

300 millilitres (½ pint/1¼ cups) semi-skimmed milk

50 grams (2 ounces/¼ cup) caster (superfine) sugar

1 teaspoon vanilla essence (extract)

2 teaspoons ground nutmeg

1 Preheat oven to 160ºC/325°F/Gas Mark 3. Grease a deep 20-centimetre (9-inch) pie dish.

2 Cut malt loaf slices in half to make 2 triangles. Arrange so that they cover the bottom of the dish.

3 Sprinkle the slices with the dried fruit.

4 In a bowl, beat eggs until well mixed. Add milk, sugar, and vanilla essence. Beat together.

5 Slowly pour over the bread, making sure it's all well soaked.

6 Sprinkle with nutmeg and bake for 45 minutes.

Tip: *This recipe works best if you can make up to stage 5 and allow it to sit for 30 minutes before cooking.*

Per serving: *Calories 446 (From Fat 72); Fat 8g (Saturated 4g); Cholesterol 170mg; Sodium 277mg; Carbohydrate 83g (Dietary Fibre 4g); Protein 13g. Approx. Salt (g) 0.7.*

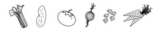

Tips for Eating Out

Statistics show that people are eating out more and more for a variety of reasons. Eating out is not necessarily wrong but if you use it as an excuse to overindulge and you're eating out on a regular basis, you may be storing up trouble for yourself. Another problem when eating out is that you may not realise how much fat or salt the chef is using. Both ingredients tend to be used liberally to enhance the flavour of food. Fortunately many chefs now realise that consumers prefer not to have food laden with fat or salt and are adapting their style accordingly.

There's no harm in having a word with the restaurant beforehand to ask if the chef can make a particular dish with less salt and/or fat. If more people did this, restaurants would make their food offerings less calorie laden and salty.

Here are some top-tips to follow when eating out:

✔ Ask for smaller portion sizes and share your starter or dessert with a companion.

✔ If possible, avoid foods that say they are au gratin, crispy escalloped, or sautéed, because they are high in fat.

✔ Ask the chef for details if a dish says it's pan-fried or stuffed, and avoid the dish or ask for it to be modified if it seems high in fat. For example, you may want the dish to be grilled, oven baked without extra fat, or poached.

✔ Go for dishes that involve steaming, boiling, baking, grilling, or poaching because these methods don't usually involve the addition of fat during cooking.

✔ Avoid high-salt foods – these tend to be ones that include pickles, are in a cocktail sauce, smoked, au jus, or with soy or teriyaki sauce.

✔ If in doubt, you can always ask for any dressings, gravies, or sauces on the side. This applies to desserts as well. That way you can avoid them or just add a little if it seems fatty, over sugary, or salty.

Table 9-1 has some tips for choosing the best options from some different types of restaurants, and what you should avoid.

Table 9-1	Safe and Sorry Food Choices	
Type of Cuisine	**The Sorry Choice**	**The Safe Choice**
Chinese	Fried rice	Steamed rice
	Oyster, bean, and soy sauce	Sweet and sour sauce, plum or duck sauce
	Dishes with fried meat	Dishes with lots of vegetables and stewed or baked meat
	Crispy fried noodles	Boiled noodles
Indian	Beef or lamb dishes	Chicken or seafood dishes
	Food prepared with ghee (clarified butter)	Food cooked with vegetable oil or no oil at all.
	Curries made with coconut milk or cream	Curries with vegetable or dhal base

(continued)

Table 9-1 *(continued)*

Type of Cuisine	The Sorry Choice	The Safe Choice
Indian	Samosas (fried turnovers filled with seasoned vegetables or meat)	Papadum or papad (crispy, thin lentil wafers)
	Pakoras (fritters dipped in a spicy chickpea batter)	Tikka or Tandoori dishes
	Fried or stuffed bread	Chapati or naan breads
Italian	Pasta or meat with cream-based and cheese sauces	Pasta or grilled or baked meat with tomato-based sauces
	Pizza with lots of meat and cheese	Pizzas topped with lots of vegetables
Fast food	Burgers topped with cheese, mayo, or bacon	Burgers topped with extra pickles, onion, tomato, peppers, or mustard
	Fried chicken sandwiches	Grilled chicken sandwiches or chicken fajita pittas
	Baked potato with butter, full-fat sour cream	Baked potato with baked beans or low-fat sour cream
	Cookies or cakes	Frozen yoghurts, low-fat muffins
Thai	Deep fried dishes	Stir fried dishes
	Food cooked in coconut oil or lard	Food cooked in vegetable oil
	Dishes cooked in coconut milk	Fresh spring rolls
	Fried rice	Steamed rice
Greek	Deep fried starters and those made from filo pastry	Tzatziki dip (yoghurt with cucumber and garlic purée) with crudités or Horta (greens steamed or blanched and made into salad)
	Moussaka	Baked stuffed vegetables or Stifado (beef and onion stew with red wine and cinnamon)
	Baklava (filo pastry layers with nuts, sugar, syrup, and cloves)	Figs with a little Greek yoghurt

Part IV
Other Helpful Stuff for PCOS

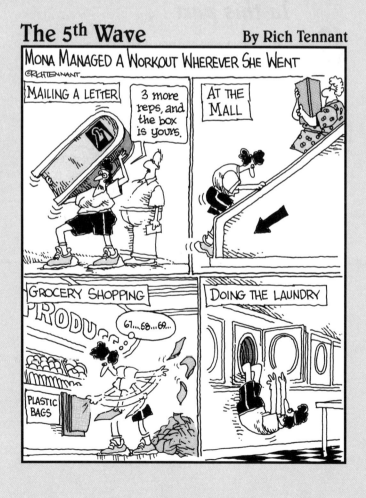

The 5th Wave   By Rich Tennant

MONA MANAGED A WORKOUT WHEREVER SHE WENT

MAILING A LETTER   3 more reps, and the box is yours.

AT THE MALL

GROCERY SHOPPING   67...68...69...

DOING THE LAUNDRY

PRODUCE

PLASTIC BAGS

In this part . . .

*B*esides diet, what else can you do to help alleviate your PCOS? This part covers it all. You'll find advice on how to be physically active (vitally important to everyone, but particularly if you have PCOS). I share info on what your doctor might prescribe for you to help your PCOS symptoms. You can find advice on what supplements, complementary treatments, and herbals may help you. This part also deals with how you can maximise your chances of having a healthy baby.

To help you on your journey, this part dishes out some advice on how to prepare yourself psychologically for some of those lifestyle changes you need to make to keep your PCOS under control.

Chapter 10

Let's Get Physical

*Y*ou may believe that you simply don't 'do' exercise. Perhaps you feel that you're too big, you're too busy, or that exercise makes you feel too uncomfortable. But, alongside watching your diet, exercising is the best way to improve your PCOS symptoms and improve your general health. Exercise has the added benefit of making you look and feel better about yourself. So what are you waiting for? Read on and discover that everyone can get more physically active – you may even start to enjoy it!

Reasons to Get Physical

Researchers keep finding out more and more about the benefits of exercise; from preventing certain cancers to making you feel happier! Obviously, exercising helps you burn calories, but for those with PCOS, it also reduces the symptoms of PCOS, such as insulin resistance, which then has the knock-on effect of improving skin, reducing hair loss, avoiding diabetes, and increasing fertility.

Although uncommon to be told that you can't exercise for medical reasons, you may be advised to start slowly and perhaps do one form of exercise rather than another.

 Always tell your doctor before you embark on any sort of exercise routine; he or she is sure to welcome it as great news but may need to give you some specific advice on how to start and what to do or not do when you make the first move!

Helps burn off the calories

Your weight is, essentially, the difference between the energy you bring in minus the energy you use up. Exercise is the energy-out part of the equation; the food you eat is the energy-in part. When energy out is greater than energy in, you lose weight.

Your body burns up fuel (which is what the energy-out side is all about) in two ways:

- **Your resting metabolic rate** is the energy you burn up by just trying to stay alive. Digesting food, breathing, and thinking all use up energy. You burn up this energy regardless of whether you're active at all. Medical experts call this the *basal metabolic rate*.

- **Your activity level during the day** is the energy you use up by moving around. It includes the energy you use up doing your chores, walking to the bus stop, cleaning your teeth, and so on, plus any energy you use up doing formal exercise.

You don't have as much control over your basic metabolic rate, but you can have a lot of control over how active you are. Ideally, your exercise regime should include formal exercise – a particular activity that you do for a specific amount of time on a regular schedule – and general activity throughout the day.

Compared to 30 years ago or so, people are now undertaking more formal exercise sessions, such as going to the gym, but are doing less and less physical activity in their everyday lives. Researchers believe that the everyday general lack of activity is as least one cause for the rapid rise in obesity levels. Formal exercise sessions are good and help boost your fitness and overall calorie burning in the day, but you also need to stay active throughout the day.

Think about it: If you go for a half-hour walk everyday, you aren't making much difference to your overall energy burning over the course of 24 hours – especially if you believe you have done your exercise for the day and behave like a couch potato for the rest of the day. That half-hour can help to keep you fit and have health benefits, but it's not going to contribute much to your daily energy output. Keeping active as much as you can all day long helps you burn up calories better than a short sharp burst of activity followed by little else.

Formal exercise

So how much formal exercise should you do every day?

> ✔ The American National Academy of Sciences recommends you do 60 minutes of physical activity daily. This level of activity may help offset that gradual gain in weight that tends to creep on over time.
>
> ✔ For maintenance of heart health and other benefits to the body, '30 minutes exercise on most days of the week' is the mantra supported by the UK government and the British Heart Foundation.

The exercise needs to be something that gets you slightly breathless, such as brisk walking, digging a garden, cutting the grass, swimming, and cycling. For example, if you do 30–35 minutes of moderately intense exercise (such as jogging or cycling), you burn up an extra 300 calories a day. If you do this for 5–7 days a week you can burn off the equivalent of an extra 1500–2100 calories in a week. This expended energy is equivalent to burning off a whole day's calorie intake in just one week.

General activity

If you engage in some type of formal exercise regime, great. But what about working on your general level of activity for the rest of the day?

Facts and figures on exercise and weight loss

Research done by the National Weight Control Registry (a register of around 4000 people who have successfully maintained a minimum 15 kilograms weight loss for at least one year) has shown that:

✔ Around 90 per cent of people registered used both diet and physical activity to lose weight; only 9 per cent of successful weight losers used diet alone. However only 1 per cent managed to lose weight using exercise alone. What this means is that the combination of physical activity and watching your calorie intake is more effective for weight loss – and maintenance of weight loss – than cutting calorie intake alone.

✔ A common factor that predicted the successful maintenance of weight loss was participating in a high level of physical activity. In fact the registrants appear to do 60–90 minutes of moderately intense physical activity a day (equivalent to brisk walking, cycling, or jogging at a rate of around 250–350 calories an hour), amounting to around 2500 calories a week being expended.

✔ Amongst the registrants, walking appeared to be the most popular form of physical activity, but most people also engaged in some other planned exercise sessions too. In fact only 28 per cent used just walking as their exercise whereas about 50 per cent combined walking with another form of planned physical activity, such as aerobic classes, cycling, and swimming.

✔ A sample of the registrants were fitted with a pedometer to find out how much they walked a day: They walked 5½ to 6 miles a day or 11,000 to 12,000 steps.

Here are some ideas on how you can get more active everyday:

- ✔ Take the stairs rather than the lift.
- ✔ Abandon the remote control for everything that uses them in your home so that you have to physically get up and move to the machine you're controlling.
- ✔ When watching TV, try to incorporate some sort of exercise, such as using a resistance band (a stretchy rubber tube with handles either side) so that you give your muscles some resistance training.
- ✔ Household chores can burn up extra calories, especially when done with a lot of elbow grease; so get polishing, vacuuming, and stretching up for those cobwebs; don't think of it as a chore, but as a mini-workout!

To prove how being more active during your waking time can make a real difference to your weight, you just need to look at twitchers. Twitchers are people who just can't keep still; they're always doing something like jiggling their leg while sitting down or wriggling around in their seat. Twitchers tend to be lighter than those who sit perfectly still. So although you don't need to become a twitcher (too much twitching can annoy others!), you do need to try to invent ways to expend more energy during your waking day, especially if your job is sedentary.

Calorie cost of various exercises

To lose half a kilogram in weight, you have to be in negative calorie balance by around 3500 calories. For this reason exercise alone is unlikely to burn up enough calories for you, unless you're working out intensely every day, which is impractical for most people and not necessary to maintain health. This equation works in reverse too, so that to gain half a kilogram in weight you need to eat an extra 3500 calories.

Table 10-1 gives you an idea of what you can burn up by performing the activities listed. The figures listed are for a woman weighing 64 kilograms and performing the activity for 30 minutes.

You burn up more calories if you're heavier to start with because it takes more work for you to move your body around.

Table 10-1	Energy Costs of Various Activities
Activity	*Energy Cost (Cals per 30 Minutes)*
Leisurely walking	80
Very brisk walking	200
Low impact aerobics	185

Activity	Energy Cost (Cals per 30 Minutes)
High impact aerobics	235
Rowing machine, moderate	235
Stationary cycle machine	235
Weight lifting	101
Bicycling 12–14 mph	269
Skipping (jump rope)	336
Running 5 mph	267
Boxing/sparring	302
Golf (carrying clubs)	185
Tennis	235
General housework	118
Mowing lawn with push hand mower	185
General gardening	151
Shovelling snow by hand	202

Pumps up the metabolism

The energy you use up maintaining all your metabolic functions while the body is at rest accounts for the largest amount of your overall calorie expenditure.

When you exercise, you not only burn up calories during the exercise, but you also keep your metabolism going at a slightly higher notch for an hour or so after you have worked out.

Muscle is far more metabolically active than fat. So part of your exercise routine needs to try to build up more muscle (see the 'Resistance work' section later in this chapter) and convert some of your fat to muscle. Muscle is heavier than fat, so that you can actually lose a lot of your body fat but not register any weight loss on the scales; you may, however, notice it in your dress size and how toned you generally look. The more muscle you have on your body, the higher your metabolic rate is, and the faster your rate of burning calories, even when asleep!

As you get older, you tend to lose muscle mass as a natural consequence of ageing, especially from the upper body. Muscle tends to turn to fat and congregates around your middle, just where you don't want it! But you can fight back; by exercising regularly and combining that with working your upper body with a few weights, you can offset that muscle loss.

Losing weight, especially if it is done rapidly, can result in muscle tissue being lost as well as fat. Your scales may register a weight loss, but don't believe it's all good news! If you don't concurrently exercise while losing weight gradually, you lose a lot of your muscle and consequently lower your metabolic rate too. If you subsequently put some weight back on, it goes back on as fat and then if you lose this again by dieting and not exercising, you lower your muscle mass and metabolic rate even more, hence making it harder to avoid further weight gain.

Invest in some body fat measuring scales so that you can keep an eye on what's happening to your body fat level as you lose weight. See Chapter 5 for more details on how to interpret these scales.

Makes you look great

Having PCOS may make you feel unattractive, but exercise can help. By exercising, you get:

- ✔ A warm glow to your face and your skin looks less sallow.

- ✔ More definition and sculpturing of the body as your muscles develop, even if you don't lose weight. Women don't tend to build up bulk in their muscles like men, but their muscles definitely become more defined.

- ✔ More of a defined waist as your waist circumference decreases, which is a great PCOS symptom-reducer. Clothes hang much better on your more sculptured frame.

- ✔ Improved moods, confidence, and feelings of well-being. When you feel good inside, you look better on the outside too!

Makes you feel great

After about ten minutes of the kind of exercise that gets you slightly out of breath, the body starts to produce hormones called endorphins which give you a natural high and happy feeling. In fact you typically feel more energised after you've exercised than before (unless of course you've overdone it!). Getting active is now known to overcome depression and generally lift mood, both side effects of PCOS.

Other health benefits

Here are some other positive health effects of exercise:

- ✔ Reduces the risk of osteoporosis (brittle bones).
- ✔ Reduces the risk of getting certain cancers including breast cancer.
- ✔ Raises the level of 'good' cholesterol (HDL) in the blood and so helps to protect you from heart disease.
- ✔ Generally reduces the risk of developing heart disease and strokes.
- ✔ Lowers blood pressure.
- ✔ Makes you feel less tired and lethargic when you do regular exercise, and you may find that you can get away with needing less sleep.
- ✔ Helps your bowels to stay regular and be less sluggish; hence, you're less likely to get constipated.
- ✔ Helps you to look and feel younger, and may also help you live longer!
- ✔ Generally raises feelings of well-being and reduces stress and anxiety levels.

Being active protects from a variety of cancers

People with the lowest cancer risks are those who have healthy body weights and who engage in the most physical activity. Not moving around enough increases your risk of colon and breast cancer: Being very active can probably halve your risk of colon cancer. Physical activity protects against breast cancer in women both before and after their menopause. But scientists have seen the greatest risk reductions in women who are active early on in life before menopause. As with bowel cancer, physical activity probably reduces breast cancer risk by lowering levels of insulin, hormones, and growth factors. Some evidence exists that physical activity can alter oestrogen metabolism to produce weaker versions of this hormone and so reduce the cancer-promoting effect that oestrogen can have on the body.

Inactivity may also be linked to cancers of the womb and lung. A recent analysis of several studies found that high physical activity reduced the risk of lung cancer by about 30 per cent. Being active may reduce lung cancer risk by improving the lung's efficiency. This may reduce the time that cancer-causing chemicals spend in the lung, as well as lowering their concentration.

Being overweight and obese can greatly increase your risk of cancer, and if you have PCOS you're more likely to carry some extra weight. So you're adding to this already increased risk if you're also inactive. For reduction of cancer rate, the amount of exercise suggested is 30 minutes of moderate physical activity, five times a week.

Regular exercise reduces fatigue

Frequently feeling listless and tired is a symptom of PCOS, but the good news is that recent research in the US shows that regular exercise plays a significant role in increasing energy levels and reducing fatigue.

When you're feeling tired and fatigued the last thing you want to do is exercise, but if you're physically inactive and tired, being just a bit more active helps. Health professionals encourage regular exercise to prevent or improve symptoms of conditions such as diabetes, heart disease, and obesity. In addition, the latest scientific evidence shows that regular exercise works even better than drugs in people suffering from fatigue.

A review has shown that nearly every population group, from healthy adults to cancer patients, to those with chronic conditions such as diabetes and heart disease, benefit from exercise. Although it seems counter-intuitive that expending energy through exercise increases feelings of energy and reduces fatigue, the drop in fatigue levels is probably due to the marked increases in the levels of energy-promoting and mood-enhancing neurotransmitters such as dopamine, and serotonin.

Reduces the symptoms of PCOS

Being physically active can help reduce most PCOS symptoms, mainly by reducing insulin resistance.

Insulin resistance occurs fairly commonly in PCOS. Most of the resistance occurs mainly in the muscle. This means that muscle tissue is unable to properly utilise insulin so that more insulin has to be pumped out by the pancreas before it can start to have an effect. Being physically inactive further aggravates the insulin resistance. So by incorporating plenty of physical activity you get these benefits:

✔ You make your body more receptive to the effects of insulin. Thus less insulin is required to be pumped out.

✔ You increase the rate at which glucose gets used up (to help generate energy for the muscles). This means that less insulin is needed to bring down blood sugar levels.

✔ Lowered insulin levels lead to a more regular menstrual cycle, and so to better fertility and fewer symptoms such as acne and hirsutism.

✔ If you are at risk of developing type 2 diabetes, increasing your exercise level (even if you don't actually lose weight) can lower your likelihood of developing full blown diabetes.

In addition, accumulating fat around the tummy is what PCOS women seem to do well. And having fat around this area makes it more likely that you develop insulin resistance and all the PCOS symptoms that go with this, such as acne and hirsutism, as well as more seriously increasing your risk of having type 2 diabetes and heart disease.

The good news is that research has shown that exercise may be especially helpful in reducing the size of fat cells around the waistline and more so than diet alone. Among a group of obese women who were placed on a regimen of calorie cutting alone or diet plus exercise, those who exercised showed a reduction in the size of fat cells around the abdomen. Women who only dieted showed no such change. However, both groups trimmed about the same amount of fat cells from the hip area. So exercise was targeted at the waist – the most dangerous place to be carrying fat.

Ground Rules Before You Start

In the same way that you have to plan before embarking on a diet, you need to think about a strategy before you start on a new exercise regime. Lack of planning, and not thinking realistically about what you are hoping to achieve, is one of the major reasons for failing to sustain any lifestyle change.

First, visit the doc

If you have a medical condition, such as PCOS and are overweight, tell your doctor whenever you plan to join any classes or engage in more taxing exercise.

Your doctor may want to check your heart and lungs. If you've had any joint problems or are quite severely overweight, he or she may advise you which exercises to avoid to start with.

Overcoming common barriers

Unfortunately 50 per cent of people who start on an exercise programme drop out within six months, and this seems to be more the case in people who are carrying extra weight. The good news is that if you can keep up an exercise routine beyond the six months, you'll have well and truly got that routine licked and are likely to retain it for the long term.

Table 10-2 lists common barriers to doing exercise and how you may be able to overcome them.

Table 10-2	Barriers to Physical Activity and How to Overcome Them
Common Barrier	*Possible Solution*
Lack of time	Time can always be made, even if it is only 20 minutes a day. You can always build exercise into your everyday routines and possibly save money. For example if you jump into your car to get to the station but always get held up in rush-hour traffic, why not cycle to the station instead (and save on carbon emissions too!).
Lack of money	Getting active doesn't have to cost money. You can do lots of things for nothing such as taking a brisk walk or even a jog. You can even make a jumping rope out of practically any old rope you find.
Lack of support	Embarking single-handed on an exercise regime can be daunting, so get a support network around you before you begin. Exercise with a partner, friend, or kids, and get your friends to encourage you along, or even start off with a few sessions with a personal trainer.
Accessibility	You don't need to be within easy reach of a gym or have access to a car. You can work out in your own living room with an exercise DVD. Or the big outdoors is only a few paces away with the opportunity to walk briskly. What about some skipping or trampolening indoors or out?
Previous negative experience	Many of you may have been put off exercise from your school days. Or you may have recently joined an exercise class and felt humiliated. But you can rise above that; find some friends who enjoy working out, and find out what they do and try it yourself.
Feel too embrassed because of appearance	You need to try to rise above this. If you want to join a class, realise that everyone else is typically too intent on their own efforts to be looking at you! Don some exercise gear that makes you feel good. Go with a friend for added confidence. If you feel really embarrassed by your appearance, start off at home and build up to more public exercise when you feel more confortable and confident about exercising.
Feel so unfit that you don't even think you have the energy to start	Everyone can start somewhere, however unfit. You'll be pleasantly surprised if you stick with it at how quickly you notice a change in fitness level, mood, and appearance. So start with 10 mins and build up. Maybe concentrate more on gentle exercise to start with such as yoga, pilates, or other stretch classes to get your body used to moving about first, before you introduce the huff and puff stuff!

Tailoring your workout

Bear these points in mind when choosing what exercise to do:

✔ Take heed of any advice your health professional may give you. If he or she suggests that you avoid certain exercises or begin with others, keep these restrictions in mind.

✔ Think realistically about how much time you can devote to working out. Don't sabotage your success by trying to do too much too fast.

✔ Plan exercise around your daily routine, such as walking to places rather than taking the car or other transport, or even cycling to the station or to work. Doing so helps you stay active throughout the day, an important component of a healthy lifestyle.

✔ If you have children, plan a physical activity you can all do together. Children learn by example but they also respond best if you can do things as a family. This can be swimming at the weekend or taking a long walk in the country on a Sunday.

✔ If you respond best to competitive sport, consider joining a netball, hockey, or even badminton club.

✔ If you respond best to working out in company rather than being a solitary exerciser, choose group activities such as cycle rides with friends or swimming with your partner at designated times in the week.

✔ You can exercise for free or pay for classes or a gym. You may want to mix and match: Attend a bums and tums class twice a week and then do a dance video twice a week too.

✔ Perfect the art of combining exercise with your social life! Why not go dancing and meet some new people too; check out your local adult education facility or town hall for dance classes. You don't even need to go with a partner for ballroom, salsa, or jive classes.

✔ You can find out about self-defence as well as getting fit by joining a martial arts class, such as Taikwando, or something like kick boxing which is very energetic!

✔ You do need some motivation, but if you know you're likely to run out of it very quickly then why not invest in a personal trainer and have some regular pre-planned sessions with him or her.

Remember you can only keep up regular physical activity if you enjoy it and it fits in to your daily life.

Not All Exercise Is the Same

To get the full benefit of being active, and especially to have the biggest chance of reducing your PCOS symptoms, you need to do a mixture of three different types of exercise to get the full body benefit:

✔ Aerobic exercise

✔ Resistance training

✔ Gaining and maintaining flexibility

These types of exercise are sometimes known as the 3 Ss: Stamina, Strength, and Suppleness respectively. Each different form of exercise has different effects on the body and exerts different benefits. Ideally you need a combination of all three types of exercise during the week. The amount of exercise that you should do for each type each week is as follows:

✔ Do aerobic exercises every day if possible, but at least for five days of the week and for half-an-hour minimum each time. Don't forget that you can do your aerobic exercise in 10 minute bouts throughout the day.

✔ Do resistance exercises 2–3 times a week but leave a day between each session if you can, or exercise a different set of muscles if you're training on consecutive days.

✔ Stretch after every aerobic work out.

✔ Do some flexibility exercises as part of your stretching after each aerobic work out. If you find it relaxing do a pilates, t'ai chi, or similar class (see the later section 'Maintaining flexibility'); you can then do one of these once a week or every day if you prefer.

Aerobic exercise

One definition of aerobic exercise is: 'Sustained exercise that uses large muscle groups and places demands on the cardiovascular system.' In other words, the type of exercise that gets your heart pumping and gets you a bit breathless.

Here are some reasons why you need to undertake some aerobic activity if you have PCOS:

✔ It improves the condition of your heart and lungs.

✔ It reduces insulin levels and insulin resistance.

✔ It lowers blood sugar levels.

✔ It helps lower blood pressure.

✔ It lifts your mood.

✔ It speeds up your metabolism and makes you burn up more calories, both during and after exercise.

Aerobic exercise explained

Any exercise that gets you slightly breathless and warms you up can be called aerobic, including walking (if done briskly enough), jogging, running, digging the garden, and dancing.

Experts recommend that as a minimum, you do at least half-an-hour of some sort of aerobic activity, five times a week. If you haven't done any aerobic exercise for a while, you may need to start slowly and visit the doctor before you start.

If getting the time to do a solid half-an-hour of aerobic exercise is difficult, doing it in bouts of 10 minutes is fine. This can include things like walking briskly to the bus stop, taking another brisk walk at lunch-time, and cutting your lawn or pushing the vacuum cleaner around the house briskly for 10 minutes in the evening.

Fit yourself with a pedometer

Pedometers are a little gizmo which you fit to your waist band that measures how much you walk in a day (it actually tells you how many steps you take each day).

Thinking that you're more active and walk farther or longer than you actually do is common. Pedometers can give you a more accurate picture of how active you are. You may find that you spend much of your day behind a desk, in front of a computer, or otherwise sitting down. You may be shocked to find out how few steps you take in a typical day.

Taking a minimum of 10,000 steps per day is recommended.

Pedometers can be a great motivational tool as you see your step count climb. A quick check lets you see at a glance how active you've been, and spur you on to get in a few more steps. Keeping a log of your steps may help motivate you to keep it up. The steps can also be translated into actual distance and calories burnt, and your pedometer instructions should be able to help you do this. The instructions should also tell you how to wear the pedometer properly so that it records your steps accurately.

Use the first week with your pedometer to establish a baseline for future comparison. That is, go about your normal daily routine while wearing your pedometer but don't change your activity pattern. After you see what you've been doing, you can determine if you need to be more active. Set a goal that you can reach, for example, an additional 200 steps per day. When you have established this new level of activity, you can set a new goal for yourself.

Walking as a form of aerobic activity

Walking is cheap, easy, and good for you. If you're a PCOS sufferer who's carrying around some extra weight, walking is an ideal exercise that doesn't put too much stress on your joints. Walking is the least likely of all forms of exercise for people to give up on as they get older.

A regular walking programme can result in some of the following benefits:

- ✔ Lowered resting heart rate (which is a sign of general fitness)
- ✔ Reduced blood pressure
- ✔ The expending of calories
- ✔ Reduced stress levels
- ✔ Increased muscle tone

Obesity and high blood pressure are symptoms of PCOS and can lead to a heart attack or stroke. A walking programme can help reduce the risk of these serious complications.

Walking is a fantastic way to start introducing some exercise into your life, especially if you're a PCOS sufferer who has never done much or any exercise before, because you can start really slowly! Walking is a simple way to exercise that doesn't require a lot of equipment or a special place. You can keep up your exercise programme even when you're travelling.

Experts recommend that you try to work your way up to about 45 minutes three to four times a week. That should be the goal, not something you do right away. Shorter distances and less time are the watchwords when starting out.

Resistance work

Resistance training includes weight training, weight machine use, and resistance band workouts.

Technically resistance training literally means working against a weight, force, or gravity.

Advantages of resistance training

Resistance training:

- ✔ Increases your strength, muscular endurance, and muscle size.
- ✔ Helps boost metabolic rate and thus fat burning capacity. Muscle tissue is estimated to be up to 70 times more metabolically active than fat – really important if you have PCOS!

✔ Helps reduce insulin resistance, which is vital to reduce PCOS symptoms.

✔ May help lower blood pressure, which has a tendency to be higher in PCOS.

✔ Helps offset osteoporosis (where bones become brittle and fracture easily), because bones are strengthened by bearing weight and by the pull of active muscles.

✔ Helps offset lower backpain and other muscular problems.

✔ Improves your balance and stability.

✔ Keeps your muscles primed and ready for action (with muscle strength and fuctionality it tends to be a case of 'if you don't use it, you lose it').

Research indicates that virtually all the benefits of resistance training are likely to be obtained in two 15 to 20 minute training sessions a week.

Practical aspects of resisting

Sensible resistance training involves precise controlled movements for each major muscle group and doesn't require the use of very heavy weights. You can incorporate this kind of exercise into your exercise routine in several ways:

✔ **Using your own body weight such as doing bent-knee sit-ups or abdominal curls, push-ups, and chin-ups.** Using your own body weight is convenient and free. However, once you're strong enough to cope with your own body weight, you can't add any more resistance without turning to devices such as resistance bands or free weights.

✔ **Using resistance bands which are like giant rubber bands.** The bands are portable and can be adapted to most workouts. For example, to work the biceps you step on the band and hold the other end in your fist and curl up and down. Unlike free weights, the bands provide continuous resistance throughout a movement. However, bands don't exert as much force on the muscle as a free weight, which means they may be better suited for gentle shaping and toning.

✔ **Using free weights such as dumbbells or barbells.** Free weights can be used to target every muscle in the body. Generally, you need a gym membership or a set of weights at home. However, beginners can use everyday household items for dumbbells, such as a couple of soup cans.

✔ **Using weight machines.** These machines are devices that have adjustable seats with handles attached to either weights or hydraulics. Weight machines are helpful for beginners because they guide the movement and ensure good form. However, you can't always adjust a weight machine to get the perfect fit for your body size and shape.

Getting started on your walking programme

Here are some ground rules before you embark on a walking programme:

✔ Wear a good pair of shoes; a sturdy heal support is imperative.

✔ Dress appropriately for the time of year, in layers so you can shed layers if you get too warm.

✔ Walk in daylight or well-lit areas at night.

✔ Wear reflective clothes if you do walk at night.

✔ Walk with someone else if at all possible.

✔ Don't wear headphones. They can prevent you from hearing a car or other forms of danger.

Most fitness experts suggest that you use weights that you can lift 8 to 12 times. You may then repeat this whole set 2 to 3 times. A good idea is to get some advice about which of these, or a combination, would be best for you and how you do the exercise. If done incorrectly weight training can end up doing you more harm than good! Leave an interval of 24 to 48 hours between resistance training sessions for a particular set of muscles. However, you can work on a different set of muscles within that time.

Maintaining flexibility

Being supple and flexible improves your posture and balance and allows you to maintain full movements throughout your body. Although this isn't essential to helping with PCOS symptoms, being flexible is part of the whole getting fit package that helps you to look and feel better about yourself.

Stretching

To maintain suppleness and prevent muscles and joints from stiffening up always stretch out your muscles before and after an exercise session, whether you're doing resistance training, aerobic training, or both. Here are some of the advantages of stretching:

✔ It enhances physical fitness.

✔ It can increase mental and physical relaxation.

✔ It can help reduce the risk of injury to joints, muscles, and tendons.

✔ It helps prevent or reduce muscular soreness.

✔ It helps to increase suppleness by stimulating the production of chemicals which lubricate joints.

✔ It may even help to reduce the severity of painful menstruation.

Never over-force yourself into a stretch or bounce yourself into it; you need to just let your body relax into the stretch or otherwise you may do yourself an injury. Again, get advice from a qualified fitness instructor, or a good DVD. If you have any injuries, muscle, or joint problems, certainly don't go ahead without seeking some professional help.

Flexibility exercise

Like muscle use, putting the various joints of your body through their paces and reminding them of the movements they should be able to do helps prevent you seizing up for good.

Lots of classes are offered that build in a high degree of flexibility, including:

- **Yoga:** a system of exercises aimed at helping you control your body and mind as well as improving your breathing and focusing the alignment of your body.

- **Pilates:** a form of exercise which aims to help develop body awareness, improve posture, and alignment as well as increase flexibility and ease of movement.

- **T'ai chi:** combines movement, meditation, and breath regulation with the aim of enhancing the flow of vital energy in the body, improving blood circulation, and enhancing immune functions. In China, around 200 million people practice t'ai chi everyday.

Pumping iron slows middle-aged spread

Research has shown that a twice-weekly strength training regimen slows down the accumulation of so-called middle-aged spread which tends to occur as you get older. And in women with PCOS, it tends to be something that happens without needing to be middle-aged!

Researchers took a group of women aged between 25 and 44, who were overweight or obese, and put them into two groups: One group was given advice about diet and told to exercise moderately to vigorously for 30 minutes on most days of the week (but no checks were made on whether they carried through any of the advice). The other group were given supervised robust resistance training by trained instructors. Both groups were told to keep their weight steady.

The body fat was measured using Computerised (Axial) Tomography scan (CT or CAT scan) at baseline and then after two years.

After the two-year period both groups had not changed their body weight, but visceral fat (the fat around the middle) had increased by 20 per cent in the group told to exercise and given dietary advice, whereas those that were trained to pump iron only gained 6 per cent visceral fat. Thus the weight training helped the women to avoid gaining too much weight around their middle as they got older.

Such classes also help to improve your posture, balance breath control, and reduce symptoms of stress. If you have PCOS, they're a very gentle way to start exercising and still give you a bit of a workout without getting too puffed. But when you start finding that moving about is a bit easier, go for some more aerobic stuff too, to have a real effect on those PCOS symptoms.

Exercise in pregnancy

Here are some general guidelines about exercise during pregnancy, which apply to all women, whether they have PCOS or not:

- ✔ If you have been physically active prior to becoming pregnant then carrying on as before is fine, providing the exercise is moderately intensive and doesn't go beyond about 30–40 minutes. So running marathons is probably out!

- ✔ Avoid exercise that involves long durations of intense training.

- ✔ Exercising aerobically 3–4 times a week is probably the limit during pregnancy, for no more than 30–40 minutes at a time.

- ✔ Non weight-bearing exercise such as gentle cycling or swimming is particularly recommended (although in late pregnancy you may want to stick to an exercise bike, as you're less likely to fall).

- ✔ Avoid any exercises in the first 3 months that involve lying flat on your back.

As soon as you know you're pregnant, check out with your doctor whether carrying on exercising is okay. If you have not been exercising before, check with your doctor what sort of things you can try to keep yourself flexible and fit but not add too much strain to your body! As someone with PCOS, you may have had problems with miscarriage in the past. Get some advice from your midwife or doctor about what particular exercise you can do, and what you should avoid.

Eating for Exercise

Unless you're training to be an elite athlete, you don't have to worry too much about what you eat to get the best out of your physical activity sessions. Just continue to follow the dietary advice throughout this book to help you with your PCOS. If you're following the low-GI balanced diet which is advocated for PCOS and following the guidelines laid out in Chapter 3, you're doing alright!

Here are some basic guidelines that can help you to maximise the benefits of your physical activity programme but which also provide you with a balanced diet suitable for your PCOS.

- Eat a wide variety of foods to ensure that you have all the nutrients your body needs to function at its peak.

- If you drink alcohol, drink in moderation but avoid drinking before or immediately after exercise.

- Make sure that you're well hydrated before you exercise.

- If you sweat during exercise, remember to drink extra water to compensate for the fluid lost in sweat.

- Eat plenty of low-GI carbs. Because the energy release from low- to medium-GI foods is more sustained, this type of food may help you to exercise more efficiently without running out of steam.

- Eat at least five portions of fruit and veg every day.

- Eat less fat and replace saturated fats with unsaturated ones.

- Eat moderate amounts of protein.

- Eat two portions of fish a week; one of which should be oily.

- Don't exercise on a full stomach or after a big meal.

- If you undertake regular exercise every day, eating smaller main meals with snacks in between is best.

Fuelling your workouts

What you eat before exercise can make the difference between an energetic, perhaps even peppy, workout and a tired, looking-at-your-watch-every-five-minutes workout. Follow these basic guidelines for fuelling your workouts.

Early morning workouts

If you like morning workouts (before your body has a chance to protest), try to nibble on something to avoid feeling dizzy and hungry. Make sure that you allow enough time for your food to digest so that you avoid a side-stitch or, worse, nausea. Try the following:

- If you're exercising within an hour after you wake up, eat around 200–300 calories before your workout.

- Avoid too much fat because it can hang around in the stomach for a while waiting to be digested and so make you feel uncomfortable when you work out.

Good food choices for early morning workouts include bagels, raisins, bananas, or a blended fruit and milk-based drink. Or try a couple of slices of granary bread with mashed up banana and a little peanut butter.

Lunchtime workouts

By lunchtime, breakfast is probably a faint memory. In order to avoid hunger pains and fatigue during your lunchtime workout, have a low-GI and low-fat carbohydrate rich snack one or two hours before your workout. Good choices include a milk shake, wholegrain crackers with peanut butter or hummus, yoghurt, fruit (fresh or dried), or a small bowl of a low-GI cereal. Also make sure that you eat a balanced meal after your workout!

After work workouts

The workday's done, you're on the way to the gym, and you're *hungry.* Does your steering wheel mysteriously turn your car in the direction of the nearest burger bar? That's because lunch was a long time ago and your body is out of fuel. You need to follow the same advice given for those who work out at lunch: Have a low-GI and low-fat carbohydrate rich snack one or two hours before your work out. Why not try some of the ideas given in our snack chapter (Chapter 8)? And, eat a balanced meal afterwards.

After the workout

When you're finished exercising, you need to replace some of those calories you burned; if you've worked out intensely, your glycogen reserves are likely to be low and need replacing.

Glycogen is your body's easily accessible source of fuel which gets converted rapidly to glucose during activity. Failing to replace your glycogen reserves (which are stored in the liver and muscles) means that you have very little energy reserves left for the next time you need to do anything even slightly energetic.

To replace your glycogen reserves, simply ensure that your after-workout meal is a good source of carbs. Having some protein with those carbs may further enhance the body's ability to restock glycogen.

Don't wait too long after exercise before you grab yourself a meal or a snack, otherwise you may find yourself flagging!

Chapter 11

Other Solutions: The Good and Bad

*P*COS was first named as a condition in 1930 and is now known to be one of the top reproductive endocrine disorders in the world. Diagnosing the syndrome remains problematic, because you can have so many varied symptoms. No final cure exists, but doctors do now know how to treat PCOS to keep symptoms at bay. Much of the treatment lies in your hands, because by adopting a holistic approach (following the right diet and lifestyle), PCOS can become virtually symptomless.

However, the growth in understanding of the condition is not helped by people trying to claim wondrous cures which at best can disappoint you and at worst do some real harm. This chapter looks at alternative treatments that have been advocated for PCOS including the low-down on whether they're helpful, or dangerous, or likely to do nothing. The chapter also looks at some of the medical treatments available for PCOS and considers what new stuff medical research has thrown up – or is likely to throw up in the near future – including on-going research regarding low-GI diets.

Eating a Vegetarian or Vegan Diet

People who avoid meat appear to have better health generally, live longer, and suffer less heart disease and cancers than meat-eaters. A possible reason may be that non-meat-eaters are generally more aware of their diet and strive to eat a healthy diet and take more exercise. Another explanation may be that a meat-free diet tends to be high in fruit, vegetables, nuts, and seeds; higher in fibre; and lower in saturated fat. Avoiding meat also puts less of a strain on the kidneys and may help to offset kidney damage which can occur if diabetes goes on for a long time without being adequately controlled. You don't need to cut meat out altogether – have a few meat-free meals now and then and use beans or pulses to provide your protein. Chapter 9 provides you with plenty of meat-free recipes that are quite easy to make.

A low-fat vegan diet improves glucose control

A recent study of some 99 individuals, half of whom followed a vegan diet and the rest the type of diet advocated by the American Diabetes Association (ADA), produced some interesting results. After 22 weeks on these diets the researchers found that:

✔ 43 per cent on the vegan diet had been able to reduce their diabetic medication compared to only 26 per cent of those on the ADA diet.

✔ The overall diabetic control, measured by the amount of glucose circulating in the blood over a number of weeks, improved by twice as much in the vegan group compared to the ADA group.

✔ Body weight decreased by 6.5 kilograms in the vegan group compared to 3.1 kilograms in the ADA group.

✔ Cholesterol levels decreased by 21.2 per cent in the vegan group and 10.7 per cent in the ADA group.

So the vegan diet followers appeared to do twice as well as those following the ADA advice, but both diets achieved success. However a vegan diet is quite tough to follow, and great care needs to be taken that it contains sufficient nutrients, especially iron and calcium. What this research shows is that, as well as following a healthy balanced diet, there may also be some merit in consuming more veggie meals or even meals that are just based on beans, pulses, grains, nuts, and seeds (because vegans don't eat any animal-derived products, their diet also excludes eggs, milk, and milk products, such as cheese.)

Avoiding Alternative Diets

Alternative diets are 'niche' diets that claim to eradicate your PCOS symptoms. They may not follow the usual rules on healthy eating, which is to eat a variety of foods, to have low-GI carbs, and to limit fat and salt. This section helps you to analyse these diets for what they are.

Low-carb diet

A low-carbohydrate diet contains a much smaller percentage of calories than the 50 per cent recommended by bona fide experts (see Chapter 3). On these diets you have to cut down or cut out foods such as potatoes, pasta, rice, and bread, along with foods containing sugar, and possibly fruit too.

As far as weight loss is concerned, some short-term success may be gained in following a low-carb diet, but no real data show the long-term success of such diets. The reasons these diets may work short term are:

- By following such a diet you're cutting out a large food group and thus restricting the number of foods you're allowed to eat, which means you eat fewer calories. Naturally you get bored eating fewer kinds of food, eat less of them, and lose weight!

- By cutting down carbs you tend to eat more protein (along with more fat). Some evidence exists that a higher protein intake helps to curb your appetite.

- On such a diet you tend to produce high levels of ketones as a result of the body trying to metabolise fat, especially in the first two weeks of the diet. High ketone levels can lead to feelings of nausea and subsequent loss of appetite.

But the real reason you shouldn't follow a low-carb diet is that the disadvantages (from your health point of view) outweigh the advantages. Here are just two of the disadvantages:

- You eat a lot of fat on such a diet which may increase your risk of getting heart disease.

- Ketones are highly toxic to newly-conceived babies so if you become pregnant on such a diet you're putting your baby at risk.

Here are some of the names of some low-carb diets for which you should get medical advice before committing yourself – some of them are more severe and therefore potentially more dangerous than others:

- ✔ Atkins diet
- ✔ Carbohydrate addicts diet
- ✔ Protein power
- ✔ Sugar busters
- ✔ The Zone

Detox diet

The detox diet is claimed to be the answer to everything these days and carries with it some magical air (probably because no one really knows what it's all about or how it works other than the diet somehow rids the body of stuff that ought not to be in there!).

Detox diets tend to involve only eating a very narrow range of foods. Limiting the range of foods consumed can lead to some weight loss, but you shouldn't stay on this sort of diet for more than a few days; the gains to your health and weight loss tend to be small. PCOS sufferers with big appetites who regularly feel the effects of low blood sugar, are likely to feel, frankly, awful on such a restricted diet.

The body has organs that deal with waste and toxins: The kidney filters and cleans the blood perfectly well in most people and the liver does a great detoxifying job providing we don't overload it too often (such as with regular bouts of binge drinking). However, the body prefers not to have to cope with unnecessary problems so don't imbibe too much alcohol and stay off any unnecessary drugs. If you do overtax your liver, a detox diet is unlikely to be the solution to reverse the damage.

Avoid products that claim to detox, especially if they claim to enhance the immune system, relieve pain, flush out toxins, and stimulate circulation. These products are very unlikely to have undergone proper medical tests, and such claims are only allowed after rigorous medical testing. In the UK, it is a criminal offence under the Medicines (Advertising)

Regulation Act (1994) to advertise a product in such a way unless it has been awarded a proper licence that proves it can deliver what it says and is safe to use. However, certain brands of foods or supplements sometimes still do try it on and advertise themselves with wild claims. They do eventually get caught and prosecuted, but in the meantime may have deluded many hopefuls!

Organic or additive/caffeine/ alcohol-free diets

Some diets work by making you feel guilty for eating ordinary food bought from the supermarket which may not have been organically grown, and may include the odd cup of tea or coffee and the occasional glass of wine. Just to reassure you, nothing's wrong with doing so!

Many of the books and articles on PCOS contain 'information' to make you feel very guilty. For instance, some diets insist you have to go organic and avoid every last E number or additive. Even that nice cup of tea or the odd glass of wine are guaranteed to evoke guilt! Most of these diets don't do you any physical harm (just mental anguish!), but they're unlikely to do you any good either. They're more likely to increase your stress and leave you unable to cope. Thinking about trying to eat a balanced diet and avoid weight gain is hard enough, let alone having to make sure that everything you have is additive-free and organic.

For a start organic food is expensive and not always readily available. Most nutrition experts claim that eating organic doesn't make you any healthier, but feel free to buy some if you think it tastes nicer (or if you have strong desires to support sustainable farming). Similarly the additives in food are often there for good reasons, such as keeping food fresh and reducing bacterial growth. Before being used in food, additives have to undergo rigorous testing and so come with a clean bill of health with regards to human safety.

Of course your diet is probably more nutritious if you buy as many fresh ingredients as possible and don't rely too much on ready-made meals which often contain excessive salt, sugar, and trans-fats. (That's why this book has so many recipes to choose from!)

Supplements: Taking Care Not to Over Do It

The best way for you to achieve peak vitamin and mineral status is by eating a wide variety of foods. However, if your diet has been poor or restricted to less than 1500 calories for some reason, you may need a full-spectrum multi-vitamin and mineral supplement. In the case of calcium and iron, a little extra in the diet in the form of a supplement may be beneficial in PCOS.

Supplements don't act as a cure but having an adequate vitamin and mineral status forms part of your overall armoury to fight PCOS. However, even with something as seemingly innocuous as supplements, you must take care not to overdose. Just because a little does you good, doesn't mean that even more does you more good. Treat supplements exactly as you do drugs, because they can have powerful effects on the body. With some supplements the difference between a level that is just right (the recommended daily amount or RDA) and a toxic level can be quite small.

Vitamin A

Vitamin A is necessary for the maintenance of healthy skin and hormonal balance which has led some people to claim that taking vitamin A in the diet, or as a supplement, helps with some PCOS symptoms. The evidence is still lacking, but you do need to make sure that you're getting an adequate amount in your diet, and this aim is best achieved by ensuring you take a good range of the products listed below.

Good sources of vitamin A include:

- ✔ Liver (but avoid if planning to get pregnant or are already pregnant)
- ✔ Carrots
- ✔ Green, leafy vegetables
- ✔ Yellow and orange fruits

Carrots, green, leafy vegetables, and yellow and orange fruits are sources of carotenoids such as betacarotene, some of which are converted into vitamin A in the body. They are a safe source of vitamin A because you can't as easily overdose on carotenoids – and if you do the consequences aren't so serious (you may, however, turn orange!)

If you decide to take a supplement containing vitamin A, never exceed the RDA because high-dose supplements taken long term can lead to osteoporosis (brittle bones). Furthermore, high doses taken at around the time of conception have been shown to increase the risk of birth defects in the baby. So make sure that you have enough vitamin A in your diet, but not too much.

Vitamin B6

Traditionally, B6 is the vitamin used to treat PMS symptoms. Vitamin B6 has also been used to treat PCOS, especially for symptoms such as acne. However, the doses recommended were at levels up to 100 times the RDA. Experts now say that a maximum of 10 milligrams a day of vitamin B6 should be consumed but such a dose is unlikely to have any effect on the symptoms of PCOS. Only take doses greater than 10 milligrams per day under medical supervision, because of the risk of nerve damage with high doses.

Calcium and vitamin D

Some evidence suggests that altered hormone levels in PCOS can lead to a loss of calcium from the bones. This loss is similar to that in women who have gone through the menopause (either naturally or due to having their ovaries removed).

Recent evidence has also shown that women with a high intake of vitamin D and calcium appear to have a lower risk of developing type 2 diabetes. Both nutrients seem to play a role in improving insulin production and sensitivity.

To get the calcium you need, drink 3–4 helpings of milk-based foods every day; a helping is:

- 125grams/5 ounce pot of yoghurt or fromage frais
- 175 millilitres/⅓ pint of milk
- 25 grams/1 ounce cheese

You have loads of low-fat dairy products on the market to choose from:

- Yoghurt
- Fromage frais
- Milk
- Milkshakes made with low-fat milk

And you can generally find lots of lower fat versions of normally high-fat products such as cheese, cream cheese, and crème fraiche.

Nothing is wrong with using some full-fat cheese if you want to add calcium and/or protein to a dish. Use a strong flavoured cheese and grate to make it go further.

Don't avoid dairy products with the mistaken belief that they are high in calories. However, if you need to avoid milk and milk products for allergy reasons you can use soya alternatives, providing you buy the versions fortified with calcium. If you really don't like these then you're going to need to take a calcium supplement daily which provides you with 100 per cent of your RDA.

Vitamin D sources are more limited but can be found in:

✔ Oily fish (or fish oil supplements)

✔ Eggs

✔ Fortified spreads

✔ Fortified breakfast cereals

Iron

Although absent or infrequent periods are common in PCOS, you may be one of the less common PCOS sufferers who unfortunately experience very heavy, prolonged, or more frequent than monthly, periods. If this is the case you may find that such loss of blood causes a drain on your iron reserves, and you therefore need to take care that you're getting enough iron in the diet; otherwise, you may become lethargic and anaemic.

Iron supplements can give rise to constipation and stomach upsets. So getting your iron from food is best unless your doctor tells you to take a prescribed supplement. Good sources of iron include:

✔ Offal

✔ Beef

✔ Pork

✔ Sardines

✔ Fortified breakfast cereals

✔ Beans

✔ Lentils

✔ Green vegetables

✔ Dried fruit

To absorb the maximum amount of iron from non-meat sources, eat it with a source of vitamin C such as fruit juice, a green veg, or citrus fruit.

Zinc

Zinc is thought to help hormonal-related acne and is believed to work best when coupled with adequate vitamin A in the diet. Some researchers believe that a lack of zinc in the diet leads to an increased production of androgens. Zinc is best obtained from dietary sources because zinc supplements may interfere with the absorption of other minerals from the gut because they tend to compete for absorption. Dietary sources of zinc include:

✔ Beef

✔ Pork

✔ Lamb

✔ Peanuts

✔ Brazil nuts

✔ Wholegrain cereals

✔ Pumpkin seeds

✔ Yeast

Chromium

Overt chromium deficiency produces symptoms of diabetes and insulin resistance. Modern diets, with their reliance on refined grains, especially if also high in sugar, may result in marginal chromium deficiency. You may read claims that chromium supplements help with weight loss and muscle build-up but such claims have never been proven in mainstream research. Chromium helps insulin to work efficiently and an adequate amount in the diet may help in reducing insulin resistance.

Chromium supplements on their own (rather than in a multi-vitamin) aren't recommended because a fine line exists between taking a safe amount of chromium and overdosing. Some cases have been reported where people taking regular doses of a supplement that provided more than the recommended intake developed liver and kidney failure.

To be safe, all you need to do is follow the balanced low-GI diet advocated in this book. This diet provides you naturally with plenty of the foods that are high in chromium, such as:

- Beef
- Liver
- Eggs
- Chicken
- Wholegrains
- Bran cereals
- Wheat germ (found in granary and wholegrain bread)
- Green peppers
- Tomatoes
- Onions
- Apples
- Bananas
- Spinach

Essential fatty acids

Essential fatty acids are deemed essential because your body needs them but can't make them on its own. If you eat a balanced diet that includes a wide variety of food you normally get these essential fatty acids from oils that you consume in your diet.

You actually require two types of fatty acids: One is an omega-3 called alpha linolenic acid, and the other is an omega-6, called linoleic acid. After these get into the blood stream they are converted into a myriad of important chemicals in the body. When incorporated into the diet oils containing a high level of essential fatty acids are believed to help reduce insulin resistance and improve glucose metabolism. Some people claim they can even help acne because they have a balancing action on hormones. Sources of these include vegetables, nuts, seeds, oils, and oily fish. You need to have a varied source of these every day in your diet. Getting adequate omega-3 fatty acids can be hard if you don't eat oily fish, in which case you may need a fish oil supplement.

Taking a Leaf from Herbal Medicine

A lot has been claimed for herbal medicines in the treatment of PCOS. The truth is that the evidence is still very sparse. If they were that fantastic then they would be recommended by doctors everywhere and news about them would travel like wildfire amongst PCOS sufferers. If you want to try them, stick to the ones listed below. Other herbal supplements may actually do more harm than good, and cases of liver damage are not unheard of with some dodgy herbal preparations.

See a qualified medical herbalist if you want to try out some herbal remedies. If you're on any other medication or are trying for a baby or are pregnant or breastfeeding, double check with your pharmacist or doctor that taking the herbal supplement is safe.

Agnus Castus

Agnus Castus is also known as chasteberry (because it was used by monks to reduce any horny feelings they may have had!), monk's pepper, or Abraham's balm. Agnus Castus is the dried berry extract from a densely branched shrub which grows in the Mediterranean and central Asia. You can easily buy the supplement in chemists or health food shops these days, and it is available as a powdered form made into tablets or capsules, or as a concentrated liquid herbal extract. This herbal extract is believed to help relieve many PCOS symptoms, including restoring periods when they have stopped.

When you take Agnus Castus, a whole cascade is set into motion:

1 First the extract exerts a hormonal effect via the pituitary gland in the brain.

2 Then the pituitary gland releases a hormone which stimulates the ovaries to produce more luteinising hormone and less follicular-stimulating hormone.

3 The result is that the balance of oestrogen to progesterone is changed in favour of progesterone.

Agnus Castus is also effective in reducing PMS symptoms. In Germany it has a medical licence for the regulation of hormone levels, and so something may really be in this herb that works.

The recommended dose is 40 milligrams dried extract, 40 drops of liquid extract, or 175–200 milligram capsules daily.

Don't worry, no evidence exists that it helps promote chastity in women!

Saw Palmetto

Saw Palmetto may help reduce hirsutism, but the evidence is still weak. Saw Palmetto supposedly reduces the level of circulating testosterone (an androgen) which reduces hirsutism. Traditionally this herb is used as a boost to the male reproductive system and as a treatment for prostate problems, but don't let that put you off! No side effects have been documented with this herbal, but also no long-term research on it.

Other herbals

Other herbals that may be advocated for used in PCOS include:

- ✔ False unicorn root
- ✔ Sarsaparilla
- ✔ White peony combined with liquorice
- ✔ Chinese angelica/Dong quai
- ✔ Blue cohosh
- ✔ Motherwort
- ✔ Nettle

A progestogenic action in the body to counter high androgen levels is claimed for some of these herbals, whereas others are meant to improve the skin or help the liver efficiently metabolise hormones. However, evidence for these herbs actually achieving these functions tends to be anecdotal.

Using Complementary Therapy in PCOS

Complementary therapies complement or offer an alternative to traditional medical practice and treatment and are unregulated by medical authorities. If nothing else, complementary therapy can be relaxing and act as a real feel-good factor in your armoury against PCOS. Unfortunately, evidence on the success of complementary therapies in PCOS tends to be anecdotal rather than science-based. Of course the defenders of complementary therapy may tell you that is because research money is only available for testing drugs, because testing is paid for by the big pharmaceutical companies who have little interest in testing 'natural' therapies which hold little profit margin for them. So the debate rages on!

Complementary therapy should be used as an adjunct to mainstream treatment. Don't shun the medical profession and just seek help from the complementary side, because you may not get adequate treatment for certain symptoms which, if left unchecked, can lead to long-term problems. These problems include uncontrolled blood sugars, which can result in blindness and kidney damage if not treated, and absent periods which can give rise to endometrial cancer.

Some complementary therapies, and what they claim to deliver, are shown in Table 11.1.

Table 11-1	Complementary Therapies Claimed to Be Helpful in PCOS	
Therapy	*What It Claims to Offer*	*What to Watch Out For*
Acupuncture		
(The insertion of small needlesat various key points on the body.)	Kick-starts periods.	Requires that you are treated for one week or more every month.
Aromatherapy		
(Involves using essential oils to massage into the body and sometimes additionally burning in a vaporiser.)	Balances the hormones.	Long-term treatment is usually advocated.
Herbalism		
(Using certain medical herbs to treat symptoms of PCOS.)	Encourages hormonal balance and is a treatment of many PCOS symptoms. May be that harm. Do not use advised as an adjunct to diet and lifestyle changes.	Seek out a properly qualified herbalist or you may receive herbs as an alternative to proper medical treatment.
Nutrition Therapy		
(Advocating dietary changes and use of supplements.)	Claims to match your diet to your unique problems and circumstances.	Nutritional therapists are not dieticians and have rarely received the same standards of training. They usually advocate supplements, often in doses that are far too high.

(continued)

Table 11-1 *(continued)*

Therapy	*What It Claims to Offer*	*What to Watch Out For*
Homeopathy		
(The use of almost undetectable amounts of chemicals which are meant to stimulate the body to heal itself.)	A homeopath takes a detailed history and chooses a unique treatment for each individual. Individual PCOS symptoms can be targeted.	Long-term treatment is advocated as it may take up to 6 months to see a lessening of symptoms.
Reflexology		
(The stimulation of specific reflex points in the foot which are thought to link to energy channels throughout the body.)	Claimed to help regulate the menstrual cycle and aid relaxation.	No downside except for cost and may set up false hopes.

Following the Current Medical Approach

Unless your PCOS is mild and fairly symptomless – or you have managed to get your weight right down and are regularly undertaking physical activity – recommended treatment normally consists of a course of drugs plus exercise and advice on losing weight. The types of drugs you need to take depend on your symptoms. However, some drugs help several PCOS symptoms whereas others are more specific. Although the majority of this book focuses on diet and lifestyle changes you can make to help reduce symptoms, the following section explains some of the medical treatments and drugs you may be given.

Table 11-2 lists some of the common symptoms of PCOS and which drugs may be prescribed for them. The following sections go into more detail.

Table 11-2	**PCOS Symptoms and Treatment**
Symptom	*Treatment*
High cholesterol levels.	Statins.
Insulin resistance/reducing blood sugar levels.	Metformin, thiazolidinediones, acarbose.
Poor development of the uterus lining (the endometrium.)	Natural or synthetic progestogens/ progesterones.

Symptom	Treatment
Irregular periods.	Oral contraceptive.
Lack of ovulation/ infertility.	Clomid and chorionic gonadotrophin, follicle-stimulating hormone (FSH).
Depression.	Anti-depressive agents such as selective serotonin reuptake inhibitors (SSRIs.)
Excessive hair growth (hirsutism) and acne.	Anti-androgens, aladactone (anti-testosterone diuretics), topical anti-hirsutism cream, statins (new evidence emerging).
Obesity.	Orlistat, sibutramine, rimonabant.

Taking prescribed medication is not an easy way out to escape the hard work of exercising or dieting. Drugs tend to have side effects and can interact negatively with each other. Use them only if diet and exercise aren't having the desired effect on symptoms which require immediate attention.

Treating insulin resistance

Metformin, an insulin sensitising agent, is used in treating PCOS because it has been found to help in:

✔ Reducing insulin resistance and therefore high blood insulin levels.

✔ Losing weight.

✔ Reducing male hormone (androgen) levels.

✔ Restoring normal blood fat levels.

✔ Reducing the high long-term risk of heart disease in PCOS.

✔ Improving regularity of menstrual cycles.

✔ Improving fertility.

Doctors and PCOS medical experts are split on how effective metformin is in the treatment of PCOS. One of the problems with the drug is that it can give rise to an assortment of gastro-intestinal effects.

Other insulin-sensitising agents include the thiazolidinediones. These drugs do help to improve insulin sensitivity but some have been reported to screw up your liver and so are not always used as the first line of defence! They tend to be used more for slim PCOS sufferers who don't tolerate metformin very well.

Reducing blood glucose levels

Acarbose is a drug that stops carbohydrate being broken down into glucose in the gut. Unless carbs are broken down to their simple sugar state they can't get absorbed into the blood stream. The most common simple sugar broken down from carbohydrates is glucose. Once absorbed, it requires insulin in order for the cells to use or store it. Taking acarbose can give rise to some digestive side effects (basically wind) which are due to bacterial fermentation of undigested carbs sloshing around in the gut.

A recent study shows that treatment with acarbose in women with PCOS leads to reduced acne, better insulin response to a glucose load, and more normal androgen levels.

Regulating periods

Birth control pills are usually recommended to women with PCOS who don't want to become pregnant in order to regulate their menstrual cycle and perhaps to improve some of the PCOS-related symptoms. In women with PCOS who experience absent periods, the progestogen also helps protect their womb lining from changes that may eventually lead to endometrial cancer.

Many doctors are prescribing a fairly new pill on the market called Yasmin to women with PCOS because it contains an anti-testosterone agent which can help alleviate some PCOS symptoms.

Not all women can tolerate birth control pills; some women experience serious adverse reactions when they take them, especially weight gain and mood swings.

Drug treatment for acne and hairiness

Acne or excessive hairiness where you don't want it (hirsutism) are usually due to your body producing too many male hormones (although all women make some!). Oral contraceptive pills seem to work well for acne and hirsutism providing they contain an anti-androgen component, such as Yasmin. If you don't really want a contraceptive agent, ask your GP for anti-androgen pills on their own.

Because metformin helps to reduce the levels of male hormones, it may also be useful in reducing hirsutism in PCOS.

New research has shown that statins may help to reduce androgen levels as well as correcting some of the metabolic symptoms associated with PCOS such as elevated blood cholesterol levels. However, more research is needed in this area before they are generally prescribed for their testosterone-reducing properties.

Stopping build-up of endometrium

Medroxyprogesterone acetate is a progestin, a synthetic progestogen, that triggers a period (or menstrual cycle). The role of progesterone and progestogens is to maintain the healthiness of the womb lining, preventing it from getting too thick, which can lead to endometrial cancer if left unchecked.

Common side effects include depression, breakthrough bleeding, breast tenderness, mood swings, and changes in weight. For women not having regular periods, synthetic progestogens are a good way to induce regular periods in order to maintain good menstrual health, or to help start a cycle during fertility treatments.

Some women can't tolerate synthetic progestogens and do better on natural progesterones which can also be prescribed.

Treating infertility

Infertility is generally managed initially through lifestyle measures (diet, exercise, and weight reduction). If this fails the next step may be the use of clomiphine citrate along with something called chorionic gonadotrophin. When combined, these two drugs stimulate the proper development of the follicles in the ovary and thus proper ovulation. Ovulation is the release of an egg, and this has to occur before you can get pregnant.

Laser treatment of the ovary is being looked at and early indications are that it can lead to the development of normal ovarian follicles. The pregnancy rate among women who received this experimental treatment increased.

Medical treatment for weight loss and obesity

The idea of drugs for weight loss is that they can give you a boost in helping you overcome a weight-loss plateau. They can't be taken indefinitely, so sooner or later you always have to go back to dieting or keeping the weight off the hard way by exercise!

Orlistat

This drug stops you absorbing about one third of the fat that you eat. Because fat is so energy-dense (9 calories per gram) you can stop a lot of calories being absorbed using this drug. However, don't expect to be able to carry on eating lots of fatty food, oh no! Unless you also cut down on the amount of fat you eat, the unabsorbed fat simply leaks out of you in a rather embarrassing and smelly way! The gut can cope with passing a little undigested fat, but not too much! You may lose some of your fat-soluble vitamins such as vitamin A, D, and E with this drug too, so your diet must supply adequate amounts of these vitamins.

Even a low dose of this drug can be effective if combined with a weight loss diet. As well as significant weight loss, you may experience a resultant drop in blood pressure and a decrease in the harmful blood fat levels.

Normally you can't keep on it for longer than two years.

Sibutramine

Sibutramine is a serotonin-noradrenaline re-uptake inhibitor. Basically this drug helps you to feel more satiated; you don't feel hungry as often, or think about food as much, and you're less tempted to overeat. It may also boost your metabolic rate so you burn more calories.

This drug is contraindicated if you are taking certain other drugs, and you're not normally allowed on it if you have high blood pressure. Normally you can take this drug only for a maximum of a year.

Rimonabant

Rimonabant, an anti-obesity drug, is now being claimed as a wonder drug. It helps you lose weight, quit smoking, and protect your heart. It may even help you cut back on alcohol. Trials have shown that 33 per cent of people on Rimonabant lost 10 per cent of body weight and kept their weight down for two years. The second 33 per cent lost 5 per cent of body weight and also kept it down.

Rimonabant is an *endocannabinoid receptor blocker*. In their normal state, endocannabinoids act as nerve modulators (in other words, they can change the pattern of transmissions that go backwards and forwards in the nerve fibres of your body) and are produced when they are needed and then quickly deactivated. However, in conditions such as obesity, endocannabinoid receptors can be over-stimulated for long periods due to overproduction or not being deactivated quickly enough. This over-stimulation contributes to excessive food intake and fat storage, which can lead to obesity. So blocking the endocannabinoid system can counter obesity and help people to lose weight.

Some endocannabinoid receptors exist in the brain and fat cells. These receptors tell the body to overeat (and keep smoking). Rimonabant blocks the signals these receptors give out preventing them from telling you to overeat. Overeaters and addicted smokers have very active receptors of this kind. By blocking the signals, the overeater or nicotine addict doesn't have the same urge to eat or smoke. What the medicine appears to do is help people stick with diets, and there's an independent effect on fat cells that helps you to lose weight.

Because Rimonabant also seems to improve glucose tolerance and insulin resistance, lower certain bad fat levels, and encourage weight loss around the danger middle area, it may become the ideal drug for PCOS.

Rimonabant acts on the brain, and early indications have shown that side effects may include an increase in anxiety and irritability, but also an increase in libido, which can't be bad!

If your doctor feels that you may benefit from taking a weight loss drug, he or she should discuss the best option with you. You can't buy weight loss drugs over the counter and need to have them prescribed. Your doctor can also offer lifestyle advice so that the drugs act as a kick start and boost, rather than a main feature of your weight loss strategy.

Weight loss preparations you can buy

You can, of course, buy all sorts of slimming preparations. The harmless ones are meal replacement drinks where you have some sort of shake instead of a meal. However, avoid non-prescribed slimming pills or herbal preparations. Although many of the dangerous ones have now been banned, you may still find them turning up for sale in some places and some out there may still be dubious. The banned ones were based on dangerous drugs such as amphetamines and ephedra (also known as ma huang); both drugs can lead to heart problems and death. Recently some of the weight-loss herbals have been found to lead to liver toxicity.

A recent article in a scientific journal claimed that the use of performance-enhancing and weight-loss supplements is prevalent in the United States. These drugs are the kind taken by athletes to keep their weight down and their athletic ability high. However, they can equally be taken by someone just desperate to lose weight. The article reports much concern about the side effects of such supplements, and that the particularly dangerous ones to look out for are the caffeine-based herbal supplements because they can cause blood pressure to rise to dangerously high levels.

Bariatric surgery

Bariatric surgery is a term derived from the Greek words for 'weight' and 'treatment'. Although probably the most extreme measure for weight loss, bariatric surgery is now being recommended for women with PCOS who are obese and have tried hard and failed to lose weight. Bariatric surgery is not an easy option, even if you're obese. It is a drastic step, and carries the usual pain and risks of any major gastrointestinal surgical operation. Bariatric surgical procedures are major gut operations that:

✔ Seal off most of the stomach to reduce the amount of food you can eat.

✔ Rearrange the small intestine to reduce the calories you can absorb.

Several different types of bariatric weight loss surgical procedures exist, but they are known collectively as bariatric surgery. They are an extreme solution for when it is imperative for health that weight is lost and when all other routes of less drastic weight loss have been tried. Surgery is always associated with risks and the procedure leaves you with a lot of pain and discomfort afterwards.

Bariatric surgery works by compelling people who have had the surgery to change their eating habits radically, and makes them very ill if they overeat. After bariatric surgery is performed, patients remain at a lifelong risk of nutritional deficiencies. So this surgery is not an easy choice for weight loss, but one to be considered with care after weighing up the pros and cons.

Chapter 12

Balancing Mind, Body, and Spirit

- -

In This Chapter

▶ Psyching-up for the job ahead

▶ Thinking positively

▶ Keeping a holistic outlook on life

▶ Asserting your needs

- -

*T*o achieve maximum results when attempting to improve your health, you need to balance the whole body both mentally and physically. Looking at diet and exercise without paying attention to the state of your mind, such as worries or stress levels, can't give you the results you seek.

This chapter looks at how you can psych yourself up for the challenge ahead of reducing your PCOS symptoms as much as possible. This chapter helps you to motivate yourself to keep to a diet and exercise regime while staying stress free.

Psyching-up for the Task Ahead

Like any task you're about to embark on, changing your diet and lifestyle isn't something that you can launch straight into. You have several stages to go through before you get on with it. Listed below are the eight steps of a cunning plan to help you achieve your goal of changing your lifestyle in order to help reduce your PCOS symptoms.

Following the eight-point plan

Here's a quick eight-point plan, and some of these issues are picked up again later in the chapter:

1. **Decide why you feel that you need to change your diet, lifestyle, or both.**

2. **Decide what changes need to be made.**

3. **Make a list of advantages of changing compared to the disadvantages.**

   Do the advantages outweigh the disadvantages? If the answer is yes then proceed and when you feel at a low ebb later on you can refer back to the list and see just why you need to stick to your plan! If no, you may need to go back and re-think the list in a few weeks time, because you are likely to fail if you embark on change at this stage or in your present mindset!

4. **Check when the best time to embark on your positive changes is likely to be.**

   Your doctor may have told you that you need to do something immediately for the sake of your health. But you may want to put it off until you have prepared yourself or until that weekend away, or that wedding, or whatever, is over. But don't put it off longer than a week or so if you've been told to do something urgently or if you really feel that something needs to be done.

5. **Put together all the 'tools' you need for the job ahead.**

   The tools can include having the knowledge about what to do, getting rid of foods in your house that aren't conducive to the new diet, and getting in suitable alternative ingredients (such as the store cupboard lists in Chapters 6, 7, and 8).

6. **Improve the skills you need for the job ahead.**

   For example, if you are useless at cooking, find out how to cook (it can be fun, honest!): You can get more practice from books, from television cooking programmes, or you can sign up for a course. Do you know what exercises suit you best? If not, sign up with a personal trainer and have a read of Chapter 10. Even a one-off session with a trainer can point you in the right direction.

7. **Make plans and contingency plans.**

   You need to set out what your daily routine is going to be and when you plan to fit in your exercise. You also need to have some sort of a diet plan to follow. Make sure that you plan out your food intake and recipes at least two to three days in advance, and then make sure that you have the necessary food ingredients for each meal. You even need to think about what you want to do when you're invited out for dinner, have a holiday, or a special occasion to go to.

8. **Think about providing yourself with motivational support.**

    This can be telling friends and family how you'd like them to support you (such as asking them not to buy you chocolates!). You may need to plan certain rewards for each milestone (such as a massage, new jewellery, or clothes). You may want to plan to diet with a friend so that you can motivate each other. If you really struggle on your own, you may need to employ the services of a regular personal trainer or some sort of motivational counselling sessions. It may be that a slimming club or a private dietician is the best way for you to stay on course.

 Before embarking on any sort of diet or exercise regime, talk to your doctor first about what you plan to do. He or she may be able to refer you to a suitable therapist (such as a dietician, occupational therapist, or physiotherapist) who can give you some tailored advice about what is best for you.

Staying positive

Before you can be successful, you have to start off knowing that you are going to succeed! That's why you need to go through the eight-point plan outlined in the preceding section before you embark on any change in your life.

Following are some motivational tips.

Break a big task down into small manageable chunks

Whatever your goal is – to lose 15 kilograms or to get to the gym three times a week – it can seem like a mammoth task. Keep two things in mind as you deal with the huge mountain you have to climb that's looming in front of you:

- ✔ **You have to take the first step.** A Chinese proverb says that in order to take a journey of a thousand miles you have to take the first step. After you've made the first step, the next one is easier to make, and then the next one, and slowly the journey is well on its way.

- ✔ **You need to break up the task into bite-size pieces and then reward yourself for achieving each bit.** Set some realistic time lines of when you expect to achieve each small goal. With a weight loss of 15 kilograms you can just aim for 2 kilograms at a time. Your reward needs to be something that helps you to feel good about yourself (such as a hair cut or facial) or that you enjoy (such as a a trip to the cinema, or a new piece of jewellery). Avoid rewarding yourself with food!

Don't let failure keep you down

Because you're human, you make mistakes and fail from time to time. The secret of coping with failure is to understand that it does happen and to not let it drag you down for long. You need to shake yourself down mentally, and start again. Table 12-1 has some common causes of failure and advice on how you can overcome them so that you don't lose motivation.

Table 12-1	Ways to Stick to Your Weight Loss Goals
Problem	**Solution**
Having very daunting goals that seem impossible to achieve, such as a total of 50 kilograms to lose.	Break up the task into bite-size chunks, each with an achievable milestone which doesn't take longer than a month.
Feeling disappointment and demotivated when you have followed your diet carefully and done your physical activity, yet no weight loss results.	Weight does plateau from time to time and you should see it falling again soon. If it doesn't then you may need to write down everything you eat very carefully, being honest with portion sizes and every last nibble. Take a good hard look to see if you really are sticking to the diet you set out to follow. From time to time, it may also be worth ringing the changes of your exercise routine so that you give your body a kick-start again.
Drifting back into your old comforting ways of eating what you like and doing no exercise.	Look at the reasons you wrote down for why you wanted to improve your diet and lifestyle. Don't let a few lapsed days put you off track. Just shake yourself down and get back on track!
Repeatedly slipping up and failing.	Check that you haven't been too rigid with your goals and setting yourself up for failure.

Keep a journal

The act of writing the things down that you want to achieve, and how you can achieve them, is psychologically very positive. After your objectives and plans (both short-term and long-term) are committed to paper, you'll feel that you are well on your journey. Keep a log of your progress, such as what exercises you have done, your weight, your waist measurement, and so on; this log enables you to see your progress, or if you are going through a negative patch, you can see how well you've done in the past and how you encountered hard times before and came through them.

Chapter 5 explains how to keep a food diary: This record is where you list absolutely everything that you eat and drink, when and where you ate them, and how you felt when eating them. This kind of record-keeping enables you to build up a picture of why you eat and whether a pattern emerges that may need to be broken. For example a bad day at work may result in your raiding the biscuit tin when you get home!

Clear out the negative energy

You don't need negativity in your life because it tends to drag you down with it. Negativity comes in several guises:

- ✔ Avoid friends who get jealous because they may not want you to succeed and may try to bring you down if they see you doing well. Some friends and loved ones may be worried that you're going to change from the person they know if you are successful. You need to talk to them honestly about what it means to you to make these changes.

- ✔ You don't need to get all fanatical about feng shui; but the idea behind this philosophy makes a lot of sense. Create a sense of space around you and have your surroundings obey some kind of order. You may find that when you de-clutter your surroundings you have more energy, are less stressed, and are able to concentrate more on the job in hand. See for yourself how freeing and motivating a weekend clearing out the junk can be; you may find that you then want to clear out the junk from your own diet and lifestyle. And don't make it just a one-off exercise – take steps to ensure it doesn't build up to the same level of clutter again!

- ✔ Make sure that your doctor or any therapist you use isn't filling you with frightening thoughts, or trying to lecture to you about what you should be doing. You need someone who can fill you with hope and inspiration. Try having a word with them or simply ask to see someone else.

- ✔ Lack of money can be a very negative influence so try to sort out some sort of budget so that your income doesn't exceed your outgoings. If necessary see a financial adviser.

- ✔ Lack of time is another negative influence and continually chasing your tail is very stressful. Making time for yourself is a bit like physically de-cluttering your life; you need to think about what you do each day and each week and whether anything can be dropped. You may need to become more self-centred and say no to certain things.

- ✔ If other worries are playing on your mind, you aren't going to be in a positive mood for moving ahead on your diet and lifestyle plan. Writing down your worries or sharing them with someone else can help. Part of the new you is to tackle your worries and concerns head on and see if they can be overcome. Don't do this all at once but prioritise your 'worry' list and deal with the top priorities first.

Talk nicely to yourself

According to recent research, approximately 87 per cent of people talk to themselves as if they were their most despicable enemy! They call themselves 'stupid'; if they drop something they call themselves 'clumsy', and so on. This is no way to carry on! This sort of speak develops into a self-fulfilling prophesy! Start to talk positively about yourself and then start to give yourself permission to succeed so that you probably can; for example, 'I have strong will-power so can resist that gooey cake with my coffee!' Even if no one else has faith in you, you must have faith in yourself, and in doing this you may find that others catch on to your positive attitude about yourself.

When the challenge seems too much and you feel daunted, have some positive affirmation statements that you can repeat to yourself and have some of them posted in large writing around your house and work. Following are some examples:

- ✔ 'I'm looking and feeling good.'
- ✔ 'My diet is healthy and doing me good.'
- ✔ 'I like exercising because it makes me feel good.'
- ✔ 'Every day I'm one step closer to my goal.'

You can create your own affirmations, but they have to be positive and they have to be in the present tense.

Being realistic

No one should pretend that changing your diet and lifestyle is going to be easy. No change is easy. When you do something in a particular way for a period of time, your neural pathways get 'set' into doing things a set way, and the longer you spend doing them a certain way, the more entrenched those patterns become and the harder it is to change them. So if you always have a biscuit when you have a cup of tea or coffee, you almost get to depend on having that biscuit and you really notice the loss when you don't have it!

To break out of this cycle you have to re-programme the pathway to go a different route. The longer you do something in a different way, the more the old links get broken and you find doing things the new way habitual. This can work from not piling your plate with food and not having a dessert to always walking up the stairs rather than taking the lift.

Of course, things aren't that simple, because other factors come into play; for example, if you start cutting down on food and get ravenously hungry mid-morning, no amount of neural re-programming is going to convince you not to have that custard cream with your mid-morning cuppa!

The Holistic Balancing Act

The term *holistic* means being concerned about the whole person, rather than just focusing on different parts of the body or mind. You need to bear in mind how PCOS affects your whole body, including your state of mind, rather than looking at each symptom in isolation. In PCOS the symptoms are all related and often have a common cause that you can tackle when you see the bigger picture!

You can't isolate what's going on in one part of your life from the rest of your life. Although putting certain aspects of your life on hold for a while is fine (for example, forgetting about that blazing row with your partner when you need to focus at work), sooner or later you have to deal with this part of your life. So if something isn't quite right in one part of your life, whether it be physical or emotional, it can affect the rest of you and your body. Equally, if something is going really well in one bit, it can give your whole body a lift. Have you noticed that you can be feeling really awful one day, and then you get some really good news and suddenly life is rosy again and you feel physically so much better?

The next few paragraphs show you how you can balance the physical along with the mental parts of your life.

Physical wellbeing

You may feel that the physical manifestations of the PCOS symptoms are turning you into a physical wreck but you can do a lot to improve your physical wellbeing right now, including your physical external appearance:

- ✔ **Take a long hard look at what's in your wardrobe.** The general rule is to prune out anything you haven't worn for a year. If something is too small for you it does no good to say that you're going to keep it until it fits, because all it does is serve as a constant reminder of how you've failed. All your clothes in your wardrobe need to flatter you physically. If they don't, go shopping. You don't need loads of clothes, just some good quality separates that you can mix and match that work for you. If you're not sure what does suit you, see an image consultant. Go with a friend if it all seems too scary!

- ✔ **Always stand tall and be aware of your posture.** Good posture is flattering to your figure and stops you from getting odd aches and pains in your back, and so on. Like any new habit, the more you practice good posture, the more it becomes second nature.

- ✔ **Do some physical activity whenever you get the chance.** Even short bouts of 10 minutes that get you slightly out of breath are beneficial. You immediately feel physically and mentally better.

✔ **Change your image.** You don't have to go in for the full make-over thing, although having advice from an image consultant is a great treat, but you may want to try a new hair cut, or try wearing an outfit you wouldn't normally wear. You can even invest in some snazzy glasses or sunglasses.

✔ **Finally, get treatment for your PCOS.** Don't put it off. If you feel the treatment isn't working, ask the experts why not and what you need to be doing instead.

People with medical conditions often feel they're powerless and that their lives have been taken over by visits to doctors, being monitored, given drugs, and so on. However, with PCOS you can do a lot to help yourself, and indeed this is the most powerful thing you can do to help alleviate the symptoms. So don't be a spectator on your own treatment; take back the reins yourself and feel empowered and motivated by what you can actually do for yourself. Don't forget that all you're actually doing is to try to eat healthily and take some exercise, something everyone should be doing!

Perceiving that your physical appearance doesn't live up to what you think society expects women to look like today can be a real cause of low self-esteem, particularly in teenagers and younger women. If you feel under this pressure, don't resort to extreme tactics such as starving yourself. Extreme behaviour tends to give rise to more extreme problems. Bulimia nervosa is more common in women with PCOS than in women without it. For information on eating disorders and PCOS, refer to Chapter 5.

Mental wellbeing

Self-esteem is a vicious circle: the less you have of it, the less likely you are to pull yourself up by your boot straps and work on yourself so that you can improve your self-esteem. On the other hand, if you do make a start on making some changes, you get positive feedback; so making gradual improvements to your diet and health makes you feel better about yourself and that makes you want to continue to make those changes that make you feel good!

Here are some tips on how to psych yourself up mentally into believing in yourself and feeling good about yourself:

✔ Think about what you're good at, and not only work-related stuff. Write them down. Perhaps you're good at painting; being a good listener; remembering people's birthdays. When you next need a reminder about who you are and what you can achieve, have a look back at this list.

✔ Ask people you know well and trust to write out a list of what they think you shine out at and why they like you. This can sometimes give you some pleasant surprises. However, don't ask them to write out a list of your less pleasant attributes, at least not until you have an ego the size of a planet!

✔ Find out how to be assertive so that you can say what you mean clearly and can communicate your needs without being whingy, aggressive, or argumentative. Loads of assertiveness courses are available, and most work-places offer them too.

✔ Stop comparing yourself with other people; you can never be like anyone else because you're original and unique. On the other hand, do try to work out how some people achieve things in their lives, and take a leaf out of their book; this can act as an inspiration.

✔ Smile and never lose your sense of humour!

✔ Don't label yourself, or let other people label you as being ill, or some-what different. Feeling marginalised is enough to put anyone in a mental slump. You are you, and still able to reach goals and function very effectively in society, PCOS or no PCOS.

Stress: Know your limit

Some stress is good; it can motivate you to do things and give you a buzz about life. What you need to avoid is distress, and that's when stress gets pushed too far for you. Different people get stressed over different things and so situations that would send you berserk are what other people thrive on! However, coping with long-term ill health or uncertainty about how an illness changes or progresses is a recipe for stress in most people.

When you feel stressed you release a hormone called *cortisol*. A high level of this hormone has been associated with many of the same symptoms as PCOS such as:

✔ Increasing the likelihood that you're going to gain weight round your middle.

✔ Increasing insulin resistance.

Emotional speak

Here are some statistics about what women feel about themselves, and this is not women with PCOS in particular:

✔ 64 per cent are plagued by unhappy thoughts about their weight and shape.

✔ Over 50 per cent of women feel guilty about eating anything.

✔ 41 per cent are in a constant battle between dieting and exercising, bingeing, and giving up trying.

So having PCOS doesn't make it your unique pre-rogative to worry about such issues! Even so. the secret is to try to do something about your well-being without being totally hung-up about it 24/7.

Although acute and intense stress, such as becoming bereaved, can make you lose your appetite, chronic stress – when you're at a constant stressed-out state over a period of time – often leaves you reaching for food as a comforter.

The following sections offer ideas you can try to limit the impact of stress.

Getting enough sleep

Different people need different amounts; the average is around seven hours sleep a night, but if that still leaves you yawning and dopey the next day, up it by half-an-hour until you reach your ideal. When you get into the swing of regular sleep you find that you are more able to cope with the odd late night or sleepless night without it completely knocking you for six. You are also more able to cope with stress when you aren't tired. Don't forget that stress can tire you out in the first place and make you less likely to have a good night's sleep. If you're stressed, a wind-down bedtime routine is essential, such as:

- Having a bath.
- Having a hot milky drink (without caffeine!).
- Stopping work at least an hour before you go to bed.
- Avoiding exercise at least an hour before bed.
- Getting stuck into a good book before you turn the light out so that your mind isn't dwelling on the cares of the day.

Staying active

Do something physically active as exercise reverses the negative effects of stress hormones. This doesn't have to be a formal exercise session but may be a bout of spring cleaning or a brisk walk. Chapter 10 has some more ideas on how you can get more physically active.

Using relaxation techniques

Try some relaxation techniques. You can pick up CDs that take you through a relaxation exercise and show you how to breathe in the right way to help you calm down. Many people tend to hyperventilate when stressed which leaves them feeling dizzy, light-headed, and with tingling in hands and feet. Proper breathing can help you avoid doing this.

Keeping things in perspective

Put things in perspective by imagining your current situation and the worst thing that can happen in that situation. Try to imagine yourself coping with that situation. Also try to think how you're going to feel about your current situation in three months' time. These imagining techniques often help to put things in perspective and stop you making mountains out of molehills.

Maintaining a balanced diet

Your body doesn't cope with stress very well if it feels deprived of food or fluid. Make sure you drink plenty of fluid during the day, and not too much caffeine if you are prone to stress or don't sleep too well. Eating regular low-GI meals also helps your body to maintain a regular blood sugar level which helps you cope better with stress.

Don't use props to cope with stress such as caffeine or alcohol. They may help you feel better in the short term, but payback time comes eventually and when that happens you feel ten times worse coping with caffeine- or alcohol-fuelled sleep deprivation.

Strict dieting or eating an unbalanced diet is going to add extra stress to what your body already has to put up with. The best diet for de-stressing is to keep everything in moderation. If you need to cut the calories to reduce weight, the food you eat needs to be of good nutrient quality so that you don't lose out on your vitamins and minerals just because you're cutting back on the calories.

Other stress busters

The list goes on and on for what you can do to beat stress. Below are a few more examples – they won't all suit you, but you may find that one of them is just the ticket!

- ✔ Join a choir or take singing lessons! The breathing exercises you discover and the act of actually singing helps to reduce stress levels.

- ✔ Have a good laugh; they often say laughter is a good medicine and this saying contains some truth. Keep a few DVDs at hand that are guaranteed to bring a smile to your face and dig them out when you feel stressed or gloomy and see how much better you feel afterwards!

- ✔ Make plenty of time for yourself everyday. Use it to do something you enjoy doing. Now and then book yourself some indulgent time which doesn't centre around food. This can be a massage or just a long walk in the country.

Are you feeling happy? Dealing with depression

Being down is not going to help you to move on with your life; you may tend to want to wallow in it all! Depression can be something that hovers over you like a dark cloud for an afternoon or it can go on for months. If your depression is of the latter sort, you may need to get some medical help. Although everyone hates taking medication, you may need some sort of anti-depressants to help give you the impetus to sort the rest of your life.

Have a nice cup of tea

Recent research from University College London shows that having a cup of tea after a stressful situation actually brings down the level of stress quickly. And it isn't just the act of sitting down and having a cuppa. The researchers took two groups of people and gave them both drinks that tasted the same, but one group actually had ordinary black tea in their drink, whereas the other group didn't. The researchers then subjected both groups to a stressful situation and gave them the drinks. Those that had the drink with the tea in it were found to recover from the stress significantly more quickly than those who had the 'dummy' drink, and this was thought to be due to levels of the stress hormone, cortisol, being lowered more quickly in the tea drinkers.

Even short bouts of depression if they happen often enough can hinder your progress in tackling changes in your diet and lifestyle. Here are a few things to start doing – and a few to stop doing – in order to avoid bouts of depression:

- ✔ **Get enough sleep:** Lack of sleep can leave you feeling tired and unable to cope.

- ✔ **Don't take on too much:** This may be work, or helping out other people. You may need to cultivate some degree of selfishness in order to have the motivation to deal with your own challenges ahead.

- ✔ **Don't drink too much alcohol:** Although your cares may seem like they float away for a while, they can come crashing back down on top of you worse than ever the next morning and leave you feeling anxious and depressed.

- ✔ **Eat a good balanced diet:** Have plenty of food variety to ensure that your body gets all the nutrients it needs. Being properly nourished and free from any nutritional deficiencies, however slight, maximises your chances of not succumbing to depression.

A few promising studies of late have shown some benefit of eating plenty of oily fish or taking fish oil supplements to alleviate depression.

- ✔ **Don't isolate yourself:** If something is getting you down, try to talk it through with someone. This special someone can be your mum, your best friend, or even a trained counsellor. Sometimes sharing worries with other people who know what you're going through can be good, and so joining a PCOS network may help. With some of these networks you may be able to share concerns online and attend regular meetings where you can meet with other sufferers.

- ✔ **Treat yourself from time to time.** Massage or aromatherapy sessions are good stress-busting treats.

Excuses, excuses

You may always be able to find a reason for not adhering to your chosen self improvement plan. Life is so frantic and so full of snares that finding a good excuse for not getting down to something is easy. But at the end of the day you're only fooling yourself; you simply can't avoid the issue and bury your head in the sand! You may have some really good acute reasons which genuinely make you incapable of applying yourself to any self-improvement plan, such as a major family trauma of some kind. However, if you are just experiencing some of those chronic everyday stressors in life which simply have to be endured as part of life, you can still engage in some healthy eating and exercise. Indeed following a good diet and doing some exercise makes you better able to cope with everyday stress.

As well as having too many other stressors in your life, Table 12-2 has some other common excuses as to why you're unable to adopt a healthy lifestyle – and why they just don't wash!

Table 12-2	Excuses and Solutions
Excuse	*Solution*
I don't like many healthy foods.	Keep trying lots of different fruit and veg and less salty, fatty, and sugary foods, and after a few weeks your taste buds readjust.
I have to buy and cook different foods for the rest of the family and then I get tempted to eat their foods.	Why inflict less healthy food on the rest of the family? They can also benefit from a healthier diet; so tell everyone it's a family effort.
Other people frequently cook for me and when they have made something that shouldn't be part of my plan I don't like to refuse because it's rude.	If someone else cooks for you, tell him or her about your new regime and why following it is important. Kind cooks should understand. Give them some of the recipes from this book to try; they are mostly quick and easy.
Once I start eating, I can't stop!	Go for quality and not quantity. Don't let yourself get too hungry because this state can trigger a binge. Eat several small low-GI meals so that blood sugars stay on an even keel.
Food is one of my great pleasures in life.	Then enjoy it, take time over it, ensure it's delicious, and again go for quality and not quantity. Also work on some of those other pleasures of life, such as relaxing with a good book or going for a country walk.

(continued)

Table 12-2 *(continued)*

Excuse	Solution
Food calms me down and de-stresses me.	Somewhere in the past you started to use food as a comfort. This behaviour can be broken by using other ways to calm yourself down such as yoga, a brisk walk, a hot bath with essential oils, or just some simple breathing exercises.
I can't exercise because I was no good at it at school.	Very few people, except for those picked for teams, enjoyed school physical education sessions. Exercise is so much more than gym, hockey, or netball. What about dancing, swimming, or even fencing? Find some activity you enjoy and do it energetically.
I am simply not fit enough to exercise!	Then start somewhere, and build up your fitness levels slowly. Everyone can get fitter but if you don't use it, you lose it!
I don't have the time or money to exercise.	Fit in exercise around everyday activity. This approach may include cycling somewhere that involves a short journey rather than taking the car. This way you save money too!

Talking About It

Keeping shtoom about your worries and concerns is not the way to move ahead. Different people can help in different ways; some things can be shared with your mother, some with your girl friends, and some with your partner, but some may require some professional advice.

Use your friends and family

Talk to friends and family, especially when you're feeling low and lacking in confidence. Avoid friends who drain you or who always try to go one better than you. Instead, surround yourself with friends who have no ulterior motives. Being part of a friendship means that you confide in each other and share your worries and concerns. If you keep things to yourself all the time, people may think you are an 'ice-maiden'.

You can't always be the one who shares problems; to be a friendship, things have to work both ways. Sometimes offering a listening ear and support to your friend's problems can bring you out of your own slump or at least help to put yours in perspective.

Bring in the professionals

Sometimes if a problem is deep-rooted or doesn't seem to be resolving itself, or you just can't bring yourself to talk it through with even your nearest and dearest (and indeed they may be the root of your problem), it may be time to bring in a professional counsellor. Your workplace may have a counselling service, or you may be able to get some advice from your doctor on which professional you need to see. In the UK your local Citizen's Advice Bureau (www.citizensadvice.org.uk) can give advice on where to go. If you have got yourself into such a state that you need to ring up someone urgently to talk to, the Samaritan service (call 08457 90 90 90 or visit www.samaritans.org.uk) is always there to lend an ear and offer further advice.

Fanaticism versus Staying in Control

When do you cross the line from staying in control to becoming a control freak or even a downright fanatic? You need to be able to stay in control but not make having control rule your life and your every waking (and often sleeping) moment. When exerting reasonable control in your life becomes a fanatical behaviour pattern, that line has been crossed.

Eating disorders are the extreme end of something that many of you may struggle with, which is trying to stay in control without being fanatical.

People who suffer with eating disorders spend their whole lives obsessing about their diet and food. They impose a very rigid regime on themselves as a way of trying to stay in control. And for the short term, they follow this regime and feel powerful and confident. But they always set themselves an impossible regime to follow and soon end up slipping from it – which leads to a huge amount of self-loathing and stress for themselves. Sufferers try to get back on their strict regime only to slip again and feel even worse, and so the pattern continues until ill health forces them, or those close to them, to seek help to break the cycle.

So how can you avoid falling into the fanatics' trap? Following are some simple tips:

✔ Don't set yourself up for failure by expecting too much of yourself. Make your goal achievable and realistic. For example, 500 grams to 1 kilogram weight loss a week is probably achievable, whereas 1.5 to 2 kilograms is not; getting to the gym three times a week may be achievable, whereas every day may not be.

✔ Don't think of yourself as either on a diet or not on a diet. Feeling that you are 'on the wagon' is enough to make you want to jump off! Instead, just think of yourself as having chosen to eat a sensible diet in order to make yourself feel better. Don't forget that this new regime is probably something you're going to want to follow for life (with a few less calories if you are actively trying to lose weight). If you return to your old style of eating you may end up back where you started in quite a short space of time!

✔ Allow yourself to indulge occasionally. This indulgence can be allowing yourself to slouch around in your dressing gown all day rather than sticking to your exercise routine; or it may be to allow yourself an indulgent pudding now and then. However, grant yourself that indulgence without seeing it as the beginning of the end. Know that you need to be straight back to your usual routine the next day, or the next meal.

✔ Staying in control means being organised, but this degree of organisation doesn't mean being inflexible if something unexpected crops up. If too many things are happening that stop you following your chosen path – say you find that you can never get to the gym – you may have to rethink your plan and perhaps clear some space for the gym by saying no to certain things. Or you may need to find a way to exercise outside the gym environment, closer to home.

Chapter 13

Preparing for a Baby

. . . .

In This Chapter

▶ Maximising your chances of getting pregnant and having a healthy baby

▶ Taking positive steps for a healthy pregnancy

▶ Avoiding the danger areas that can harm your future baby

▶ Working as a team with your partner

▶ Overcoming disappointments and frustration

. . . .

*F*or some of you, the diagnosis of PCOS may well have been made when you went to see your doctor because the baby you were planning just wasn't happening. Infertility is a common and distressing symptom of PCOS and extra help is often needed before you can hear the patter of tiny feet. 90–95 per cent of women who attend fertility clinics due to lack of ovulation are believed to be PCOS sufferers. However, experts believe that women can do a lot to help themselves, so that a visit to a specialist clinic may not be required.

This chapter looks at how you can maximise your chances of falling pregnant. Also, because the so called 'pre-conception' period is as important as the actual pregnancy as far as the health of the baby is concerned, this chapter also looks beyond the fertility issue to how you can maximise your chances of having a bouncing baby.

Maximising Your Chances: Things to Do Before You Conceive

Infertility is not inevitable in PCOS but even if you are having trouble conceiving, you can increase your chances of getting pregnant by following some basic lifestyle rules. Changing your lifestyle just a bit may be all it takes to make the difference between being able to fall pregnant or not.

Getting fit and healthy doesn't happen overnight. You need to concentrate on a healthy lifestyle for three to six months before you start trying for a baby. Although this doesn't guarantee a problem-free pregnancy or birth, it may increase your fertility and the chances of having a healthy baby, while reducing the risk of a premature birth or a low birth-weight baby.

Weighty issues

Being able to conceive is very much affected by your overall percentage of body fat; being both underweight and overweight can reduce fertility. However, the risk of infertility rises if a tendency to store weight around the middle is present. This 'apple' shape type of obesity is very common in PCOS because it is a result of insulin resistance. In turn, this insulin resistance has an effect on the reproductive hormone levels in the body. If these are disrupted, the viability of the egg you release (which would need to become fertilised by sperm if pregnancy were to take place) is reduced.

Your fertility rate is therefore going to improve if

✔ You can lose some weight.

✔ You can lose the weight around your midriff.

Diet can help you lose weight, but to target weight loss specifically around your middle you also need to get physically active. Exercise can help you lose weight around the middle. Your doctor may also prescribe you the drug metformin which helps to reduce insulin resistance and thus helps to restore fertility.

Being overweight or obese prior to and during pregnancy is associated with several pregnancy problems, and the risks increase with the increasing amount of excess weight you carry:

✔ Even if you're not diabetic now, the stress of pregnancy is more likely to bring it on if you are also carrying excess weight.

✔ You're more likely to develop high blood pressure.

✔ You're at higher risk for developing pre-eclampsia (when blood pressure rises so high it can endanger the life of you and your baby).

✔ You're more likely to experience abnormal labour which may require an emergency caesarean section.

✔ Your baby is more likely to be born prematurely and be at risk for health problems associated with being born too early.

✔ You're more likely to give birth to a baby with congenital problems.

Fertility: Some hormone facts

Hormones play a huge role in getting pregnant and pregnancy, and because all the hormones seem to influence the action of each other, the issue is complex. If your body is resistant to the effect of the insulin (itself a hormone) that the pancreas is producing, the body has to pump out even more insulin in order to achieve the desired effect. This high insulin level unfortunately has a knock-on effect on other hormones, notably androgens. Now androgens are normally thought of as a male hormone, but women produce them too. In fact, they are produced by the ovaries. The follicles in the ovaries also contain the eggs, and normally, once a month, an egg is released from a follicle. However, in PCOS, the high level of androgens produced when the insulin level is high stops the egg from being released. This follicle, which has not released an egg, goes on to become the characterisitc cyst seen on the ovaries of PCOS sufferers. So no egg release means no baby. The key is therefore to reduce the level of insulin in the body.

Dieting to lose weight is not advisable during pregnancy; therefore, if you are overweight or obese, losing the weight before you try to conceive is important.

Eating right: Balance and variety are best

As well as addressing the weight issue, looking at the quality of the diet is important. All the nutrients need to be present and in sufficient amounts. Women who conceive while on a slimming diet are more likely to have low birth-weight babies. These babies are much more likely to have immediate as well as long-term health problems (see the sidebar 'Low birth-weight babies are at risk' later in this chapter).

At the embryo stage, which represents the first few weeks after fertilisation, your baby is at its most vulnerable as this is when its cells are dividing rapidly and differentiating themselves into the various body organs. Most organs, although very small, have already been formed by 3–7 weeks after the last menstrual period. And at this stage you probably don't even know you're pregnant! Any abnormalities that happen now can't be corrected at a later stage.

So improving the balance of your diet *before* you are likely to conceive is vital.

Variety in the diet is essential to ensure that every nutrient is covered and to provide little Bert or Bertha with the best environment in which to develop.

As a guide to healthy eating, make sure that you have foods from each food group (head to Chapter 3 to find plenty of information to help you maximise your intake of all the right nutrients and in the right proportions).

Having a balanced diet before conception is important, so if food allergy is causing you to eat a diet devoid of several foods or food groups, see a dietician to make sure that you are getting all the nutrients you require. For example, if you are milk-intolerant your body may become low on calcium and so you need to ensure that you get calcium in other ways, such as from fortified soya milk.

Fruit and vegetables

A minimum of five portions a day is recommended. This includes dried, tinned, and juiced. You can't include the same fruit or vegetable twice, and potatoes don't count. Try to get as many different colours of fruit and vegetables in your diet as possible, because the variety of colours assures an assortment of antioxidants which protect you from cancers and heart disease.

When having a meal, about 40 per cent of the food on your plate should be made up of vegetables or salad.

Starchy foods

Starches are your staples and include potatoes, rice, pasta, bread, cassava, and sweet potato. Try to have the wholegrain variety which contains more fibre. The number of helpings of these starchy foods depends on your overall energy requirement. When having a meal, they should make up about 40 per cent of the quantity of food eaten. An average woman requires about four to five portions of starchy foods a day. Carbohydrates should make up 50 per cent of the calories from your diet.

Starchy foods help to fill you up without providing too many calories. Wholegrain and unrefined starches are more likely to have a low glycaemic index (GI) which helps normalise insulin secretion (which in turn can improve fertility). More details on how to follow a low-GI diet are found in Chapter 4.

Protein

You only need two portions of this group a day which includes meat, fish, cheese, eggs, nuts, and beans. When having a meal, the protein part should only take up about 20 per cent of the plate. Proteins should make up around 15 per cent of the calories from your diet.

Dairy

You need three to four helpings of these foods a day to ensure that you get sufficient calcium in your diet. If you can't tolerate milk products, you need to seek advice from a dietician regarding appropriate alternative foods. This group includes cheese, milk, and yoghurts. A portion is equivalent to 1 small pot of yoghurt (150 millilitres or 5 fluid ounces), 28 grams (1 ounce) of cheese, and 190 millilitres (⅓ pint) of milk.

Fats/oils and sugars

These foods include pastries, oils, jams, sweets, sugary foods, margarine, and butter. All these foods need to be kept to a minimum because they can lead to weight gain, but add little nutritional value. Excess sugar can also contribute to dental caries, and excess fat can contribute to heart disease. Fats should make up no more than 35 per cent of the calories from your diet.

Some oil is needed in the diet, but not a lot. Oils and fats can provide essential fatty acids and fat soluble vitamins. Although weight-for-weight all oils and fats contribute the same number of calories, and are very calorie dense, some are better for heart health than others and, in small amounts, may positively protect against heart disease. Such oils include the mono-unsaturated fats found in olive oil, rapeseed oil, nuts, and avocados. Fish oils are also beneficial to health, as are some seeds and rape seed oil which contain a high percentage of omega-3 fats.

Trans and saturated fats found in cheaper margarine, cakes, and pastries, and fats derived from animal products, are particularly harmful to the heart and health. During pregnancy, trans fat can bring unique health risks because of the way trans fat interferes with the body's use of omega-3 fats. These fats are essential building blocks for the brain and the eyes of a developing baby so a high trans fat diet during pregnancy (or indeed during breast-feeding) can affect the growth of these organs in the baby.

Supplements

If your diet has been poor and you're thinking of trying to conceive, taking a multivitamin and mineral supplement may be worthwhile.

Taking supplements can never replace an adequate diet because the diet provides all kinds of other non-nutrient substances that are beneficial to health, such as fibre, and antioxidants called flavonoids. The combination, and the form, of nutrients found in food also means that the nutrients in food work more efficiently in your body.

However certain stipulations apply about what this multivitamin should and shouldn't contain:

- Although the requirement of some vitamins are increased during pregnancy, it is not by a huge amount, and so any supplement you take shouldn't contain much more than 100 per cent of the recommended intake for any of the vitamins and minerals it contains, except for folic acid. High-dose nutrient supplements may do more harm than good. Multivitamin and mineral supplements designed especially for pregnancy are usually OK, but check that they don't provide huge doses of any one nutrient.

- The supplement shouldn't provide vitamin A from retinol, but from betacarotene, a safer source if you do fall pregnant.

- The supplement should contain 400 micrograms of folic acid.

A recent study published in the respected medical journal *The Lancet* showed that high doses of vitamin C and E taken during pregnancy actually increase the risk of having a baby with a low birth-weight. The researchers however confirmed that doses of these antioxidant vitamins taken in the amounts found in a multivitamin supplement didn't pose a threat.

Once you do fall pregnant, your doctor may prescribe some supplements if he or she believes that you're deficient in anything. Typically your doctor may prescribe a supplement at higher levels than you would find in a general multivitamin and iron supplement. This is perfectly safe because it brings your very real depleted nutrient levels back to normal. The most common supplement a doctor prescribes is iron if he or she finds that you're anaemic. This can happen if you have had heavy periods for a while.

Adopting a healthier lifestyle

Even if you have your diet licked (no pun intended), thinking about the rest of your lifestyle, mainly physical activity and stress, is still worthwhile.

Weight loss itself may not mean the end of carrying stubborn weight around the abdomen, which is the area that predicts the likelihood of having insulin resistance and therefore infertility. Physical activity can help to redistribute fat and move it away from the abdomen area. Physical activity also increases your general wellbeing and general stamina – all important factors for pregnancy.

Exercise such as 30–40 minutes of brisk walking, or half an hour of swimming 5–6 times a week, should be enough to help reduce some abdominal fat, providing that you also keep an eye on your diet!

Stress can lead to infertility, which in itself can lead to stress, which then makes it even less likely that you're going to conceive. So discover how to chill out and do the best you can to get your body in the best shape it can be. This maximises your chance of a double bonus – freedom from PCOS and a beautiful baby! Why not join a yoga or meditation class, or have a massage, or just make sure that you take some time out for just you!

Ticking off the boxes of do's and don'ts

As the preceding sections make clear, the main things you can do to maximise your chances of falling pregnant are to lose weight if you are overweight, to eat right, and to exercise. Even a 10 per cent weight loss can be enough to stimulate a normal menstrual cycle in which an egg is released. And having a healthy, varied, and balanced diet ensures an adequate intake of energy and nutrients. The following sections list some other things you want to do to get your body ready for pregnancy. Of course, there's also a list of things *not* to do – or to *quit* doing – if you want to get pregnant; these things are listed too.

Get enough iron and folic acid

Take particular care on getting enough iron and folate-rich foods. You require an extra 400 micrograms of folate a day before pregnancy and up to week 12 of pregnancy. After this period, an additional 100 micrograms of folate is required. Tables 13-1 and 13-2 list sources for these vital nutrients.

In addition, if you are planning to conceive you should take a 400 micrograms folic acid supplement to protect against the possibility of having a baby with a neural tube defect such as spina bifida.

Table 13-1	Food Sources of Iron		
Food	**Amount (milligrams) per 100 grams**	**Portion Size (grams)**	**Amount (milligrams) per Portion**
Bran Flakes*	24.3	30	7.3
Rye bread*	2.5	50	1.3
Brown rice, raw*	1.4	100	1.4
Spinach boiled*	4.0	100	4.0
Peas, frozen boiled*	1.6	100	1.6
Curly kale, boiled	2.0	100	2.0
Baked beans*	1.4	225	3.2
Lentils, green or brown, dried, boiled	2.4	100	2.4
Dried apricots*	4.2	50	2.1
Beef, mince, cooked	2.7	140	3.8
Egg, boiled	1.9	1 medium (60)	1.1
Sardines, canned in tomato sauce	2.9	100	2.9

* These sources of iron are called 'non-haem' sources of iron because they aren't derived from meat or similar. If the food itself doesn't contain any vitamin C you need to have a good source of vitamin C, such as orange juice, with it in order for your body to absorb the iron from the food.

Low birth-weight babies are at risk

As well as having problems with fertility, not adopting a healthy lifestyle before you conceive puts you at risk of having a low birth-weight baby. Low birth-weight is defined as under 2500 grams or 5½ pounds. You may wonder what is wrong with having a baby with a low birth-weight. Well, a low birth-weight infant is at risk from the following:

✔ Congenital malformations, particularly of the central nervous system.

✔ Low intelligence.

✔ Behavioural problems.

✔ Reduced immunity.

✔ Increased risk of developing allergies.

✔ Some experts believe that being born light may predispose your baby to diseases such as high blood pressure and diabetes.

Table 13-2	Food Sources of Folate		
Food	*Amount (micrograms) per 100g*	*Portion Size*	*Amount (micrograms) per Portion*
Yeast extract	2620	Thin spread on bread	26
Fortified breakfast cereals	111–333	30 grams	33–100
Granary bread	88	Medium slice	32
Raspberries	33	60 grams	20
Oranges	31	Medium orange	50
Orange juice	18	160 millilitres	29
Brussels sprouts	100	90 grams	90
Sweet potato, cooked and mashed	23	200 grams	46
Asparagus, boiled	173	125 grams (about 5 spears)	216
Peas, frozen, boiled	47	70 grams	33
Beef, mince, cooked	17	140 grams	24
Semi-skimmed milk	9	250 millilitres	23

Have a check-up and sort out any medical conditions

Have a check-up with your doctor or Well Woman Clinic; you may want to ask about:

✔ Medication. Don't take any medications – even over the counter medications and herbal supplements – without first checking with your GP that they are safe to take when planning to get pregnant.

✔ Genito-urinary infections.

✔ Birth spacing. Studies have shown that the ideal birth spacing is 18 to 23 months after a full-term birth before conceiving again. This birth space is important because pregnancy can deplete the body of nutrients and it takes a while for these levels to optimise again. Close birth spacing can increase the risk of having a low birth-weight baby.

✔ Immunity to rubella.

✔ Diet and exercise.

If you are suffering from any other medical problem, get it sorted. Sexually transmitted infections (STIs) can particularly play havoc with fertility and possibly affect the baby if you do fall pregnant. Chronic conditions such as diabetes and asthma should also be optimally treated before conception. Some experts believe that even food allergies and intolerances can have an effect on fertility and pregnancy. Reviewing any medication you are on is important if you're trying to get pregnant.

Avoid supplements containing vitamin A and foods containing liver

Although having enough of the essential vitamins and minerals in the diet is important, taking excessive amounts of some of these can be harmful to you and to a potential baby. One such vitamin is Vitamin A.

Vitamin A in the diet is derived from two sources:

✔ As vitamin A precursors called carotenoids which are found in many fruits and vegetables.

✔ As retinol, which is a preformed form of vitamin A and is found in some animal products such as dairy products, liver, and fish liver oil.

Recently it has been found that animal livers contain very high levels of retinol. (This is thought to be because retinol is added to the animal feed to enhance productivity, reproduction, and immune status). Therefore experts advise women who are pregnant, or may become pregnant, to avoid:

✔ Liver and liver products (such as pâtés)

✔ Supplements containing retinol (including high-dose multivitamins)

✔ Cod-liver oil supplements

Only the pre-formed variety of vitamin A can be a danger, because high amounts are toxic to the developing baby and can cause birth defects. The same is true if you take high-dose supplements of retinol, and so experts have set a limit of 3000 micrograms a day.

Watch that booze

Too much alcohol drunk during the very early stages of pregnancy and before conception can lead to problems:

- ✔ It can reduce your chances of conceiving.
- ✔ It can reduce the ability of the embryo to survive early on in pregnancy.
- ✔ If the embryo does survive then alcohol drunk in excess can cause congenital problems which include mental retardation.
- ✔ It can reduce valuable nutrient stores in the body, including folic acid, and so make the embryo more vulnerable to damage.

In order to maximise your chance of conceiving and having a healthy baby, many experts recommend cutting right back on alcohol both before and during pregnancy. To be safe, most experts recommend that you avoid alcohol altogether for at least the first twelve weeks of pregnancy.

Cut back on the caffeine

The evidence for harmful effects from drinking a lot of coffee before or during pregnancy is not clear. To be on the safe side experts recommend that women who are pregnant, or planning to become pregnant, limit their caffeine intake to about 300 milligrams of caffeine a day which is around four cups of coffee. But don't forget that other drinks also contain caffeine. Table 13-3 details the caffeine content of some popular drinks.

Reducing the chances of having a baby with spina bifida

Congenital diseases such as spina bifida and anencephaly are called 'neural tube defects', and they can be the result of having too little folate (one of the B vitamins) in the diet. The neural tube is formed well before a woman realises she is pregnant; neural tube defects occur when the brain and skull and/or the spinal cord and its protective spinal column don't develop properly within the first few weeks after conception, and so having enough of this vitamin is critical before conception and during the first twelve weeks of pregnancy. To safeguard the baby, women who are planning a pregnancy are told to take a 400 micrograms supplement of folic acid – the manufactured form of the vitamin which is easily absorbed by the body and acts in the same way as folate in food. In addition, women should also consume plenty of folate-rich food, as well as food fortified with folic acid such as breakfast cereals (refer to Table 13-2).

Table 13-3	Caffeine Content of Popular Beverages	
Drink	*Serving Size (millilitres)*	*Caffeine Content (approx. milligrams)*
Instant coffee	190 (1 cup)	75
Filter or percolated coffee	190 (1 cup)	100–115
Decaf coffee	190 (1 cup)	5
Tea	190 (1cup)	50
Drinking chocolate	200	1–10
Energy drinks containing caffeine or guarana	250	30–90
Cola (regular or diet)	330 millilitre can	10–70

Do be aware that caffeine is also found in a number of prescription drugs and over the counter medicines such as headache pills and cold and flu remedies.

Protect yourself from food poisoning

Food poisoning is an unpleasant experience for anyone, but if you're trying for a baby and become pregnant, some food-borne diseases can harm the baby before you are even aware that you are pregnant. Furthermore, a food-borne disease can lurk around in the body for a long while and it can take up to three months to establish adequate immunity from these diseases; which means that your newly conceived baby is left unprotected.

Here are some general rules on food hygiene which are good to follow generally but particularly if you are planning to get pregnant:

- Store food as directed by the food manufacturer.
- Eat food by the 'use-by' date.
- Make sure that your fridge and freezer are at the correct temperature (0–5 degrees Celsius for the fridge and minus 18 degrees Celsius for the freezer).
- Store cooked food above raw food in the fridge.
- Keep food wrapped or covered.

✔ Wash your hands carefully before preparing food and protect cuts and wounds with a plaster.

✔ Wash utensils and work surfaces thoroughly with a household detergent especially after preparing raw food.

✔ Use a separate chopping board for raw and cooked food.

✔ If you use a microwave, make sure that you know the power rating and follow the cooking instructions, and the stirring and standing directions, carefully.

✔ Cook all food thoroughly and avoid eating shellfish or raw or under-cooked fish, meat, eggs, or poultry.

✔ When re-heating food, make sure that it's piping hot all the way through. Don't re-heat food more than once.

✔ Cooked food that is not eaten straight away should be cooled as rapidly as possible, and then stored in the refrigerator.

✔ Avoid unpasteurised milk and milk products.

✔ Avoid foods that carry a high risk of being contaminated with listeria. These include:

- Soft ripened cheese such as Brie, Camembert, or blue vein cheeses.

- Fresh meat pâtés.

- Pre-packaged supermarket salads.

- Salads in dressings from 'deli' counters.

A special warning about cats

Toxoplasmosis is a particularly nasty parasite which can be carried by household pets, in particular cats. If you become infected with this parasite in the very early stages of pregnancy or just before you fall pregnant, this can lead to blindness and other problems in your baby. However, you can take some simple actions to avoid picking up this parasite:

✔ Avoid changing cat litter, or wear rubber gloves and disinfect them afterwards.

✔ Wear gloves when gardening because the parasite can live in soil where the cat has defaecated.

✔ Wash your hands after handling pets.

What your other half can do

As well as being supportive, men can take some positive steps (along with avoiding some things) in order to maximise the chance of you conceiving and having a beautiful bouncing baby.

You don't just have to think about diet and exercise. The best sperm is produced by men in their prime so this means being in good shape, fit, and eating well. Drugs (medicinal as well as recreational), alcohol, and cigarettes all take their toll on sperm quality. If your man works with certain chemicals, he needs to check whether they are known to have an effect on sperm quality too.

Here's a list of some other factors which can have an effect on sperm quality as well as reduce male fertility:

- ✔ Fever: Flu, or even a severe cold, can cause a high fever, which adversely affects sperm production and quality. These changes usually recover over a few weeks.

- ✔ Diabetes: In the longer term, this can cause problems with erection and ejaculation.

- ✔ High blood pressure: Can cause problems with erection, either directly or as a side effect of medication.

- ✔ Arterial disease: Can cause problems with erection. This can be due to generalised hardening of the arteries, in the penis as well as the heart, or to drugs used in the treatment of heart problems.

- ✔ Neurological disorders: Such things as multiple sclerosis, spinal injury, or a stroke can all cause problems with erection and ejaculation.

- ✔ Kidney disease: Can result in a build up of waste products in the body adversely affecting sperm quality and fertility. It can also cause erection problems.

- ✔ Cancers: Can affect the genital tract or endocrine (hormone-producing) systems and may directly reduce fertility. Otherwise, drugs and radiation used to treat cancer may severely reduce sperm production or even stop it altogether.

- ✔ Alcoholism: Alcohol is toxic to sperm and overuse of alcohol can reduce sperm quality and fertility.

- ✔ Stress: Causes several hormonal changes in the body that can affect fertility.

Coping with Disappointment

Disappointment may occur because you are unable to get pregnant or you miscarry. Unfortunately a greater chance of both exists with PCOS. By following the advice in this book, and the particular pre-conception advice in this chapter, you are maximising your chances of getting pregnant and lessening your chances of losing the baby. However, if you still have few or no monthly periods, you are very unlikely to get pregnant as this is an indication that no egg is being produced to be fertilised. If you are having regular periods, reasons other than the PCOS may be causing the infertility and getting your partner checked too is always worthwhile. In cases such as this, medical intervention is required.

When nothing happens

A diagnosis of infertility is made when you have tried for a baby for a year and still haven't fallen pregnant. If you have PCOS and your symptoms aren't under control, the fact that you haven't conceived within the year is not surprising. Getting older delays the process too and age 35 is taken as a cut-off where fertility is known to decline significantly. But, if you are experiencing infertility even though you are within your healthy weight, eat correctly, and keep fit (and your partner is in tip-top shape too), you need to consider other possible problems.

Medical intervention

If you do need to visit your doctor for infertility, he or she may need to refer you to a specialist. A number of standard procedures exist for treating infertility in PCOS, after weight reduction through diet and exercise have been tried first. These procedures are:

- A six-month trial on a drug called clomid (clomiphene citrate) which stimulates ovulation.
- Injection of follicular stimulating hormone which encourages an egg to be released from ovarian follicles.
- A course of the drug metformin which increases the chance of spontaneous ovulation and enhances the effect of the drug clomid.
- Ovarian drilling/diathermy or laser treatment.
- Other ovarian surgery including a procedure called 'open wedge resection'.

Surgery is a last resort to encourage ovulation if all else fails. Your doctor or specialist can explain which procedure suits you best, if indeed you need to go this far.

Where to go for further help

This section contains a pick of many, many organisations in the UK and USA that can offer advice and support if you're struggling with fertility issues, have had difficult pregnancies, miscarriage problems, or carried a baby that has had problems.

Family Planning Association (UK only)

The fpa (formerly The Family Planning Association) is a registered charity working to improve the sexual health and reproductive rights of all people throughout the UK. The Web site address is: `www.fpa.org.uk`. Helpline staff provide a confidential advice service for the public answering over 100,000 enquiries a year. The helpline number is: 0845 310 1334 (Monday to Friday 9 a.m. to 6 p.m.).

Foresight

Foresight calls itself the Association for Pre-Conceptual Care. Foresight offers a thoroughly researched pre-conception care programme, which identifies and addresses various areas of concern in the health of any pair of prospective parents. The objective is to optimise the health of both prospective parents well before conception occurs so that a pregnancy can be started with a normal, strong sperm and ova and the embryo can implant and develop under optimum conditions in a healthy uterus, with no danger of damage from nutritional deficiency, toxins, or disease. You can find foresight at: `foresight-preconception.org.uk`. Their address is: Foresight Preconception, Mead House, Littlemead Industrial Estate, Alfold Road, Cranleigh, Surrey. GU6 8ND, UK. Telephone: 01483 869944.

Preconception.com

Preconception.com is part of iParenting.com which covers all aspects of parenting. Preconception.com offers information on couples trying to conceive. The Web site can be found at `www.preconception.com`.

Predicting fertility

You can buy kits from the chemist which tell you when and if you are ovulating. This involves a simple urinary test that measures the surge of lutenising hormone (LH) which occurs at ovulation. In particular, you can buy an antimullerian hormone test over the Internet which predicts fertility from the eggs left in the ovaries.

You should use the test a day or so before you expect to ovulate and if you want to get try and get pregnant, you need to have intercourse when the test kit shows a colour change, which indicates ovulation is happening.

Ovulation can be monitored by ultrasound, but this requires a trip to a hospital and so is reserved for if you need to have more complicated fertility treatment.

The Infertility Network

The Infertility Network is a non-profit making organisation providing information about infertility and the work of infertility support associations within Europe and the rest-of-the-world. Their mission is to provide quality up-to-date information and news on assisted human reproduction, infertility, getting pregnant, and other aspects of infertility. Their address is: Woodlawn House, Carrickfergus, Co. Antrim, Northern Ireland. BT38 8PX. Tel 07885 138101 or email webmaster@ein.org. Their Web site is www.ein.org.

NetDoctor

NetDoctor offers discussion and support on many medical conditions including women's health, PCOS, and fertility. NetDoctor attempts to break down the medical language barrier between the doctor and the patient. Over 250 of the UK's and Europe's leading doctors and health professionals write, edit, and update the contents of NetDoctor. In addition to creating written content for the patient, these same health professionals respond to users' questions and concerns regarding general health matters. The Web site is www.netdoctor.co.uk.

American Society for Reproductive Medicine (ASRM)

ASRM is interested in all aspects of the reproductive life-cycle. They provide information on infertility, menopause, contraception, reproductive surgery, endometriosis, and other reproductive disorders. ASRM can provide patients with fact sheets and questions on topics related to reproductive health. You can find them at www.asrm.org. Their address is: American Society for Reproductive Medicine, 1209 Montgomery Highway, Birmingham, Alabama 35216 2809, USA. Tel: + 001 205 978-5000.

International Council of Infertility Dissemination (INCID)

The International Council on Infertility Information Dissemination (INCIID – pronounced 'inside') is a non-profit organisation that helps individuals and couples explore their family-building options. INCIID provides current information and immediate support regarding the diagnosis, treatment, and prevention of infertility and pregnancy loss, and offers guidance to those considering adoption or childfree lifestyles. The Web site is www.inciid.org. Their address is: PO Box 6836, Arlington, VA 22206, USA. Tel: +001 703 379-9178.

RESOLVE

The mission of RESOLVE is to provide support and information to people who are experiencing infertility and to increase awareness of infertility issues through public education and advocacy. Their Web site is www.resolve.org and address is RESOLVE, 1310 Bradway, Somerville, MA 02144, USA. Tel: +001 617 623-0744.

Hormone disturbances and miscarriage in PCOS

Although some researchers believe that the link between PCOS and miscarriage is due to insulin resistance, other studies find links between miscarriage and high levels of luteinising hormone (LH). This hormone stimulates ovulation and can be high in women with PCOS. If LH levels are found to be high, drugs can be taken which keep the level of this hormone down.

Other studies suggest that high androgen (male hormone) levels may contribute to the problem; another hormone that is high in women with PCOS.

However, levels of both these hormones become elevated due to insulin resistance, so controlling insulin resistance is key.

Fertility Research Foundation (FRF)

Established in 1964, the FRF provides fertility counselling and treatments. You can find them at: `www.frfbaby.com`. Their address is Fertility Research Foundation, 877 Park Avenue, New York, NY 10021, USA. Tel: +001 212 744-5500.

Doing your best to avoid a miscarriage

Miscarriage is the spontaneous ending of pregnancy by loss of the baby before the 24th week of pregnancy. The average for miscarriage is one in every six pregnancies, and the majority happen before 24 weeks.

Studies suggest that PCOS is associated with a higher incidence of miscarriage than that quoted above, and this is thought to be linked with the high levels of insulin that occurs in PCOS sufferers. So when you do become pregnant, the best thing you can do is to be diligent about the following:

✔ See your doctor as soon as you realise you are pregnant.

✔ During your pregnancy, report anything that seems unusual such as bleeding, cramping, or a sudden loss of the pregnancy symptoms you've had.

✔ Eat well (but there's no need to eat for two).

✔ Keep yourself active but don't start any new form of activity you've not done before, and avoid dangerous sports. Your doctor or midwife can advise you on the best type of activity.

However if miscarriage does happen even after you've taken the advice above, blaming yourself is pointless. Bear in mind that even after a miscarriage, including more than one, you still have a very good chance of carrying a child to term. Saying all this may not help much when you are currently going through the emotional strain of miscarriage. Your doctor should be able to refer you (and your partner if you want) to a trained counsellor who can help you come to terms with the emotional toll caused by such a loss.

As well as ensuring your PCOS symptoms are under control, doctors can prescribe certain drugs such as metformin which reduces insulin resistance and can help to reduce the incidence of miscarriage.

Part V
The Part of Tens

The 5th Wave   By Rich Tennant

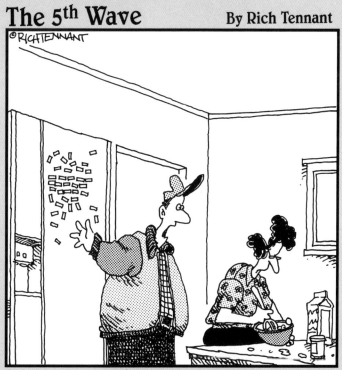

"It's been two months since your diagnosis, and I know you're reluctant to talk about it. But we've got to start discussing it in some way other than messages left on the refrigerator with these tiny word magnets."

In this part . . .

This part is where you get loads of concise and helpful tips. Each chapter in this part inspires you and makes you realise you can do an awful lot to help yourself overcome your symptoms.

And if this book didn't quite give you all the support and help you needed (well, it did try), you can find a list of organisations guaranteed to offer a further helping hand.

Chapter 14

Ten PCOS Symptoms You Can Take Action On

In This Chapter

▶ Giving you an overview of the PCOS symptoms you can do something about

▶ Motivating you to take action to shrink away those symptoms

*T*aking control of your diet and lifestyle really helps you to lessen some of the unpleasant side effects of PCOS, as well as reduce your risk of getting even more serious medical conditions, such as diabetes and heart disease. This chapter lists ten (okay, eleven) PCOS symptoms that you can ameliorate just by being proactive with your health.

Frumpy and Unfit

The answer to feeling frumpy and unfit is easy on paper: You need to tighten up on your diet and do some exercise! Of course, real life is more difficult than that. However, even if you start off just by getting more physically active, you can go a long way towards feeling more toned and fit. Although exercise alone is unlikely to lead to weight loss, it can make weight loss easier, help you maintain a certain weight, and offset further weight gain. Exercise can offset feelings of frumpiness by:

✔ Making you feel more energetic for the rest of the day. Feeling frumpy is harder when you feel energised!

✔ Lifting your mood and giving you a more positive outlook on life.

✔ Toning up your whole body, so that even if you're the same weight, you look slimmer and clothes hang on you better.

✔ Getting you fit. You notice this when you don't get so out of puff walking up the stairs or walking briskly to the shops.

✔ Helping to reduce your tummy, which is a real problem area if you have PCOS.

You also need to address frumpiness with diet. The diet you follow should be a calorie controlled one of around 1,500 calories. Sticking to low-GI eating (where you eat mostly carbs that have a low Glycaemic Index) is also recommended, unless you have been advised differently by a health care professional. Do not follow a diet (or exercise regime) that hasn't been approved by a qualified nurse, dietician, or doctor.

A steady weight loss of ½ to 1 kilogram (1–2 pounds) a week is fine. It may seem frustrating to be losing weight slowly, but you'll get there in the end. The combination of a balanced diet, that isn't too strict, coupled with exercise, helps to ensure that you don't lose muscle as well as fat mass and that the weight stays off.

No Patter of Tiny Feet

PCOS is often diagnosed when you've been trying to get pregnant but haven't been able to. The good news is that losing even 5 per cent of your current weight (if you're overweight) can trigger a return to fertility. The reason you may be infertile if you have PCOS and are overweight is due to a cascade of factors:

1. Increased weight leads to the muscles becoming resistant to the effects of insulin.

2. More insulin is produced in order to have the same desired effect on the muscles.

3. You end up with a condition, called hyperinsulinaemia, where high levels of insulin are circulating in your blood.

4. The high insulin levels affect other hormones in the body, and your ovaries overproduce testosterone.

5. Too much testosterone leads to abnormal production of the hormones LH and FSH.

6. Abnormal production of LH and FSH causes the ovaries to underproduce oestrogen, produce abnormal levels of progesterone, and continue to overproduce testosterone. The result is that the follicles in the ovary (which contain your eggs) don't reach maturity. This means that no egg is released.

7. Without an egg being released, there can be no period and no egg to fertilise.

In order to restore fertility, you need to stop the whole cascade from happening at the very start. This means losing weight, which then reduces the over production of insulin and reduces the hormone imbalances. The final effect is that the ovaries release an egg that can be fertilised. A low-GI diet also helps to lower the level of circulating insulin.

Diabetes and Its Complications

Gaining weight, particularly around the middle (which is what tends to happen in PCOS), triggers the production of a hormone that can trigger the muscle cells to be insensitive to the effects of insulin. And as mentioned in the previous section this triggers the pancreas to push out more insulin. However, what happens eventually is that the cells that produce the insulin get exhausted and can't keep up with the amount of insulin needed to bring blood glucose levels down to normal level. When blood glucose levels start to exceed the normal range, this is the point where type 2 diabetes develops. A person with type 2 diabetes whose blood sugars aren't controlled adequately has an increased risk of developing several complications, such as:

- Heart disease and stroke, which are mainly caused by damage to the arteries.
- Renal (kidney) damage, which leads to kidney failure.
- Damage to the back of the eye (retina), which can lead to blindness.
- Nerve damage.
- Increased risk of developing gangrene in the feet, which may result in having to have a foot amputated.

To prevent type 2 diabetes developing, and to lessen its impact if it has already occurred, you have to lose weight and take up exercise. Even a small weight loss of 5 per cent can have a significant effect. If you have type 2 diabetes or insulin resistance, following a low-GI diet helps you to:

- Have better blood sugar control in the short and long term.
- Reduce the diabetic medication needed to control your blood sugar.
- Lose more weight.
- Reduce the risk of developing heart disease and other complications of diabetes.

The 'C' Word: Cancer

The relationship between PCOS and cancer in general is not completely clear, although women who are overweight are more likely to get some kind of cancer. Also, in general, women who are infertile (whether they have PCOS or not) are more likely than fertile women to get a cancer of the reproductive system.

The strongest link between a cancer and PCOS is endometrial (lining of the womb) cancer. A few studies have suggested a correlation between PCOS and breast cancer, whereas others have not. No relationship seems to exist between PCOS and ovarian cancer.

Breast cancer and endometrial cancer are described as 'oestrogen-sensitive' cancers, meaning that the presence of oestrogen may cause these cancer cells to multiply.

Because PCOS causes disruptions to the normal menstrual cycle – irregular menstrual periods and the absence of ovulation – this leads to the production of oestrogen, but not progesterone. Progesterone causes the endometrium (the lining of the uterus) to shed each month, giving rise to the menstrual period. However without progesterone, no trigger exists to shed the lining and the endometrium may just keep growing which can eventually lead to changes to the cells that characterise the precursor to cancer. This pre-cancerous condition is called *endometrial hyperplasia*. If this is allowed to continue over a long period of time it can develop into full blown endometrial cancer.

So, as well as for fertility reasons, having a regular period is very important. Again, the answer here is to lose weight, and even a relatively small weight loss can help to make your periods more regular.

Acne

Acne as a teenager is bad enough, but having it as a full grown adult is just not on! Acne is a common symptom of PCOS, and is an inflammatory skin disorder that involves interactions between hormones, hair, sebaceous (oil-secreting) glands, and bacteria.

The acne brought about by PCOS can be mild or severe, but is likely to be worse the heavier you get. This is because the heavier you are, the more likely you are to have worsening insulin resistance which causes a rise in the level of androgens (male sex hormones). This androgen, a metabolite of testosterone, is called DHT (dihydrotestosterone). DHT stimulates the production of oil in the sebaceous glands of the skin, which eventually can lead to clogged glands or pores. Clogged pores, which can't release oil, allow bacteria to grow and multiply in the follicle. This leads to inflammation. Enzymes from these bacteria themselves go on to cause more damage, which then leads to a breakdown of the hair follicle and an abscess forms.

Although you can use creams and medication, which can help to lessen the acne in the short term, the most effective long-term treatment involves tackling the underlying root cause (excuse the pun!), which again is insulin resistance. So again weight loss, exercise, and a low-GI diet all help to reduce the insulin resistance.

Tired all the Time

Feeling washed out and tired is fairly common in PCOS, and has several causes:

✔ Lack of sleep is common in PCOS and affects how awake you feel the next day.

✔ The stress and anxiety brought about by having PCOS can lead to developing fatigue.

✔ Depression, which can occur in PCOS, can also cause feelings of tiredness.

✔ Because of insulin resistance, the muscles in your body can't always get enough glucose to convert to energy, which results in physical tiredness. Also, blood sugars can sometimes suddenly drop quite low, which can also result in feelings of fatigue and shakiness.

✔ Developing full blown type 2 diabetes, something you're at greater risk of with PCOS, can make you feel tired, especially if you aren't keeping it under control.

✔ If, in an attempt to lose weight, you put yourself on a diet that's too strict or restricts certain foods from your diet, you feel very lacking in energy. If you want to lose weight for your PCOS, choose a balanced low-GI diet of around 1,500 calories as advocated in this book to give you more zing, and not less!

✔ If you're taking any medication, including medication to relieve your PCOS, these can sometimes cause fatigue.

✔ If you have very heavy periods (which can happen sometimes if you have PCOS), you may have iron deficiency anaemia, which can cause fatigue.

If you do feel tired all the time, discuss this fatigue with your doctor. He or she can check out any obvious causes such as anaemia or low thyroid function, and may alter your medication.

If you follow a healthy low-GI balanced diet, which includes a wide variety of foods and is not too calorie restrictive, you can help offset fatigue. You need to couple this diet with some regular physical activity. When you're tired, exercise may be the last thing you want to do, but get started, and you usually find that getting active actually boosts your energy levels, providing you don't try to overdo it!

Heart Disease and Stroke

Researchers have found that PCOS, with its symptoms of high blood pressure, excessive fat around the abdominal area, blood fat disorders (such as high triglycerides and low HDL), elevated levels of male hormones, and insulin resistance, puts sufferers at higher risk of developing future serious, life-threatening health conditions such as coronary heart disease and stroke.

Insulin is produced by your pancreas and released into the circulatory system where it is key to the absorption of glucose by your cells. If your cells resist insulin, both insulin and glucose build up in your blood. Excess insulin leads to weight gain and high blood pressure – both precursors to heart disease. As insulin comes in contact with the interior wall of your arteries, it can damage the walls, causing the initial injury that produces plaque which 'furs up' the arteries. This plaque gives rise to a condition called *atherosclerosis*. If the arteries leading to your heart get blocked due to the plaque formation, it results in a heart attack. If the plaque builds up in the arteries leading to your brain, it results in a stroke.

Recommendations for reducing cardiovascular disease risk involve:

- ✔ Reducing insulin resistance.
- ✔ Balancing blood fat levels including reducing the level of bad cholesterol (LDL) and raising the level of good cholesterol (HDL).
- ✔ Lowering blood pressure.

You need to control your PCOS symptoms as much as possible in order to delay or prevent worsening of the underlying conditions that lead to heart disease. You can do this by being careful in your food choices (lowering calorie intake if you need to lose weight, keeping saturated fat and salt levels down, and following a low-GI diet), and taking regular exercise.

Following a diet that includes plenty of foods with a low-GI index may have a role in helping to prevent or reduce the risk of getting type 2 diabetes, according to experts at Diabetes UK, the largest diabetes organisation in the UK. Because diabetes increases your risk of getting heart disease big time, controlling your diet is obviously an important action that you can take yourself. Research has also shown that lower-GI diets can help improve levels of 'good' cholesterol and so may reduce the risk of heart disease in general.

Depression: Being a Miserable Old Cow

If you have PCOS, you're likely to feel low, depressed, and irritable some times. In fact, you may get asked if it's your time of month, because the symptoms are similar to that of PMS and indeed have the same root cause: hormonal fluctuations. The experience is compounded by the fact that you may have low self-esteem, feel downright tired, and be overwhelmed by the condition. Depression can be quite common if you have undergone long periods of unsuccessful attempts to get pregnant.

If you've been given medication for your PCOS, this may be another trigger for your irritability and depression, but get it checked out by your pharmacist or doctor, and see whether you can take an alternative drug.

If you're not sure whether what you're feeling is true depression, check it out against some of the characteristics of depression listed here:

- Feeling down for more than a couple of days in a row.
- Avoiding having a social life and preferring to stay at home by yourself.
- Crying episodes without obvious provocation.
- Persistent trouble sleeping.
- Being overly critical of yourself.
- Thinking about suicide, and feeling that the world and your family would be better off without you.

If you think you're suffering from depression, which isn't just the odd period of feeling a bit blue, you need to see your doctor to get some help. You're unlikely to be able to deal with your PCOS in an appropriate way if you are truly depressed. Of course doing some regular exercise and eating a varied, balanced diet are going to be a big factor in helping you shake it off, but you may also need to take some medication in the short term and receive appropriate therapy.

Hirsutism: The Bearded Lady

Excess hair growth is called *hirsutism*. Hirsutism affects 5–10 per cent of all women and a much higher percentage of women with PCOS. If you suffer from too much hair in the wrong place (or not enough hair in the right place), it may well be emotionally painful for you. Although not a widespread belief, our definition of feminine beauty includes smooth, apparently hairless skin. American and British women are bombarded daily by television, film, and magazine images that make it seem as though women don't have any hair at all except on top of their heads.

With PCOS hirsutism, you may find that you develop hairiness in the following places:

- ✔ Face
- ✔ Chest
- ✔ Stomach
- ✔ Back

Because physical appearance has so much to do with how people relate to each other, hirsutism can be a distressing experience. At the very least, you may be chronically stressed by the amount of time and money you spend removing unwanted hair, in a seemingly never-ending battle.

The cause of excessive hair growth in areas where you don't want it is the excess production of male hormones again, itself brought on by insulin resistance. The condition is likely to get worse the more weight you gain. Creams and cosmetic treatments are available that you can use to alleviate the problem, but to get rid of the underlying cause you need to reduce insulin resistance by losing weight, which is best coupled with a low-GI diet and physical activity.

The Balding Woman: Hair Loss

About 15 per cent of women have hair loss, also known as alopecia or baldness, but a significant percentage of those are women with PCOS and, as with hirsutism (see the preceding section), an excess of male hormones is the cause.

Normally, roughly 100 hairs are lost from your head every day. The average scalp contains about 100,000 hairs. Hair grows from its follicle at an average rate of about 12 millimetres (½ inch) per month. Each hair grows for two to six years, rests, and then falls out. A new hair soon begins growing in its place. At any one time, about 85 per cent of the hair is growing and 15 per cent is resting. But hair loss or baldness occurs when hair falls out but new hair doesn't grow in its place.

Loss of hair is more than a minor cosmetic problem. It has the potential to make you feel vulnerable and embarrassed. Women experience hair loss differently than men. In women, the main patterns are:

✔ Thinning of hair over the entire head.

✔ Mild to moderate hair loss at the crown or hairline.

Unfortunately the hair loss of female pattern baldness or severe thinning may be permanent. So prevention is essential by restoring normal hormonal levels and reducing insulin resistance.

Messed Up Periods

The name *polycystic ovary syndrome* comes from the appearance of the ovaries in some women with the disorder: large and studded with numerous cysts (polycystic). These cysts are fluid-filled sacs, known as follicles, which contain immature eggs. Because the eggs never reach maturity, periods get disrupted, or stop altogether. Irregular periods, or none at all, are the most common symptom in PCOS.

In a normal cycle, the following happens to bring about menstruation:

1. The pituitary, a gland in the brain, secretes follicle stimulating hormone (FSH) and a little leutenising hormone (LH) into the blood stream, which cause the follicles to begin to mature.

2. The maturing follicles then release oestrogen. As the follicles ripen over a period of about seven days, they secrete more and more oestrogen into the blood stream. Oestrogen causes the lining of the uterus to thicken.

3. When the oestrogen level reaches a certain point, the pituitary gland releases a large amount of leutenising hormone (LH). This surge of LH triggers the one most mature follicle to burst open and release an egg. This is called ovulation.

4. Between mid-cycle and menstruation, the follicle from which the egg burst becomes the corpus luteum (yellow body). As it heals, it produces the hormones oestrogen and, in larger amounts, progesterone.

5. 10–12 days after ovulation, progesterone levels begin to fall as a result of the corpus luteum dwindling away, its role for the month now over. This fall in progesterone level triggers the endometrium to shed its lining and menstruation begins.

6. The cycle is continuous so that another follicle gets to mature and release its egg every month.

In women with PCOS, the cycle isn't quite as smooth or continuous; a disruption in the LH and FSH levels, along with raised androgen levels, are responsible for, in extreme cases, the eggs never reaching maturity, and remaining as small cysts on the ovaries. This disruption produces some oestrogen, thereby allowing the lining of the womb to build up, but never get to release the egg or produce the progesterone. In less extreme cases an egg may get released, but the whole running operation is far from smooth and regular!

Four out of five women with PCOS have some sort of period disruption. In PCOS the periods can be messed up in several ways:

- ✔ Absent altogether – known medically as amenorrhoea.

- ✔ Irregular – known medically as oligomenorrhoea. Irregular menstruation means having menstrual cycles that occur at intervals longer than 35 days or fewer than eight times a year.

- ✔ Heavy – known medically as menorrhagia.

- ✔ Last a long time.

Sometimes spotting is present between periods, where the endometrium that has built up does break down to a certain extent, even though no ovulation has occurred.

Fertility is below par if the menstrual cycle is disrupted, because this irregular cycle is an indication that a mature egg is not being released on a monthly basis. If no period occurs, no egg is being released, and so conception isn't possible.

The answer to irregular periods is once again weight loss because losing weight enables the hormone levels that disrupt menstruation to return to normal. But bear in mind that this process works in the opposite direction too: The more weight you gain, the more irregular your periods become, and the more likely you are to cease to have periods altogether.

Chapter 15

Ten Rules for Spotting a Bad Diet

In This Chapter
▶ Knowing when not to touch a diet with a barge-pole
▶ Explaining why some diets on offer may be downright dangerous

*Y*ou have probably read, or even tried to follow, many different diets. They're everywhere – books, magazines, newspapers, celebs' life stories, on the Internet, or passed on by a friend or relative. Many of these diets seem attractive because they're a little different from the usual boring advice about diet, and also claim fantastic results; but this difference is precisely what can make them dangerous. If you have PCOS, you're very vulnerable to believing that a particular diet can really work miracles. This chapter can help you decide whether the latest rave diet is likely to work for you or not.

It Excludes Certain Foods

The key to a good diet is to eat a variety of different foods. That way you can more or less guarantee that you get all the nutrients your body needs. No one food that you eat is going to be the perfect food, containing the whole assortment of nutrients you need (unless of course it's a specially made-up formula food) and so that's why you need a whole mixture of food. Diets that stop you eating certain foods may require you to cut out foods that provide you with important nutrients. These diets are often hyped-up and claim fantastic results. They normally work by cutting out major food groups (such as carbs in the Atkins diet) so that you are unlikely to overeat on the foods that are left. Table 15-1 lists the nutrients you may get too little of if you cut a particular food out of your diet.

Table 15-1	Food Groups and What They Provide	
Food Group	**Examples of Food**	**What It Provides to the Diet**
Fats	Butter, margarine, oils, fatty meat, cheese	Fat soluble vitamins and essential fatty acids. Also allows absorption of several antioxidants such as lycopene from tomatoes.
Carbohydrates	Pasta, rice, bread, potatoes (ordinary and sweet)	Energy, fibre, B vitamins, magnesium
Dairy foods	Milk, cheese, yoghurts	Calcium, riboflavin (vitamin B2), fat soluble vitamins such as D, A, and E
Fruit and vegetables	Includes all fruit and veg but not potatoes	Fibre, antioxidants, vitamin C, vitamin A, magnesium
Meat and fish and other protein sources	Beef, pork, lamb, chicken, white and oily fish, beans, nuts, pulses	Protein, iron, zinc, and other minerals

Unless you've been told to exclude certain foods for medical reasons, such as avoiding eggs or nuts due to an allergy, don't omit any particular food from your diet. If you choose to avoid a particular food yourself, you need to make sure that you replace it with something that provides the same nutrients that the food normally provides. For example, if you cut meat out of your diet, you need to replace it with another protein-rich food such as fish or beans; cut milk out of your diet, and you can replace it with calcium fortified soya milk.

Being able to include all foods in your diet doesn't mean that you can eat as much as you like of certain foods such as high-GI foods or foods that contain a lot of fat such as pies and biscuits.

Avoid diets that tell you only to eat organic or avoid any food that has been packaged. Because such diets can be costly and time-consuming (if you need to go out of your way to shop for organic foods), you may be less likely to keep them up for long. Organic food may taste nicer, but no proof exists that organic food is more nutritious. The chemicals used to treat crops, or that are used in packaging materials, have been tested and found to be safe at the levels that most people consume. However, if your budget can afford organic and you have strong convictions about this issue, eating organic can't hurt you as long as you're still getting a nutritionally well-balanced diet.

It Only Lets You Eat A Few Foods

Some slimming diets work on the principle that they bore the weight off you! In other words, if they restrict your intake and say you can only eat certain foods, you're unlikely to overeat. This goes beyond cutting out certain foods or a particular food group – this is restriction with a capital R! For example, such diets restrict what types of food you can eat from the various food groups (such as bananas from fruit, tuna in spring water for protein, and so on), or tell you to eat certain things on certain days (such as only meat on one day, and then all the vegetables you can eat on another, but never combining them together in a proper meal).

You'll find sticking to such a diet for longer than a week very hard, because you start to have strong urges to eat the foods that you're not allowed. You may also never want to eat the foods that you are allowed again, even if it is a cream cake diet!

The best sort of diet is a varied diet. As a general rule you need to have a variety of foods from each food group, as outlined in Table 15.1. Doctors and dieticians do sometimes use a 'few food diet' and a 'rotation diet' made up of a few foods, in which individual foods are slowly added back in, but these diets are used under supervision to help identify particular food allergies, and aren't for weight loss!

It's High in One Particular Food Element

Good and bad foods don't exist, only good and bad diets. However, some foods can be eaten in larger quantities than others. Such foods include vegetables and wholegrain cereals. Foods that can be included in the diet, but only in smaller amounts, include chocolate, cheese, nuts, butter, spreads, and oils.

However, if one food, however 'healthy', is eaten to excess it means that less room is available in your diet to eat a whole variety of other foods. Also, some foods may be high in certain nutrients, which if eaten in excess can lead to unwelcome consequences, some of which can be dangerous; see Table 15-2.

Table 15-2	What Can Happen If Certain Foods Are Over Consumed
Food	*Consequence of Over Consumption*
Liver	Vitamin A poisoning.
Carrots	Skin can turn orange.
Rhubarb	The high content of oxalate may reduce calcium absorption.
Spinach	The high content of oxalate may reduce calcium absorption.
Tea	The tannins in tea can reduce iron absorption.
Milk	Can reduce iron absorption.
Egg white	Can inhibit the absorption of the B vitamin biotin.
Bran	The phytate in bran can reduce the absorption of several minerals including iron.
Pulses	The phytate in these can reduce the absorption of several minerals including iron.

It Has Too Much Protein Power (Combined with Low Carbs)

Some diets may suggest that you increase the amount of protein that you eat, for example the Atkins diet. Low-carbohydrate/high-protein plans seem attractive to many dieters because these diets set no limit on the amount of certain types of foods you can eat, may reduce hunger and appetite, and at times, produce steady weight loss, even after failure or weight gain on other diets. However a high-protein diet is not a good idea for a number of reasons:

✔ High-protein foods are likely to be high in cholesterol and saturated fats – substances that can promote heart disease and various cancers.

✔ In the absence of carbohydrate fuel, your body is forced to burn fat and protein to fulfil its energy needs. The breakdown products of burning large quantities of body fat for fuel are called ketones, which begin to accumulate in your body. A build-up of ketones in the body can cause all kinds of damage to your vital organs such as the liver and the kidneys. The build-up deranges your body's balance of acids and alkalines, causing a condition called acidosis. When the levels of ketones in your body reach dangerous proportions, you may slip into a coma, which can result in death.

✔ The accumulation of ketones in your body can leave you with unpleasant body odour and bad breath.

✔ You can lose muscle tissue as well as fat – which is not the object of weight-reduction diets. Ironically, the more carbohydrate you cut out of the diet and the more protein you eat to slim, the lower your body protein stores become, because you are burning protein foods as fuel.

✔ Not consuming a wide enough range of foods can lead to deficiency diseases.

✔ Cutting out carbohydrates can cause severe constipation because carbohydrates such as fruit, vegetables, and grains and cereals, (particularly the wholegrain varieties), are the main source of dietary fibre. Eliminating these foods in the long run can lead to diverticulitis, irritable bowel syndrome, and may even make you more susceptible to bowel cancer.

✔ Consuming a lot of red meat is associated with a raised risk of getting colon cancer.

✔ Such a diet may exacerbate gout because it may lead to a build-up of uric acid in the blood.

✔ You may experience increases in serum triglycerides and low-density lipoprotein cholesterol, both bad fats that can trigger heart disease, in particular blocked arteries and cardiac arrhythmias.

✔ Such diets have been associated with hypothyroidism (low thyroid function).

✔ In the 1960s and 1970s, liquid protein diets were associated with several sudden cardiac deaths.

✔ Low-carb, high-protein diets shouldn't be coupled with a low calorie intake because this combination can trigger severe loss of important minerals to the body, which itself can tigger sudden cardiac death.

Blood cholesterol, sugar, and triglycerides may be reduced on high-protein diets because you tend to eat much less due to loss of appetite, and sometimes nausea. In general, weight loss and health benefits are temporary because the high-protein plan is too unpleasant to continue – so you may be tempted to return to your old way of eating.

It Relies on Taking a Supplement or a Particular Substance

Although the days of fast-fix slimming pills, which were downright dangerous, are long gone, this hasn't removed the snake oil sellers from still trying to promote their wares. The 'new generation' of substances claiming to aid weight loss are not usually very dangerous, but they tend to be a load of hype that may cost you lots of money but deliver nothing. Such diets often claim that you can carry on eating as much as you like and still lose weight! Unfortunately this is just not going to be the case! Table 15-3 lists the most common substances available today, which you should avoid.

Table 15-3	Substances That Claim They Aid Weight Loss
Substance	**What It Claims to Do**
Diuretics	Diuretics make you wee more. So all you lose is body water. Unfortunately the fat doesn't get weed out. As soon as you drink more fluid, the weight returns!
Herbals	Many herbals that claim to have brought about weight loss have now been banned. Some of these actually caused serious damage to the liver and kidneys. However, other herbals that are unlikely to aid weight loss are still on the market.
Calcium (from dairy products)	Some evidence exists that a high calcium intake from dairy products can boost metabolism. In fact, other dairy components may be having the active effect. However, even if high calcium intake does do this, it is doubtful that the amount is significant.
Green tea	Green tea and extracts of green tea are believed to boost metabolism. Again the jury is out on this one.
Conjugated linoleic acid (CLA)	CLA is a naturally occurring fatty acid found in meat and dairy products. It is also a popular dietary supplement that is sold with claims of helping people lose fat, maintain weight loss, retain lean muscle mass, and control type 2 diabetes. However, CLA may also increase levels of bad fats in the blood stream. More research is needed before CLA can be promoted as a risk free and effective weight loss aid.

Only taking in fewer calories than your body actually uses is going to lead to long-term weight loss. If your diet is balanced, and as long as you don't restrict your calorie intake below 1,500 calories, you shouldn't need to take any additional supplements, because the diet still provides you with all the vitamins and minerals your body needs. A diet that suggests that you also need to take vitamin and mineral supplements is probably advocating this because it is unbalanced and inadequate.

You Have to Eat Loads of a Particular Food

Although it seems counter intuitive to be able to eat loads of a particular food when trying to lose weight, the thinking behind this sort of diet is that you only, or mainly, eat just one kind of product. If you really stick to this, you soon realise that there's a limit to how much of one product you can eat, so of course you lose weight in the short term. Not only is such a diet unbalanced, and not providing all the nutrients that your body needs, but also you are unlikely to be able to stick to it for more than a few days.

Famous examples of this sort of diet included the cabbage soup diet, the grapefruit diet, and even the Mars bar diet. The cabbage soup diet, for example, claims that you can lose 4.5 kilograms (10 pounds) in seven days. For a start, this weight loss is not a safe achievable amount in such a short period of time, and much of the weight loss is likely to be water. As well as encouraging the eating of the cabbage soup at least once a day, the diet (which should only be followed for seven days, but then what?) has you eating nothing but bananas, skimmed milk, and cabbage soup one day, just meat and tomatoes and of course cabbage soup another day, and so on. Although such a diet is meant to be a kick-start for a short period only, it is not balanced, is too severe, and is likely to cause you to regain the weight once you stop. It also doesn't re-programme your eating habits for the better.

It's Very Low in Calories

The definition of a very low calorie diet is a diet that only provides around 500 calories. Only people who are being closely monitored, such as in a hospital setting, should follow very low calorie diets. Many dangers of following a very low calorie diet exist, but sometimes it is the lesser of two dangers, for example, in the case of a very overweight patient who needs a life-saving operation but whose weight makes it a huge risk to have the operation unless she loses some weight. Such a diet should therefore only be used in cases such as this, where rapid weight loss is imperative and the lesser risk.

Here are some reasons why you shouldn't put yourself on such a strict regime:

✔ Side effects can include fatigue, constipation, nausea, and diarrhoea.

✔ As you lower your calorie intake, getting all the nutrients you need from your food becomes increasingly difficult. Lowering your diet to around 500 calories means that you're unlikely to get sufficient vitamins and minerals. You can take supplements, but these aren't guaranteed to provide you with the full range of nutrients and antioxidants, and their bioavailability (the ease at which they are absorbed into the blood stream) isn't as good as from real food.

✔ These diets can lead to muscle loss as well as fat loss, which is extremely unhealthy. To lose heart muscle, for example, is potentially fatal.

✔ These diets don't change long-established bad eating patterns and cause the body to slow down significantly, and so when the dieter returns to a more normal eating pattern the lower metabolism may lead to increased weight gain.

It Has Strict Rules on What You Can and Can't Eat

If a diet comes with too many rules, which shouldn't be broken for it to work, you're unlikely to be able to stick to it for very long. Nothing is more likely to make you crave certain foods than telling you not to eat them! Such diets may also restrict you to certain foods, which again is likely to lead to diet boredom and may mean your diet doesn't contain the full range of nutrients your body needs.

Good diets don't forbid you to eat certain foods, but they do indicate that you need to watch how much of certain foods you eat. These foods include:

✔ Foods with a high glycaemic index.

✔ Foods that are high in fat (because they tend to be very high in calories and may also contribute to developing heart disease and cancers). These foods include butter, spreads and oil, and pastry.

✔ Foods that are high in a combination of fat and sugar, as these tend to be calorie dense (you can't eat much of them before clocking up a high calorie load). These foods include chocolate and other confectionary (candy), cakes, biscuits, and sweet pies.

Foods that you can eat more freely include:

✔ Vegetables including salad veg (but watch how much high-fat dressings/ mayonnaise you use).

✔ Fruit, although going mad on this can make the calories stack-up.

✔ Beans, peas, and lentils.

✔ Low-fat dairy products.

What's important is the overall balance of the diet; you shouldn't have to agonise too much about individual foods, but think more about how they fit into your overall diet, and how often and how much of them you can eat.

Your Family and Friends Wouldn't Touch It

You don't want to have to become a recluse with your diet! Is your diet the sort that none of your family and friends would eat? If it is, why are you eating it? Part of the pleasure of eating is to be sociable and to be able to share the occasion with family and friends. Your diet shouldn't exclude you from enjoying social meals. Don't forget that your new diet isn't something you're going to follow for a week or two and then return to your usual habits. After all, those usual habits got you into trouble in the first place! Your new diet should be healthy and balanced, but it should also be based on tasty food that you, your family, and friends can equally enjoy.

Your diet should also not be based on unusual food that can only be found in specialist shops or demand hours of preparation. Unless you become an obsessive-compulsive recluse, you aren't able to maintain such a diet! Have a look at the recipes in Chapters 6 to 9: These recipes are for tasty meals and snacks that can go to form the constituents of your diet. All are tasty, balanced, and made with ingredients that are easy to buy. Furthermore, unless your friends are very fussy, they'll enjoy these recipes too!

You Can't Follow It for Life

Don't think of your PCOS diet as one you can go on for a while and then return to your past eating habits. PCOS has no cure, but you can control it so that you can reduce the symptoms or, in many cases, reverse them altogether. But this can only be achieved by permanently changing your eating habits and your lifestyle. So whatever diet you follow has to be permanent. Of course you may need to cut the calories for a bit until you get to a normal weight, but the nature and balance of the diet needs to remain the same. In order to see you through the rest of your life, a diet for PCOS needs to be:

- ✔ Based mostly on low-GI carbs.
- ✔ Low in saturated fat and salt.
- ✔ Not too restrictive in calories, and allow for three meals a day plus some snacks.
- ✔ Based on normal everyday food.
- ✔ Easy to make each meal.
- ✔ Forgiving if you occasionally slip-up and splurge.

Chapter 16

Ten Reasons to Follow a Low-GI Diet

. . . .

In This Chapter

▶ Exploring why the low-GI diet is so great

▶ Discovering how you can get the maximum benefit for just a little effort

▶ Encouraging you to adopt the low-GI diet to help alleviate your PCOS symptoms

. . . .

*T*his chapter summarises the reasons why a low glycaemic index (GI) diet is so great. Some reasons are specific to PCOS, and others relate to your general health. Reaping the rewards of a low-GI diet doesn't require a momentous effort on your part and you can be confident that it's a healthy way to eat for both you and your family. The important thing to remember with the low-GI diet is that you're not 'on a diet' – you're adopting a lifestyle that's going to change your life for the better and forever.

It's an All Round Healthy Way to Eat

The low-GI way of eating covered in this book gets a tick for all the rules on healthy eating. Low-GI eating:

- ✔ Is low in fat, particularly saturated fat.
- ✔ Ensures that most of your calories come from carbohydrate foods (carbs).
- ✔ Provides plenty of fibre.
- ✔ Provides a variety of foods that give you all the nutrients you need in the day.
- ✔ Helps to minimise extreme fluctuations in your blood sugar levels.
- ✔ Helps with weight control.
- ✔ Improves sports performance that relies on having plenty of endurance.
- ✔ Helps offset diabetes and metabolic syndrome.

✔ Reduces the chances of having a heart attack or stroke.

✔ Reduces the risk of getting certain cancers such as breast cancer.

✔ Helps alleviate certain bowel disorders.

✔ Reduces PCOS symptoms.

It's Flexible

The low-GI plan doesn't force you to eat foods you don't like, and you can still eat all the foods you do enjoy (although some moderation is called for if you can't resist chocolate and biscuits!). Furthermore, you shouldn't have to feel that you're permanently on a diet. No food is banned and you can eat at times of the day that suit you and choose what foods you have. Only four basic ground-rules apply:

✔ Eat regularly and don't leave long gaps between eating; that way you're not tempted to binge at any particular time. The ideal is to have three meals and two small snacks.

✔ Base most of your meals on a low-GI carb; this ensures that your overall meal becomes a low-GI one – simple!

✔ Don't overdo fatty or salty foods.

✔ If you need to lose weight, drop your calorie intake by about 500 calories so that you are eating around 1500 cals a day. That way you lose a steady 0.5 to 1 kilogram (1–2 pounds) a week.

The rest is up to you!

It Helps to Control Blood Sugars

Quite a lot of research has been done on the low-GI diet. Plenty of evidence shows that it can help control blood sugar levels in diabetics, and bring down insulin levels in those people with high insulin levels due to insulin resistance (which tends to occur if you have PCOS).

Here's how it works: The most common end product from starch and sugar breakdown in the body is glucose, which gets absorbed into the blood stream through the wall of the intestines. Carbs that are broken down slowly release a steady trickle of glucose into the blood stream. Carbs that are broken down rapidly release glucose into the blood stream rapidly and cause blood sugar levels to rise quite quickly.

Your body releases insulin to cope with rising blood sugar levels, but in PCOS, the insulin isn't very effective at bringing down the blood sugar levels, so higher amounts of insulin have to be pumped out. However, if you consume a low-GI meal, the blood glucose levels don't get raised quickly, less insulin is required to do the work of maintaining a steady glucose level, and so your body finds it easier to control your blood sugar levels. It also means that blood sugar levels don't swing wildly from being high, as soon as food is eaten, to crashing down low again when high levels of insulin are pumped out to cope with the sudden influx of glucose into the blood stream.

The low-GI way of eating has another bonus too: The blood sugar lowering effect of a low-GI meal can have a lasting effect on keeping blood sugars lowered after the next meal as well. So if you are mostly trying to eat low GI for each meal, every low-GI meal you eat exerts a positive additional knock-on effect to the next meal too.

Low-GI carbs get broken down slowly by the body for a number of reasons, including:

- ✔ Low-GI carbs are often rich in soluble fibre. Soluble fibre tends to increase the viscosity of the intestinal contents which slows down the ability of the digestive enzymes to get to the food and break it down.

- ✔ Some foods are low GI because a fibrous 'coat' surrounds them, such as in beans and seeds. This coat acts as a physical barrier, slowing down access by the digestive enzymes to the starch inside. You have probably noticed that some foods, like certain seeds, have such a fibrous coat that they can go through the whole digestive system unscathed, and come out the other end!

- ✔ The presence in foods of dried fruit, nuts, and seeds – common components of a low-GI diet – slows down the digestion process.

It Staves off Hunger Pangs

In theory, a low-GI diet should help to offset hunger because falling blood sugar levels are a big hunger trigger, and when a carb is broken down slowly, it releases its sugar into the blood in a slow and prolonged way. Blood sugars remain on an even keel for longer than when you eat carb foods that release their glucose quickly. So that hunger feeling that comes with falling blood sugars should take longer to happen with a low-GI carb.

The ability to keep hunger at bay for longer is one of the reasons why low-GI diets may help with weight loss, or at least weight maintenance. Well that's the theory anyway. Lots of research is still being done on the area of hunger and satiety to see if a low-GI diet is really effective at helping to offset hunger pangs. Some research has shown this is the case, but unfortunately some other studies have not backed this finding up. Remember: The body is very complex. Hunger has lots of triggers, and you may be tempted to eat for reasons other than pure hunger (including boredom or just fancying the look of that piece of cake!).

It Keeps Your Metabolism Going

Research shows that a low-GI diet may not lower your metabolic rate as much as some other diets, making you feel less tired, cold, and hungry, and more likely to stick to the regime long-term. These findings suggest that if you follow a low-GI diet you're more likely to keep weight off than if you followed, say, just a low-fat diet.

This research also suggests that not only total calories matter as far as weight control is concerned, but the type of calorie. The energy, calories, provided by a low-GI type diet may help to maintain the metabolic rate so that you burn off fat more quickly. More research is needed in this area.

A further plus point for low-GI eating is that it may help you perform better at your sport, especially with endurance sports. You can keep going for longer, thus boosting your metabolic rate even more when exercising. This benefit is believed to be due to the slow and sustained release of sugar into the blood stream that occurs when you eat a low-GI diet.

It's Good for Your Heart

A low-GI diet is good for your heart in a number of ways. A low-GI diet:

- ✔ Reduces the level of bad cholesterol (low density lipoprotein – LDL) in the blood. LDL is responsible for the furring up of arteries by depositing cholesterol-rich plaque on the artery wall. A build up of plaque can eventually cause a blockage in the artery leading to a heart attack or stroke.

- ✔ Raises the levels of good cholesterol (high density lipoprotein – HDL) in the blood. These HDL particles carry cholsterol away from the arteries and to the liver where it gets metabolised. This means that plaque formation on the artery wall is less likely.

- ✔ Lowers levels of triglycerides, another blood fat whose high circulating level is associated with heart disease.

✔ Lowers the level of *C reactive protein*, a protein associated with inflammation. Lots of disease states are associated with having high levels of this protein; diabetes and PCOS to name but two. A diet that helps lower this protein (which can otherwise cause damage to arterial walls) is good news.

✔ Normalises certain blood clotting factors. These tend to be abnormal in people with diabetic tendencies and increase the chances of a blood clot forming which can give rise to a heart attack or stroke.

✔ Help to bring down blood sugar levels, particularly after a meal. Having high blood sugar levels has been shown to be a risk factor for heart disease.

✔ Doesn't evoke a high insulin response, so that on average, circulating levels of insulin are lower on a low-GI diet compared to a normal diet. High circulating levels of insulin are also associated with heart disease.

✔ Can help prevent the development of full blown type 2 diabetes. But if type 2 diabetes has already developed, a low-GI diet can reduce its complications; one of which is heart disease.

✔ May help protect you from the increased risk of heart disease brought about by increased weight. In particular, a low-GI diet may help to reduce the excess weight carried around the middle, which is the riskiest place to carry weight as far as heart disease is concerned.

Just to show that all this isn't just based on theory, some research done in the US (Harvard University's Nurses' Health Study, to be precise, which involved thousands of female nurses) found that the women who ate diets with the highest GI had twice the risk of having a heart attack compared to women with the lowest GI, during a follow-up period of 10 years.

It's the Best Diet for Diabetics

A low-GI diet can help control/reduce the severity of all these conditions: type 1 diabetes, type 2 diabetes, gestational diabetes, insulin resistance, and metabolic syndrome:

✔ **Type 1 diabetes:** People with type 1 diabetes aren't able to produce insulin from the pancreas. This is usually due to an auto-immune disease and tends to develop in childhood or early adulthood.

✔ **Type 2 diabetes:** People with type 2 diabetes can usually produce some insulin, but it's not effective in bringing down blood sugar levels. This type of diabetes usually follows a period of insulin resistance.

- **Insulin resistance:** Also called pre-diabetes, insulin resistance is often a precursor for type 2 diabetes, and is common in PCOS sufferers who are overweight and in non-PCOS sufferers who are obese. With insulin resistance, the body pumps out high levels of insulin to make up for its inability to process blood sugars efficiently. So blood sugar levels may be pretty normal, but a blood test reveals high insulin levels, which cause a lot of havoc in the body.

- **Syndrome X:** Metabolic syndrome (or Syndrome X) tends to go hand in hand with insulin resistance and full blown type 2 diabetes and is characterised by an increased fat deposition around the tummy area, high levels of harmful blood fats, and high blood pressure. Metabolic syndrome is associated with an increased risk of having a heart attack or stroke.

- **Gestational diabetes:** Gestational diabetes occurs when the strain of pregnancy causes normal blood sugar control to be compromised. Women with PCOS who get pregnant have an increased risk of developing gestational diabetes. Although blood sugar levels do return to normal once the baby is born, women who developed gestational diabetes have an increased tendency to develop type 2 diabetes and should therefore avoid gaining weight as this can act as the trigger for diabetes to return.

A low-GI diet helps to keep blood sugar levels on a normal level. Because low-GI foods and meals release their sugar in a more gradual and steady way into the blood stream, the body doesn't need to force out loads of insulin all at once. Even when insulin has to be injected, as in type 1 diabetes and extreme forms of type 2 diabetes or gestational diabetes, the slow release of carbs makes it easier to keep the diabetes in control, and can therefore offset diabetic complications such as kidney damage and eye problems.

It's a 'People Friendly' Diet

You are spoilt for choice for recipes to follow for a low-GI diet. Even recipes not specifically identified as low-GI recipes – for example, pasta recipes – are often low GI anyway. Other recipes can be adapted to have a lower GI; for example, recipes calling for potatoes can use sweet potato, or half sweet potato and half ordinary potatoes instead. Either option brings the GI down.

The nice thing about the low-GI diet is that you don't have to feel secluded in your dietary habits because it is a normal tasty and nutritious diet that the whole family can eat. The recipes in this book are family recipes for family meals. Furthermore, the low-GI diet, and the low-GI recipes included in this book, are easy to incorporate into busy lifestyles and family budgets.

As well as being great for you, if you're cooking for any children and teenagers, the low-GI plan is great for them too as it gives them all the nutrients they need and keeps them bursting with energy. This may help offset their desire for too many sugary and fatty snacks – and it may help them to avoid gaining excess weight.

It's Bowel Friendly

Following a low-GI diet tends to mean that you eat more of the following foods which are high in fibre. Such foods help to bring down the GI of the carbohydrate food or meal they are part of:

- ✔ Bran
- ✔ Wholegrain cereals
- ✔ Peas, beans, and lentils (known as legumes)
- ✔ Nuts
- ✔ Seeds
- ✔ Most fruit (including most dried fruit)
- ✔ Most vegetables

A high-fibre diet is good news to our bowels because it can help

- ✔ Alleviate constipation.
- ✔ Reduce the risks of getting bowel diseases such as diverticulitis and bowel cancer.
- ✔ Alleviate the symptoms of irritable bowel syndrome (IBS) as it involves eating regular meals which contain plenty of soluble fibre such as oats, beans, wholegrain cereals, and vegetables.
- ✔ You feel full with very little calorie cost.
- ✔ Boost the levels of so called 'good' bacteria in the gut which help with immune function and protection from food-borne micro-organisms.

It's the Best Diet to Follow for PCOS

The root of most PCOS symptoms is the high levels of circulating insulin levels. A low-GI diet allows glucose to enter the blood stream at a slower and steadier rate than a high-GI diet. Therefore, the body doesn't need to produce so much insulin compared to what it would need to produce if a high-GI diet was eaten, which causes a rapid rise in blood sugar levels.

Some research conducted at the University of Harvard showed that insulin resistance decreased by more than twice as much with weight loss in a low-GI diet group compared to a low-fat diet group. When insulin levels start to return to normal levels, you typically experience an alleviation of several PCOS symptoms and complications, including:

- ✔ Hirsutism
- ✔ Acne
- ✔ Diabetes
- ✔ Raised harmful blood fats that can lead to heart disease
- ✔ Weight gain
- ✔ Infertility

Chapter 17

Ten PCOS Superfoods

*F*oods and food groups that fit in particularly well to the PCOS diet are highlighted in this chapter. You don't have to eat all these every day, but each one packs a lot of nutritional power so try to find room for most of them during the course of a week.

Wholegrain Breakfast Cereals

Diets that are rich in wholegrain foods have been shown to offer a number of health benefits. As far as PCOS is concerned, the main benefits are that whole-grains are believed to lower insulin resistance and help control your weight.

Experts now advise you to eat 16 grams of wholegrains 3 times a day, which gives you a total of 48 grams.

 Wholegrains are cereal grains which retain the bran (the outer layer) and germ (the seed in the middle) as well as the endosperm (the starchy bit inside), in contrast to refined grains which retain only the starchy endosperm. Wholegrain foods are those in which 51 per cent or more of the ingredients consist of wholegrains.

Wholegrain breakfast cereals are a great way to start the day for a number of reasons:

✔ They help to fill you up and stop you feeling hungry too soon before lunch because they're rich in fibre, contain some protein, and have a low GI.

✔ They provide essential fibre and lots of vitamins and minerals.

✔ They are low in fat.

Examples of wholegrain breakfast cereals include:

- ✔ Muesli or granola
- ✔ Porridge made with unprocessed oats
- ✔ Shredded wheat/raisin wheats
- ✔ Cheerios
- ✔ Shreddies/malted wheats
- ✔ Grapenuts
- ✔ Weetabix/wheat bisks

Wholewheat Pasta

Pasta is a great staple food because it has a low GI, is high in filling carbs, and provides lots of other nutrients, too. Pasta also tastes great and forms an excellent basis for many dishes. However, wholewheat pasta is even better because, as well as having the properties just described for pasta, it also provides the following:

- ✔ All the health benefits associated with wholegrains (see Chapter 3).
- ✔ Fibre (wholewheat pasta contains 4.5 grams of fibre per 100 grams compared with 1.5 grams of fibre in normal pasta).
- ✔ Vitamins and minerals including iron, selenium, magnesium, B vitamins, vitamin E, and phytochemicals that have antioxidant properties.
- ✔ An even lower GI than normal pasta: Wholewheat pasta has a GI of 37, whereas normal pasta has a GI of 41. However, both these values are classified as low.

You may not always want to use wholewheat pasta because some recipes lend themselves to the lighter, normal pasta, but experiment with it and see how you get on.

Wholewheat pasta goes particularly well if you're making soup such as minestrone.

Sweet Potatoes

Sweet potatoes are as versatile as the humble spud but for PCOS they have some advantages over ordinary potatoes. Sweet potatoes have:

✔ A much lower GI than ordinary potatoes. A baked sweet potato has a GI value of 54 whereas an ordinary baked potato has a GI of 85.

✔ A large amount of vitamins. One baked sweet potato provides masses of betacarotene, which the body converts into vitamin A, as well as being a good source of vitamin C and a significant source of iron.

✔ A rich orange colour, which means that they contain phytochemicals that act as potent antioxidants in the body.

Most recipes that stipulate ordinary potato can be substituted in part or wholly by sweet potato, but bear in mind that sweet potato generally takes less time to cook than ordinary potato (by 5 to 10 minutes). You need to experiment, but bear in mind that sweet potato does have a slightly sweet taste (hence its name!) and so, whereas this goes well with strong meat flavours and most veggie dishes, it may not go so well with fish. A 50/50 mix with ordinary potato is preferable in fish dishes. You can also use sweet potatoes in sweet recipes.

For the best food value, choose sweet potatoes of a deep orange colour and store them in a dry environment. Don't put them in the fridge because temperatures below 13 degrees Celsius can chill this tropical vegetable, giving it a hard core and an undesirable taste when cooked.

Beans

You find a lot of bean recipes in this book because beans

✔ Are versatile and tasty.

✔ Have a very low GI.

✔ Are nutritious and high in fibre.

✔ Provide a good source of protein.

✔ Are rich in antioxidants such as isoflavones.

✔ Contain anti-cancer substances called lignans. (Friendly bacteria in the colon convert lignans into hormone-like substances which scientists say may fight off breast and colon cancers.)

✔ Can help lower cholesterol levels.

✔ Count as a vegetable if you're trying to make sure you have at least five fruit and veg a day.

✔ Can help you keep away hunger for some hours after eating them due to their high fibre and low GI value. Along with their very low fat content, they may be able to help with weight loss.

Here's a list of some common beans you can easily buy in the shops with their GI value in brackets:

✔ Butter beans (31)

✔ Soya beans (18)

✔ Red kidney beans (27)

✔ Haricot beans (38) – these little beans go to make the ever-popular baked beans

With so much going for them, why not eat beans all the time? Well, they do have one small drawback, they can produce wind! However, this is usually more of a problem when you first introduce beans to your diet, and as your digestive system gets used to them, this problem typically diminishes. Maybe just don't start eating a bean dish right before that first hot date!

Most beans come as dried, and they have to be soaked and then boiled before eating. For red kidney beans, this boiling process is essential because it destroys a toxin in the bean which otherwise gives you a very nasty stomach ache.

To save time and effort you can now buy most beans in cans, which are ready to use and don't require boiling or soaking. However, because of the processing they have undergone, the GI of these beans, although classified as low, is higher than those of beans you soak and boil yourself.

Some beans can be eaten fresh such as broad beans and soya beans which can form a very nutritious vegetable side dish.

Lentils

Lentils are legumes and cousins to the pea. They can be cooked in many ways as well as being ground into a flour. Lentils are a PCOS superfood because they're:

✔ Rich in protein and carbohydrates and are a good source of calcium, phosphorus, iron, and B vitamins.

✔ Low in fat.

✔ Versatile in recipes and are particularly useful for padding out meat in a dish, contributing a low-fat source of protein.

✔ A vegetable and so count towards your five fruit and veg a day.

✔ High in soluble fibre and so can help lower your cholesterol level.

✔ Low GI (with an average GI of 27).

Many varieties of lentil are grown and eaten throughout the world, but the three most common types used in cooking are brown, red, and green.

Lentils don't require soaking. However, you can soak them for a few hours if you want to and this reduces the cooking time by about half. You can substitute one type of lentil for another, although you may need to adjust the cooking time.

Nuts and Seeds

Having been almost scorned for a long while because of their fat content, these little gems are now beginning to hog the limelight as far as health-giving properties are concerned.

Yes, they do contain oil, and their oils are often extracted to produce vegetable oils suitable for culinary uses such as salad dressings. However, the oil in nuts and seeds is predominantly mono and poly, and they are also a good source of omega-3s.

Because of their unique blend of oils, protein, low-GI properties, vitamins, minerals, and antioxidants, nuts and seeds are believed to be great for your heart, can help to normalise blood fats, and a small handful each day may even help you to control your weight.

You can sprinkle nuts and seeds on salads or add them to breakfast cereals. You can incorporate them into breads, cakes, or any form of baking. They can also be made into nut or seed butters and of course don't forget the traditional veggie nut roast. A small handful of nuts and seeds also make a great low-GI snack which can help keep away hunger until your next meal. You can roast them to give more flavour but avoid adding salt.

Examples of nuts:

- ✔ Peanut (high in protein and 50 per cent oil. Used to make low-GI peanut butter but look out for ones that don't contain hydrogenated oil).
- ✔ Almond (ground up they form the basis of marzipan and are often used to add a rich texture to baked goods and desserts).
- ✔ Walnuts (they tend to go rancid very quickly so need to be stored in the fridge or freezer).
- ✔ Cashews.
- ✔ Pistachio.
- ✔ Pine nuts (vital in pesto sauce).
- ✔ Pecan nuts (tend to be used in ice creams and desserts).
- ✔ Brazil (an excellent source of the antioxidant selenium, which can often be in short supply in today's diets).

Examples of seeds:

- ✔ Sunflower.
- ✔ Pumpkin.
- ✔ Sesame (the paste is used to make tahini).
- ✔ Linseed (particularly rich in omega-3 fats, but best ground up before consumption or they tend to pass right through! However, if eaten unground they are a useful laxative!).

You don't need to eat lots of nuts and seeds to get the benefit because they are a concentrated source of nutrients including vitamins A and E, minerals such as calcium, iron, zinc, phosphorous, and potassium, and fibre. About 30 grams is a sensible portion.

Berries

Berries really are superfoods straight from nature. You can pick them right from the garden or gather from woods and hedgerows to discover how delicious berries are. The most popular berries are naturally sweet, and don't require much effort to make them into a tasty treat. Just rinse and serve them for a healthy, easy snack or dessert.

Berries are a good source of vitamins and phytochemicals; the latter are components of fruits or vegetables that have antioxidant and other health properties when you eat them. For instance, cranberries and blueberries contain a substance that helps prevent or treat painful bladder infections. Blueberries, strawberries, and raspberries also contain powerful antioxidants which may help to keep away heart disease and cancers.

Berries also contain lutein, which is important for healthy vision, especially blueberries and raspberries. Hopefully, further research on the different phytochemicals found in berries is going to prove fruitful (pun intended!).

As well as containing health-giving substances, berries are also a great source of other nutrients – vitamin C, calcium, magnesium, folic acid, and potassium. Furthermore, they are all very low in calories at only around 45–80 calories a cup, and low GI. One cup of raspberries offers vitamin C and potassium for 64 delicious calories.

As well as eating them for dessert with some yoghurt or low-fat ice cream, berries are also great added to your favourite breakfast cereal and go a treat in a smoothie. They can also be added to baking, such as in muffins. Keep a stock of frozen mixed berries in the freezer so you can eat them all year round.

Yoghurt

What a godsend! Any low-fat cultured milk product is versatile, so you can see that a variety of types are used in the recipes in this book including Greek yoghurt, fromage frais, and plain and fruit flavour yoghurt. You can use yoghurt in both sweet and savoury dishes and in smoothies. Yoghurt is great health-wise because:

- ✔ Low-fat yoghurt is low in calories.
- ✔ Yoghurt has a low GI (around 33) so it can bring down the overall GI of dishes to which it is added.
- ✔ Yoghurt contains many nutrients including calcium and riboflavin.
- ✔ Bio or live yoghurt contains probiotic bacteria which are increasingly believed to have unique health-giving properties including aiding digestive health, offsetting thrush, and boosting the immune function.

Always have some low-fat yoghurt as a standby in the fridge: It adds a creamy texture in sauces, can be topped onto your favourite fruit as an instant dessert (going particularly well with berries), and a pot of low-fat fruit yoghurt makes a great low-fat/low-GI/low-calorie instant snack.

Green Vegetables

Your mother always told you to eat your greens for a reason! Unfortunately, our consumption of green veggies is on the decline, especially veg such as cabbage and sprouts. However, the brassica family of veg in particular needs a helping hand in being elevated to superfood stardom. Brassicas include:

- ✔ Purple sprouting broccoli
- ✔ Cabbages
- ✔ Kale
- ✔ Brussel sprouts
- ✔ Cauliflower
- ✔ Broccoli
- ✔ Chinese greens

Superbroccoli

Broccoli is one of the most popular green vegetables but lately it has achieved super-stardom status. Scientists at the University of Warwick, UK, have bred a range of Superbroccoli which they claim: helps you live longer, lasts longer on the shelves, and uses much less pesticide and fertiliser.

Broccoli is a rich source of antioxidants which have a number of health-giving properties including defending against cancers. However, broccoli's short shelf life means those important antioxidants quickly break down and can lose much of their power before being consumed. The cross-breeding programme creating longer shelf life ensures that the antioxidants remain potent for longer.

Brassicas have certain health-giving properties including the reduction of coronary heart disease and cancers. These properties are thought to be because these veg contain substances called *glucosinolates* (sulphur-containing compounds which act as anti-cancer agents). They also contain phenolic compounds which act as antioxidants. These veg are also rich in several nutrients including magnesium, folate, and vitamin C. However, if you cook these veg for too long or keep them warm for a while, you destroy some of the nutrients.

Sardines

These tasty little fish also need a boost to super-status as they are often deemed to be too humble to be of any importance! Yet sardines are an oily fish and therefore contain omega-3 oils and fat-soluble vitamins D and E. They are also a rich source of iron, and so make a good, and much cheaper, substitute for rump steaks! As sardines are very small fish, heavy metals contamination, which can contaminate large fish, is less likely.

The canned versions are great made into pâtés and of course served on toast. If you flake them up with their bones, which become quite soft when canned, they are packed with calcium and so are great for bone health. Sardines can also be purchased fresh and these are ideal for grilling on a barbecue and serving with some fresh bread and salad.

Population studies have shown that people who eat diets high in omega-3 have a reduced risk of heart disease. In basic terms, fish-eating populations are less likely to die prematurely of coronary heart disease. Current recommendations are that you need to have two fish meals a week. Oily fish are best because they are highest in omega-3 fatty acids.

Pilchards are related to sardines (they are both from the herring family) and can be substituted for them, providing similar levels of nutrients.

Chapter 18

Ten Places to Go to Get Further Information and Support

. . . .

In This Chapter

▶ Finding out where to get more help and information

▶ Seeing that you aren't alone in coping with your PCOS

. . . .

*T*en sensible, well-presented, informative, and helpful organisations that deal with PCOS and related conditions are showcased in this chapter. Some are charities that you can join to receive regular help and support and possibly meet with other PCOS sufferers. Where an organisation is based in the UK, I've added details of equivalent American organisations at the end of the entry.

Quite a few organisations claim to help women with PCOS but on delving deeper you find that they just want to sell you supplements or claim radical cures by use of crystals or avoiding electromagnetic radiation! Sometimes it seems as if we haven't come very far in the last two hundred years; so that even in the 21st century, people are still trying to peddle snake-oil that they claim cures all your ills, based on no scientific evidence! Treat with caution any organisation that offers radical cures or claims that all you have to do is take a pill or supplements. You may not be an expert, but common sense, and the advice in this book, can go a long way in sorting out the good advice from the bad!

Verity

www.verity-pcos.org.uk

Verity is one of the best-known UK charities for women whose lives are affected by Polycystic Ovary Syndrome (PCOS). You can become a member of Verity for a small fee. You then receive an information pack, regular newsletters, and invitations to Verity conferences and events. And of course you're supporting Verity in its mission to share the truth about PCOS.

Verity invites real experts and doctors working in the field of PCOS to come along to the conferences, and you always have the opportunity to ask these experts questions. Transcripts of their talks are available on the Verity Web site. Verity has produced a number of fact sheets (free to members, or non-members can pay and send off for them):

- An Introduction to PCOS
- Dealing with Excess Hair
- Dealing with Acne
- Fertility Nutrition
- Hormones
- PCOS for Teenagers
- Getting the Best from Doctors and Therapists
- Alternative and Complementary Therapies
- The Benefits of Exercise
- Long Term Health Consequences

Verity is also privileged to have the support of highly influential scientific and medical advisers. Each is an expert in their field. They all contribute to the Verity magazine, speak at Verity conferences, and keep Verity and you up-to-date with the latest PCOS research. Verity has recently begun to reach out to health professionals and bring them up-to date with the condition.

Verity's discussion board is available to members and non-members. If you join in it may help you to realise that you're not alone.

Verity is run by a group of volunteers who have PCOS themselves but are always looking for extra helpers!

Women's Health Concern

www.womens-health-concern.org

Women's Health Concern (WHC) is a charitable organisation which aims to help, educate, and support women with their healthcare by providing unbiased, accurate information. It started as an open-access clinic in London, UK, and has since expanded its services to provide women with counselling and advice through its telephone helpline and email services.

WHC employs nurses qualified in gynaecological and menopausal matters. They're backed by 21 of the UK's leading doctors specialising in the field of the menopause and gynaecology.

The helpline is managed by experienced nurse counsellors and backed up by a team of eminent medical advisers. A team of experienced nurses and medical advisers also manages the e-mail service.

A range of detailed information leaflets and fact sheets on the most common gynaecological conditions, including PCOS, is located on their Web site. You can print off this information as required.

Infertility Network (INUK)

www.infertilitynetworkuk.com

INUK is committed to providing a comprehensive support network to its members and to all those affected by infertility. As well as providing authoritative information, and practical and emotional support, INUK's mission is to raise the profile and understanding of infertility issues in all quarters, and to strive for timely and consistent provision of infertility care throughout the UK.

INUK is a membership organisation, and so some of INUK's services are available to members only. By becoming a member, you get full access to services such as access to forums and chat rooms. A dedicated daytime advice line and regional support groups are available which provide local support and group meetings. Members can also write in to medical advisers and receive independent medical advice.

INUK produces a quarterly magazine, available to members and interested organisations on application. Included in the magazine are letters from members, advice from their medical advisors, latest developments in the field of infertility, features, and useful addresses. INUK also has fact sheets on a whole range of subjects related to infertility (including PCOS) to enable people to have a better understanding of their illness.

INUK regularly runs information events, with talks by leading infertility specialists, and exhibition areas. These events are excellent opportunities to meet other members as well as the staff of INUK, and to discover the latest developments and relax and enjoy yourself in the company of people who understand where you are at. These events are held throughout the UK.

In the USA, the American Fertility Association provides reproductive information, a national newsletter, support groups, advocacy support, and research support. You can visit it at www.theafa.org.

Diabetes UK

www.diabetes.org.uk

Knowing where to start to describe this organisation and what it does is difficult. Diabetes UK is *the* main diabetes charity in the UK and also one of the largest patient organisations in Europe. Being a member of Diabetes UK offers you a lot of support and information including:

- ✔ A bi-monthly members' magazine packed with news and information.
- ✔ The ability to talk in confidence to Diabetes UK careline about any issue or aspect of diabetes.
- ✔ The chance to share experiences with other people with diabetes through the organisation's extensive network of voluntary groups.

Diabetes UK stands up for the interests of people with diabetes by campaigning for better standards of care. The organisation is the largest funder in the UK of research into better treatments for diabetes and the search for a cure, and it provides practical support, information, and safety-net services to help people manage their diabetes. Diabetes UK careline staff answer over 200 enquiries a day.

The Web site is extensive, offering information such as store tours (how to choose the best diet, read labels, and so on) and loads of recipe ideas. Information is also available about the glycaemic index. The site is great for anyone who wants to find out about eating a healthy diet because, as the organisation says on its Web site, 'People with diabetes are advised to follow the same healthy eating plan recommended for everyone – food that is low in fat, salt, and sugar including plenty of fruit and vegetables.'

Most countries have a similar national diabetes organisation because the disease is so widespread. In the USA, you can find the American Diabetes Association's Web site at www.diabetes.org.

The British Dietetic Association

www.bda.uk.com

This organisation can put you in touch with a proper qualified dietician – not someone who simply plies you with supplements and herbal remedies which, without changes to your diet and lifestyle, don't have the desired effect. The BDA's motto is: 'Trust a dietician to know about nutrition.' Registered Dieticians (RDs) are uniquely qualified to translate scientific information about food into practical dietary advice. As well as providing impartial advice about nutrition and health, dieticians also advise about food-related problems and treat disease and ill health. Many dieticians work in the National Health Service and may work in one or more specialist areas. The title 'dietician' can only be used by those appropriately trained professionals who have registered with the Health Professions Council. Those who aren't registered are breaking the law if they use the title 'dietician'. The BDA Web site allows you to check whether the person who is advising you about your diet really is an RD.

The Web site itself hosts the BDA's Weightwise campaign site which offers tips and information about weight loss. Also, the BDA has joined forces with Canned Food UK to create the world's first animated desktop 'dietician', providing consumers with regular reminders about their healthy living goals. Desktop D.A.N. (an abbreviation of Diet And Nutrition) provides free advice on diet, nutrition, and lifestyle, offering essential information from two authorities in the field of diet and food information. The BDA homepage leads you to Dan!

The BDA equivalent in the USA is the American Dietetic Association (ADA) and you can find it at www.eatright.org.

NHS Direct

www.nhsdirect.nhs.uk/articles/article.aspx?articleId=290

The Web site link above takes you to the page with information on PCOS. Everything is very logically and clearly laid out. By putting your cursor over each word that may not be completely understood, such as ovary or testosterone, a box appears which briefly explains what the word means. Quick links are also available to related topics. At the end, you can follow selected links to other organisations that can help with the particular condition.

NHS Direct also offers a phone number (0845 4647) which residents of the UK can phone to get further information on matters that may not be dealt with on the Web site.

In the USA, Med Help International is an independent organisation established to try to help patients find high quality medical information. Visit www.medhelp.org for more information.

Women's Health.gov

www.4woman.gov/faq/pcos.htm#7

This Web site connects you to The Office on Women's Health (OWH), which is part of the US Federal Government. The mission of OWH is to work to improve the health and wellbeing of women and girls in the US through its innovative programmes, by educating health professionals, and by motivating behaviour change in consumers through the dissemination of health information. OWH was established in 1991 within the US Department of Health and Human Services (HHS). OWH co-ordinates the efforts of all the HHS agencies and offices involved in women's health.

The Web site has some basic information about PCOS, but also has some great links to lead you on to other more specific sites that can give you more detail about various aspects of PCOS. As well as PCOS, the site contains masses of information and links to all sorts of women's health concerns. If you type in a subject in the search engine it provides you with the most recent information about the subject.

iVillage

www.ivillage.co.uk and www.ivillage.com

You can find a lot of down-to-earth information about PCOS based on current medical thinking on both the US and UK homes of iVillage.

You can become a member of iVillage for free and benefit from certain services, including a regular newsletter where you can specify which information you want to receive – so you don't have to have the horoscope and celeb news iVillage offers, but can opt for info on diet and fitness, women's health, and recipes.

Weight Loss Resources

www.weightlossresources.co.uk

This UK Web site offers weight loss programmes and diet tools for a healthy weight loss. A dietician has checked out this site and has given it the thumbs up of approval and declared it fad-diet free. The site offers:

- ✔ A foods calorie counter and online calorie and nutrition databases.

- ✔ Tips on how to keep a food diary – a very useful tool for helping you to make certain vital changes to your diet. The site also gives advice on keeping an exercise diary, and you can find out how many calories you burn with certain exercises.

- ✔ Tips on how many calories you need so that you can reach your weight loss goal.

- ✔ Recipes.

- ✔ A members' forum where you can share your weight loss experiences and diet tips with like-minded Weight Loss Resources members.

Membership costs from £7 a month (or $9.99) but you can take a three-day free trial. Even if you don't join, the Web site is full of tips and ideas on how to eat healthily and lose weight, including quite a bit of information about following a low-GI diet.

In the USA, a site called Free Weight Loss Resources offers a collection of free weight loss resources that can help you. Check out www.freeweightloss.com.

Polycystic Ovarian Syndrome Association

www.pcosupport.org

The Polycystic Ovarian Syndrome Association exists to provide comprehensive information, support, and advocacy for women and girls with PCOS. This American-based charity offers up-to-date educational resources, information on medical, surgical, and alternative therapies as well as lifestyle practices that may be beneficial to women with PCOS. Other services offered include:

- ✔ Support and advocacy resources for women with PCOS.
- ✔ Web services including online discussion forums.
- ✔ An online Newsletter called *Living* and other articles and information on PCOS.
- ✔ Conferences and symposia.
- ✔ Local chapters and support groups.

Being a member involves paying a fee of around $40 (around £20) but this organisation does offer you more support than simply being able to access non-membership parts of the Web site.

A lengthy nutrition section in the newsletter is written by a panel of Registered Dieticians. Many of the nutrition articles written for *Living* are available to non-members on line. Articles include titles such as 'Curb Your Carbohydrate Cravings'.

If you're not sure if you really have PCOS, the Web site has a PCOS quiz which enables you to tick your symptoms and score points. The higher your score, the more likely you are to have PCOS (the quiz is intended for educational and informational purposes only and is not a substitute for medical advice).

Index

• E •

• F •

• G •

• H •

• I •

• J •

• K •

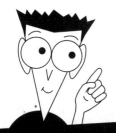

FOR DUMMIES®

Do Anything. Just Add Dummies

PROPERTY   **UK editions**

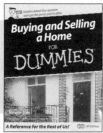 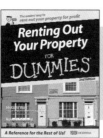 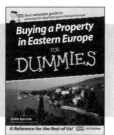

0-7645-7027-7   **0-470-02921-8**   **0-7645-7047-1**

PERSONAL FINANCE

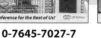

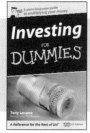 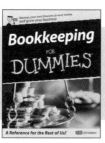 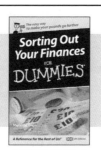

0-7645-7023-4   **0-470-05815-3**   **0-7645-7039-0**

BUSINESS

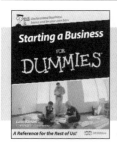 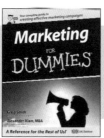 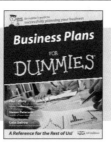

0-7645-7018-8   **0-7645-7056-0**   **0-7645-7026-9**

Answering Tough Interview
Questions For Dummies
(0-470-01903-4)

Arthritis For Dummies
(0-470-02582-4)

Being the Best Man
For Dummies
(0-470-02657-X)

British History
For Dummies
(0-470-03536-6)

Building Confidence
For Dummies
(0-470-01669-8)

Buying a Home on a Budget
For Dummies
(0-7645-7035-8)

Children's Health
For Dummies
(0-470-02735-5)

Cognitive Behavioural Therapy
For Dummies
(0-470-01838-0)

Cricket For Dummies
(0-470-03454-8)

CVs For Dummies
(0-7645-7017-X)

Detox For Dummies
(0-470-01908-5)

Diabetes For Dummies
(0 7645-7019-6)

Divorce For Dummies
(0-7645-7030-7)

DJing For Dummies
(0-470-03275-8)

eBay.co.uk For Dummies
(0-7645-7059-5)

European History
For Dummies
(0-7645-7060-9)

Gardening For Dummies
(0-470-01843-7)

Genealogy Online
For Dummies
(0-7645-7061-7)

Golf For Dummies
(0-470-01811-9)

Hypnotherapy For Dummies
(0-470-01930-1)

Irish History For Dummies
(0-7645-7040-4)

Neuro-linguistic Programming
For Dummies
(0-7645-7028-5)

Nutrition For Dummies
(0-7645-7058-7)

Parenting For Dummies
(0-470-02714-2)

Pregnancy For Dummies
(0-7645-7042-0)

Retiring Wealthy For Dummies
(0-470-02632-4)

Rugby Union For Dummies
(0-470-03537-4)

Small Business Employment
Law For Dummies
(0-7645-7052-8)

Starting a Business on
eBay.co.uk For Dummies
(0-470-02666-9)

Su Doku For Dummies
(0-470-01892-5)

The GL Diet For Dummies
(0-470-02753-3)

The Romans For Dummies
(0-470-03077-1)

Thyroid For Dummies
(0-470-03172-7)

UK Law and Your Rights
For Dummies
(0-470-02796-7)

Winning on Betfair
For Dummies
(0-470-02856-4)

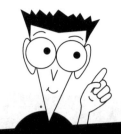

FOR DUMMIES®

Do Anything. Just Add Dummies

HOBBIES

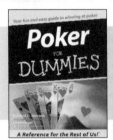

0-7645-5232-5

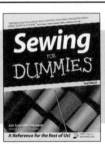

0-7645-6847-7

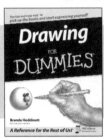

0-7645-5476-X

Also available:

Art For Dummies
(0-7645-5104-3)

Aromatherapy For Dummies
(0-7645-5171-X)

Bridge For Dummies
(0-471-92426-1)

Card Games For Dummies
(0-7645-9910-0)

Chess For Dummies
(0-7645-8404-9)

Improving Your Memory
For Dummies
(0-7645-5435-2)

Massage For Dummies
(0-7645-5172-8)

Meditation For Dummies
(0-471-77774-9)

Photography For Dummies
(0-7645-4116-1)

Quilting For Dummies
(0-7645-9799-X)

EDUCATION

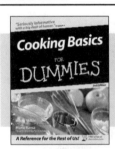

0-7645-7206-7

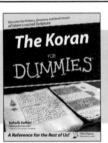

0-7645-5581-2

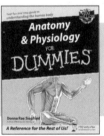

0-7645-5422-0

Also available:

Algebra For Dummies
(0-7645-5325-9)

Algebra II For Dummies
(0-471-77581-9)

Astronomy For Dummies
(0-7645-8465-0)

Buddhism For Dummies
(0-7645-5359-3)

Calculus For Dummies
(0-7645-2498-4)

Forensics For Dummies
(0-7645-5580-4)

Islam For Dummies
(0-7645-5503-0)

Philosophy For Dummies
(0-7645-5153-1)

Religion For Dummies
(0-7645-5264-3)

Trigonometry For Dummies
(0-7645-6903-1)

PETS

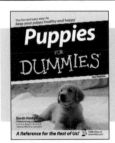

0-470-03717-2

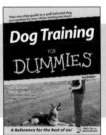

0-7645-8418-9

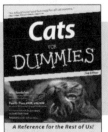

0-7645-5275-9

Also available:

Labrador Retrievers
For Dummies
(0-7645-5281-3)

Aquariums For Dummies
(0-7645-5156-6)

Birds For Dummies
(0-7645-5139-6)

Dogs For Dummies
(0-7645-5274-0)

Ferrets For Dummies
(0-7645-5259-7)

Golden Retrievers
For Dummies
(0-7645-5267-8)

Horses For Dummies
(0-7645-9797-3)

Jack Russell Terriers
For Dummies
(0-7645-5268-6)

Puppies Raising & Training
Diary For Dummies
(0-7645-0876-8)

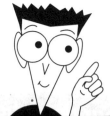
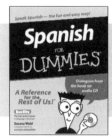
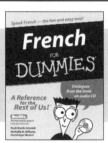
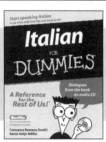
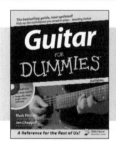
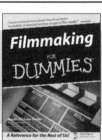
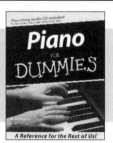
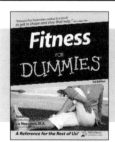
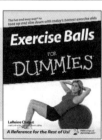
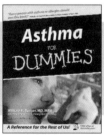

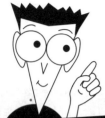

FOR DUMMIES

Helping you expand your horizons and achieve your potential

INTERNET

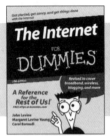

The Internet FOR DUMMIES

0-7645-8996-2

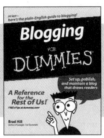

Blogging FOR DUMMIES

0-471-77084-1

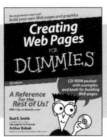

Creating Web Pages FOR DUMMIES

0-7645-7327-6

Also available:

eBay.co.uk
For Dummies
(0-7645-7059-5)
Dreamweaver 8
For Dummies
(0-7645-9649-7)
Web Design
For Dummies
(0-471-78117-7)

Everyday Internet
All-in-One Desk Reference
For Dummies
(0-7645-8875-3)
Creating Web Pages
All-in-One Desk Reference
For Dummies
(0-7645-4345-8)

DIGITAL MEDIA

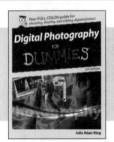

Digital Photography FOR DUMMIES

0-7645-9802-3

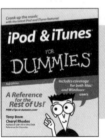

iPod & iTunes FOR DUMMIES

0-471-74739-4

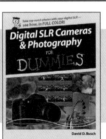

Digital SLR Cameras & Photography FOR DUMMIES

0-7645-9803-1

Also available:

Digital Photos, Movies, &
Music GigaBook
For Dummies
(0-7645-7414-0)
Photoshop CS2
For Dummies
(0-7645-9571-7)
Podcasting
For Dummies
(0-471-74898-6)

Blogging
For Dummies
(0-471-77084-1)
Digital Photography
All-In-One Desk Reference
For Dummies
(0-7645-7328-4)
Windows XP Digital Music For
Dummies
(0-7645-7599-6)

COMPUTER BASICS

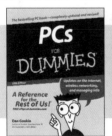

PCs FOR DUMMIES

0-7645-8958-X

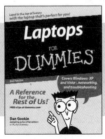

Laptops FOR DUMMIES

0-470-05432-8

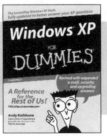

Windows XP FOR DUMMIES

0-7645-7326-8

Also available:

Office XP 9 in 1
Desk Reference
For Dummies
(0-7645-0819-9)
PCs All-in-One Desk
Reference For Dummies
(0-471-77082-5)
Pocket PC For Dummies
(0-7645-1640-X)

Upgrading & Fixing PCs
For Dummies
(0-7645-1665-5)
Windows XP All-in-One Desk
Reference For Dummies
(0-7645-7463-9)
Macs For Dummies
(0-470-04849-2)